Fundamentals of the Study of Urine and Body Fluids

John W. Ridley

Fundamentals of the Study of Urine and Body Fluids

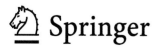 Springer

John W. Ridley
West Georgia Technical College
Carrollton
GA
USA

ISBN 978-3-319-78416-8   ISBN 978-3-319-78417-5   (eBook)
https://doi.org/10.1007/978-3-319-78417-5

Library of Congress Control Number: 2018941242

Printed on acid-free paper

This Springer imprint is published by the registered company Springer International Publishing AG, part of Springer Nature.
The registered company address is: Gewerbestrasse 11, 6330 Cham, Switzerland

To my wife, acquaintances, and the organizations to which I was unable to provide my undivided attention while completing this work. I also dedicate this book to others who encouraged me as employers, colleagues, patients, and students from whom I learned so much.

Foreword

Although I have written other textbooks during the past 10 years, this attempt focuses on a topic that differs from the previous two, although there were significant references in the previous publications to the topic of body fluids. This time around in writing this book seemed different from my previous publications even during the beginning stages. I again felt like a novice, although I have delved into fiction and nonfiction on a limited basis, but those creative manuscripts were entirely products of my experiences with life, and nothing had to be verified except by my memories and thoughts. Both were published, one with a traditional publisher and the other self-published with Amazon, so I felt some measure of pleasure at having accomplished that childhood dream. But now I was forced to completely change tracks! With this publication, *Fundamentals of the Study of Urine and Body Fluids*, everything had to be reviewed, and I wracked my brain to insure coverage of all topical material necessary to complete a book that was inclusive in both theory and practice related to body fluid analysis.

My first attempt to publish this book met with approval, but reorganization of the original publisher stymied my efforts for several years. Again, I began the mental preparation for a new manuscript and read or consulted materials from a vast number of books and the internet to insure the material I had attempted to publish was still valid and fresh. Much has been written on the topics of body fluids but all the wording in this book is a compilation of what I have experienced, know, and have studied, so any verbiage that is similar to other publications is purely coincidental. Minor changes were necessary when reviewing the original manuscript. Visits to several medical facilities to insure a product worthy of the student's education or the professional's needs as a reference were an essential part of completing this publication.

While most laboratory procedures are either fully or partly automated, it is still relevant to understand the basics of the unlimited number of procedures, as birth is given frequently to new tests and new approaches to previous methodology. When automated procedures are performed, sometimes verification or confirmation is needed, especially when test results do not correlate with the clinical picture.

Therefore, the procedures presented in this book use manual methodology, in order to give the student or professional the basics of what goes into a laboratory procedure.

Carrollton, GA, USA   John W. Ridley

Preface

For a significant number of years, the author of this book, *Fundamentals of the Study of Urine and Body Fluids*, has studied, practiced, and taught the topics presented in this textbook. Having experience with diverse backgrounds in hospital and clinic laboratories, private laboratories, and military facilities, including tertiary and field settings, I have been involved with laboratory medicine and direct medical care for more than 35 years. The significance of the characteristics ascribed to the various fluids of the body has long been a subject of interest even among ancient medical practitioners. References are made as to the "humors (fluids) and vapors (exhaled air)" in various writings of antiquity. The fluids of the body include chiefly blood by volume. However, the specialized body fluids are associated with various systems within the body and, in most cases, are derivatives of the blood plasma which is the liquid portion of the body. But the study of hematology or study of the blood requires an entirely different approach than that of the other body fluids and changes that occur during disease processes. This book undertakes the study of the clinical significance of the "minor" fluids of the body, or those other than blood.

This book is intended for use by entry level students for the diploma, associate, and bachelor's degree programs in laboratory technology. In addition, a copy of this publication would be an invaluable resource in clinical laboratories in all settings, including physician office laboratories (POLs), where test procedures for urine and other body fluids are performed. Health care professionals other than laboratory technical personnel would find this publication to be a valuable resource when seeking information related to the testing of body fluids. Pertinent information relative to all of the fluids that are routinely studied in the medical laboratory is introduced along with step-by-step procedures that can be used in writing or revising procedure manuals. Many pitfalls abound in the practice of laboratory medicine. The practitioners of this profession must develop a sixth sense that causes each laboratorian to look more intently at certain aspects of the practice, as errors are easily made while performing the multitude of repetitive and mundane procedures. This requires paying attention to sometimes intricate processes required as new tests are developed or new approaches to old tests that are developed continuously. The new discoveries and even sometimes the dusting off old procedures must be dealt with in stride for the technician, technologist, or scientist. The terminology used in identifying credentialed laboratory professionals is included in this publication.

Although the evolution of clinical laboratory medicine is rapidly expanding and changing with the advent of new research and equipment, many of the principles of laboratory medicine have remained basically the same, sometimes for centuries. References are made to the fledgling efforts of medical practitioners from the past several hundred years. Their assumptions and rudimentary procedures have been amplified and have become more complex and accurate, but with little exception their early observations have been found to be correct. This reference focuses on both manual and automated analyses to provide meaningful application of the manifold approaches to laboratory testing found in various types of laboratories and the effective training and education of those performing the procedures.

Carrollton, GA, USA   John W. Ridley

Acknowledgments

So many persons in my life, including professionals in my line of work and life in general, have often unknowingly given me the resources necessary to undertake and complete this book. My experiences began while working as a respiratory therapy assistant, and my first taste of laboratory medicine began as an Army recruit selected for a medical laboratory technician (it kept me out of the infantry) program at Ft. Sam Houston, TX.

As I moved, and sometimes advanced in my career, I learned from teachers, coworkers, other professionals, and anyone in my path who helped to complete a holistic view of medicine. Most diagnoses or confirmation of diagnoses include laboratory medicine as a tool to improve medical practice.

My wife understood the pressures of completing this manuscript replete with complex issues that required verification at each step of the way, and greatly encouraged me. In addition, I was fortunate to enlist the unstinting help of David E. Nist as an Image/Graphics editor along with help in troubleshooting some of the malfunctions of my computer mostly attributed to my shortcomings and understanding the challenges of meeting requirements by the publisher.

Contents

Abbreviations

ACTH	Adrenocorticotropic hormone
ADH	Antidiuretic hormone
ANH	Atrial natriuretic hormone
ANP	Atrial natriuretic peptide
arthro-	Joint(ed)
BMC	Boehringer Mannheim Corporation
C	Centigrade
CAPB	Cocamidopropyl betaine (derived from coconut oil)
CDCP	Center for Disease Control and Prevention
CLSI	Clinical and Laboratory Standards Institute
CSF	Cerebrospinal fluid
Cu	Cooper
dL	Deciliter (1/10th of liter)
Fe+, Fe++	Iron ions, two valences
GI	Gastrointestinal
H_2O	Chemical symbol for water
HCl	Hydrogen chloride
i.e.	"As in"
IgA, IgG, IgM	Immunoglobulins
IRIS	Brand name for automated urinalysis instrument
-itis	Suffix indicating inflammation
LPF	Low power field (microscopic)
Mcg	Microgram (one-thousandth of a milligram)
Mg	Milligram
mL	Milliliter (one thousandth of a liter)
Mm	Millimeter (one thousandth of a meter)
Mod	Moderate (estimate of a quantity)
Mosmole.Kg	Milliosmole per kilogram
MT	Medical technologist (supervisory level, medical laboratory worker)
N, N+	Sodium atom, ionized form of sodium
NaCl	Sodium chloride (salt)
Neg	Negative (not present)
Occ	Occasional (fewer than one element per microscopic field)

Pg/mL	Picogram (one-trillionth of a gram) per milliliter
pH	Potential of hydrogen to acidify based on quantity
PKU	Phenylketonuria
Pos	Positive
QA	Quality assurance, a program to determine validity of results
QC	Quality control, samples tests with samples of unknown value
RBC	Red blood cell
SCAQMD	Air pollution control agency in southern CA
SI	Standards International
Sq	Square (equal sides)
SSA	Sulfosalicylic acid
STD	Sexually transmitted disease
TCA	Trichloroacetic acid
Tr	Trace (small amount)
UTI	Urinary tract infection
UP	Universal precautions
VOCs	Sensors to chiefly determine presence of gases, i.e., carbon dioxide
w/v	Weight per volume of diluent
WBC	White blood cell
WHO	World Health Organization

Purpose of Publication

It is my desire to develop a comprehensive group of tests performed on body fluids other than blood. Urine is the major body fluid other than blood that provides valuable diagnostic values for a multitude of diseases. But other specimens of choice for procedures unrelated to urine include the "lesser" body fluids. Not all tests on the menu where urine and other body fluids are tested are included in this book, but efforts are focused toward those procedures that are commonly or at least somewhat commonly performed in clinical laboratories. With the current and growing trend toward outsourcing procedures not routinely performed in most laboratories, many laboratory professionals are never required to perform other than the most commonly requested tests.

Commonalities and differences between procedures for the various body fluids and differences in levels of analytes found in the fluids are a major focus of this book. Materials related to testing of urine samples are presented first. Since many clinical tests performed using urine as a specimen are at least in part the same as those for other body fluids, later sections provide clinical information relative to other body fluids in comparison with that of urine. References to the differences between expected results and the clinical significance of levels of analytes that vary from the normal results are presented throughout the book.

The need for sensitivity and specificity for the various analytes that are tested for and ongoing changes in methodology used for testing require that the student as well as the veteran professional remain aware of developments based on current research. The importance of accuracy and the ability to determine interferences from the environment, as well as other analytes present that might alter the results found during testing, are presented in this book. Erroneous test results that may be the result of interfering substances or physical conditions require a thorough knowledge by the testing personnel of the necessity of confirmatory testing as well as the correlation of the patient's medical condition with the results obtained. Due to the wide range of products and testing equipment, no effort is made to delineate the functions of differing equipment or to discuss the merits of any definite brand or style of equipment or supplies.

Although every effort is made to orient the student to anatomical origins of specimens and conditions related to the testing of body fluids, the student should have a working knowledge of basic anatomy and physiology. In core subjects required before acceptance into a laboratory training program, courses related to the functions of the body are necessary and are advantageous for the student to gain an advantage in becoming an effective health care professional.

Safety is paramount in the medical laboratory. Biohazards, toxins, electrical hazards, and injuries from mechanical devices require surveillance, training, and caution to avoid becoming a victim of sustaining an injury or contaminating oneself with toxins or microorganisms. Fortunately, many hazardous reagents have been replaced with safer alternatives over the years, but care must still be exercised even when using common materials. In past years, some procedures required boiling with gas equipment to achieve a reaction, but that is rare today. Sharp instruments and broken glass must be promptly and safely discarded to protect the laboratory professionals, custodial employees, and others such as patients who may be exposed to hazardous conditions. Regulatory standards, required by federal, state, and voluntary accreditation bodies, are a valuable component in the education and training of laboratory professionals. These considerations relate to quality assurance programs used to insure valid test results for body fluids, as well as safety issues necessary to provide for the safety and health of the employee as well as the patient undergoing treatment. References to these requirements based on education standards and mandated safety practices are found in this publication.

Organization of Text

The book is organized in a logical sequence from the historical introduction of the study of body fluids, progressing to the need for valid results based on standards of quality assurance. As safety is a valid concern for anyone practicing any component of medicine, particularly for those directly involved with specimens such as body fluids, a single chapter is devoted to safety in the workplace. A systematic approach to safety and the reasons for body fluid testing are not always found in many of the currently available textbooks.

The metabolic origins of body fluids, their functions in the overall organization of the human body, and the importance of these fluids as nutritive and protective substances are thoroughly discussed prior to any instruction related to testing of the materials. Constituents contained in the various fluids, some of which may be found in many of the body sites where fluids are found, are outlined to provide information related to metabolically formed components of a specimen, both of a normal and an abnormal perspective. Further steps are provided to emphasize the importance of a properly collected specimen, based on the anatomical differences of the various body sites, completes the preparatory information necessary for the practitioner to systematically incorporate this background material to the testing of body fluids.

A thorough understanding of the principles related to effective and accurate collection of fluids that may be impacted by metabolic and infectious disease processes, is necessary before body fluids testing pertinent to the various fluids and, in some cases, groups of fluids is discussed. Acceptable testing procedures are provided where necessary for each of the types of fluids found in the human body that are currently employed as manual procedures for determining the presence of disease based upon significant clinical findings in each type of specimen. A separate chapter is devoted to each of the most commonly tested fluids, and in some cases, groups of fluids with common components are logically discussed as a group.

And finally, a chapter is provided on testing of fluids and materials from the body employing some of the previously presented techniques and practices, but includes some of the lesser body fluids that are not as commonly tested for in many laboratories. A feature that is not included in many of the books related to body fluids is that of the use of the microscope in the testing of the fluids from the body. This final chapter is designed to acquaint the health care professional in the proper use and maintenance of the various types of microscopes commonly used in microscopic examinations and identification of solid constituents of body fluids.

How to Use the Textbook

This textbook should at first be used sequentially to set the stage for testing of body fluids. The initial chapters are necessary to set the stage for the student or medical professional to have sufficient appreciation for the clinical evidence body fluids provide in the adequate assessment of the patient. Properly performed procedures lead to cost effectiveness and efficiency, by providing timely and accurate clinical results for use by the medical provider treating the patient. Later use of the book as a reference can be useful in troubleshooting a procedure or determining the necessity for further testing for confirmation.

Although there is a somewhat lengthy history of diagnostic testing, laboratory testing in the recent past is becoming increasingly important in diagnosing illness and in determining the prognosis of those suffering from diseases. Clinical findings in body fluids are correlated by the physician with the physical signs observed by the medical practitioner along with the symptoms. Results of these laboratory procedures provide diagnostic information that may not even have been suspected from the initial signs and symptoms. Proper collection and handling of specimens for safety and for preserving the integrity of the samples are provided in this book. Case studies are provided and end-of-chapter tests are available for the learner and the practicing professional who wishes to refresh his or her technical expertise.

It should be understood by laboratory and other medical professionals that laboratory testing of body fluids is perhaps the single most important entity in the identification or confirmation of a specific disease and is certainly the most widely used method for these purposes. The menu of tests offered and the research leading to more tests and more refined procedures will undoubtedly grow over the years. Therefore, it is the author's wish that this book will meet the needs of the laboratory student and the laboratory professional for the foreseeable future.

Introduction to the Study of Body Fluids

1

Objective(s)

Discuss the beginnings of laboratory medicine through the examination of urine, chiefly

Demonstrate an understanding of the importance of performing examinations of body fluids

Describe the beginning studies of urine and how they evolved into a more comprehensive evaluation of urine and other body fluids

List body fluids other than blood that are examined to determine disease states of the body

Provide the three types of evaluations of urine as found in a modern laboratory

Discuss the correlation of laboratory tests and the clinical condition of the patient

1.1   History of the Analysis of Body Fluids

Initially, blood and urine were the only body fluids with which ancient medics were acquainted. The early practitioners of the healing science referred to "humors" and "vapors" when discussing clinical findings related to illness. The term "humors" has become more widely known as fluids or bodies, such as that of the *vitreous* humor of the eyeball that is now known as the vitreous body. The other major fluids of the body were not well known in early practice of medicine, but they along with urine are *ultrafiltrates* of the liquid portion of the blood called *plasma*, except for cerebrospinal fluid (CSF). Arguments occur over the site and mechanism of cerebrospinal production. The fluid contains similar chemical constituents as that of blood plasma, but at lower levels that found in the plasma, chiefly glucose and protein fractions. Studies in some instances have shown that the fluid is mostly formed by active secretion and transport by the choroid plexuses of the brain, with production of the cerebrospinal occurring in the cerebral ventricles of the brain. Urine is comprised of approximately 95% water, while some additional body fluids are more concentrated

© Springer International Publishing AG, part of Springer Nature 2018
J. W. Ridley, *Fundamentals of the Study of Urine and Body Fluids*,
https://doi.org/10.1007/978-3-319-78417-5_1

Fig 1.1 Specimen jar
called a Matula

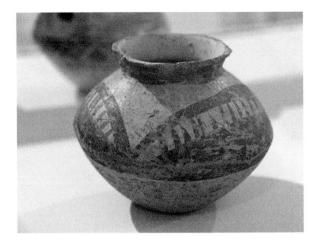

and contain *protein* along with other elements not found in detectable amounts in normal urine samples.

The earliest practice of examining the urine of a patient was called *uroscopy*, a practice that dates to ancient Egypt, Babylon, and India. Around the twelfth century, with the development of glass in Egypt and perhaps in Germany, the practice evolved into a procedure in which the specimen could more easily be visualized. The *uroscopy*, a procedure that was performed during the Middle Ages, utilized a transparent glass flask or a cup-shaped container called a *matula* (Fig. 1.1). Physicians would then visually examine the urine as illuminated by sunlight. The urine sample could be compared with a chart to distinguish levels of color, clarity, foam, and sediments. The odor of the urine was also thought to provide important diagnostic information, and in some cases probably did where aromatic materials such as acetone were present. In addition, the growth and metabolic processes of certain bacteria also imparts a characteristic odor to the urine in which microorganisms are found. Even though many research efforts were halted during the Middle Ages when many diseases were attributed to demonology, the examination of urine seemed to persist to some extent during this span of history.

Hippocrates was perhaps the first to postulate that diseases are a natural result of a malfunction of the body and was not caused by the anger of gods or by demons that possessed the victim of a disease. This belief again reared its ugly head during the early Middle Ages and almost halted any medical or other scientific advances. Hippocrates appears to be the first to venture a theory that correlates the intake of fluids with the output of urine, a basis of modern fluid balance that plays an important role in medical practice today. The weakness in this early use of urine as a diagnostic tool discounted evidence such as clinical signs and focused primarily on the appearance and physical factors associated with the specimen. But other body fluids except for "vapors and humors" were paid scant attention at that time in human history.

In early medical history, clinical laboratory tests were rudimentary and often consisted merely of a *macroscopic* opinion as to the quality of the urine. But it was not until 1694 when an actual chemical procedure was performed on urine, when Frederik Dekkers found albumin, a fractional component of protein, in urine by boiling the specimen and obtaining a cloudy color at certain temperature levels. Then almost two centuries ago, some rudimentary tests were developed for certain qualitative tests for metabolic products found in the urine of diseased individuals. A solution which is actually a combination of two solutions that are called Fehling A and B, provided a test for glucose found in the urine and the blood plasma, which prior to this time was supposedly measured by an attraction of ants to urine containing sugar, or by the taste of the urine that indicated an abnormal presence of glucose. Richard Bright in the early 1800s developed the premise that edema and protein are interrelated in certain conditions where the kidney is abnormally spilling protein into the urine.

Concurrently with some of the other developments related to the study of body fluids, Anton van Leeuwenhoek (October 24, 1632–August 30, 1723), a Dutch tradesman and scientist, unwittingly contributed to the modern examination of urine sediment as he is credited with the improvement of an older version of the microscope. His work in the observation of microorganisms and one-celled organisms undoubtedly were the forerunners of the modern *microscopic* examination of urine. The second component of a complete analysis of body fluids, following a macroscopic or visual examination of the urine or body fluid, is the *chemical analysis* of the specimen, which originally required a work-intensive individual testing for each of the basic chemical components found in a complete *urinalysis*. These chemicals are also important in varying levels in body fluids other than urine. A more efficient advancement toward the modern analysis of urine occurred in the 1950's with the development of chemically impregnated strips, which gave a quick chemical analysis without the cumbersome individual testing required for each of the constituents being tested for. This was accomplished by chemically-treated pads that react in the presence of specific constituents of the urine and provide a semi-quantitative evaluation of certain chemical components such as glucose and protein, as well as other analyses.

Today, the modern procedures performed in a urine analysis, or *urinalysis*, consists of a scientific process that includes a series of macroscopic, microscopic, and chemical tests, while uroscopy only involved a visual examination of the urine sample. But uroscopy was the forerunner of modern examinations of body fluids. Testing these fluids is helpful as a tool for providing preliminary evidence for many illnesses, particularly those that affect the urinary system such as infection and hemorrhage beginning as much as 2000 years or more ago. In modern medicine of today, three areas of examination are employed for the complete and systematic evaluation of urine as well as for various other body fluids except for whole blood.

The initial or macroscopic examination of body fluids, including urine, refers to the physical appearance of the fluid. This preliminary survey is followed by a second step, that of evaluating the urine sample for the presence or absence of metabolic chemicals., conveniently performed today by using qualitative diagnostic test strips. Initially, each chemical constituent was tested for independently by a primitive and time-consuming process. Today, these chemical constituents are quickly and easily screened for with a dipstick containing reactive pads to determine the presence of many constituents. And finally, the third step of a complete urinalysis and even that for other body fluids includes a microscopic evaluation. These three steps in a complete study of urine and other body fluids except for blood should provide a correlation between the findings during this comprehensive examination.

These three components of a complete analysis of the urine are similarly employed when examining other fluids of the body with certain procedural modifications based on a specific body fluid sample used. And today, with better analytical methods developed through research and development, the numbers and complexity of tests performed on body fluids have grown greatly. These steps are increasingly used as important tools in screening for abnormalities or for diagnosing a person's overall health and well-being. As the procedures have evolved from primitive beginnings, they continue with considerable revisions to provide valuable clinical results leading to the diagnosis of a variety of medical conditions.

1.2   Medical Application of a Complete Urine Analysis

Urine samples are most likely studied more frequently than any other body fluid, even that of blood, as a routine evaluation and will be discussed more at length than the other body fluids. A urine sample provides clues for diagnosing disease for all the organs of the body, while other body fluids generally relates to only one organ or one system of the body. As a simplistic view of urine, it is used as the vehicle for ridding the body of waste products resulting from *metabolic* processes of the body of humans and other mammals. Since urine is only a waste product, it would appear that urine is insignificant and serves little or no purpose. But it is now considered a vital specimen for providing diagnostic screening data for functions not only of the kidney but other organs and provides clues for many disease states of the body. It will be shown that a urine sample and its physical appearance and its chemical and solid constituents often yield a great deal of clinical data relative to the health of an individual.

Since a urine sample is the most commonly analyzed body fluid and appears to have been the first body fluid used for medical diagnosis, it most likely preceded any study of blood as a body fluid. The processes relevant to the analyzing of urine samples will be treated first and separately from the other major fluids of the body. Although early in the beginning of laboratory medicine, when sophisticated testing procedures were not available, certain diagnostic bits of information which are still used today were available through direct visualization. Observation of a urine sample's color and clarity, along with its smell and sometimes taste has been around for perhaps more than 2000 years. Some medical conditions incidentally discovered through using uroscopy (Table 1.1) as shown.

Table 1.1 Common diseases observed by uroscopy

Diabetes	When a urine sample was tested by the physician using a small amount of urine, a sweet-tasting urine or the ability of the sample to attract ants and other insects indicated diabetes
Jaundice	Dark yellow to brownish urine color accompanied by a foul odor was associated with liver disease
Kidney disease	The urine of a patient with kidney disease might reveal a red and/or foamy appearance
Urinary tract tumors	The detection of blood in a patient's urine indicated the possibility of a tumor in the urinary system

1.3   Urine as a Body Fluid

It is important to correlate the clinical findings that include laboratory testing versus signs (the appearance of the patient) and symptoms (subjective complaints or remarks about how the patient feels). Since symptoms presented by a patient may be misleading, objective methods such as laboratory testing which excludes any psychological aspects of a disease state must be employed. The urine of a patient is not only tested for metabolic diseases and for infectious conditions of the urinary tract, but is useful in tests of toxicology, therapeutic drugs and drugs of abuse and for appropriate physiological processes in which the kidneys are involved. Testing of urine is typically used as a convenient, cost-effective and reliable method for accomplishing the following:

1. To diagnose disease based on clinical signs and symptoms
2. To establish the prognosis for a disease under treatment and assess the appropriateness of a chosen treatment protocol
3. To screen large population groups that may be free of symptoms, which may detect hereditary or congenital diseases prevalent in various geographic regions.

1.4   Clinical Relevance of Body Fluid Examinations

Since urine is the most commonly tested body fluid and reflects many clinical disease conditions, the urinalysis will be the most practical means for screening of both individual and of large populations of patients prior to utilizing perhaps the use of blood tests, which number in the thousands. Two unique characteristics of a urine specimen enable rapid screening of all patients:

1. Urine is a readily available and easily collected specimen but must be collected properly, including timed or random specimens. Tests have now been simplified to the extent that they are suitable for screening large numbers of individuals.
2. Urinary changes that may occur will contain information about many of the body's major metabolic functions. This information can be obtained by simple and rapid laboratory tests. These characteristics fit well with the current trends

toward preventive medicine that serves to lower medical costs, a necessity for maintaining a healthy population. By offering an inexpensive way to test large numbers of people not only for renal disease but also for the asymptomatic beginnings of conditions such as diabetes mellitus and liver disease, the urinalysis can be a valuable metabolic screening procedure. However, care must be taken in the laboratory to not ignore testing standards by letting the simplicity of the procedure result in relaxing the need for due diligence. Medical care must be taken by physicians to request the tests in a cost-effective manner, since health care costs consume a large proportion of the national budget.

1.5   Use of Urine and Body Fluids as an Assessment of Health

Urine is undoubtedly the most common and most effective body fluid other than blood that is frequently analyzed to determine the health or disease state that may exist in an individual patient or a group. Other body fluids are tested for the presence or absence of similar constituents to those found in the urine and blood, but at differing levels normally. When other body fluids are tested, the symptoms and signs related to specific body fluids require more detailed clinical information. During annual physical exams, urine as well as blood is tested as an overall estimation of the general health of an individual. Body fluids other than urine and blood, the most prevalent in specimens that are analyzed routinely are analyzed for specific values related to disease that would be manifested by abnormal results found in a specific anatomic site of the human body. For instance, it would be unwise and impracticable to collect a cerebrospinal fluid (CSF) for a routine examination in the absence of clinical signs and symptoms of a neurological condition.

The urine sample is an invaluable screening tool that yields evidence of a considerable number of clinical conditions not only for diseases of the kidney or other areas of the urinary system and includes vast numbers of metabolic diseases related to other organ systems. The following chapters will provide more specific information as to the value of a complete urinalysis and follow up measures that might be required in the assessment of health of the patient. The relationship to the clinical findings of abnormalities in urine and interrelated findings from other body fluids are discussed with specific pathological conditions of the patient.

1.6   Summary

Several different major body fluids are present in the body. Blood is the chief fluid found in the body and is the origin of the other fluids that are ultrafiltrates of blood plasma and arguably a possible exception is that of cerebrospinal fluid. Depending on the site where body fluids are produced and typically found, the presence of certain chemicals or cells, if absent, increased or decreased, may provide clues for the presence of disease. In addition, body fluids may also contain metabolites that can be measured, such as toxic materials, levels of therapeutic drugs, drugs of abuse, and may be used to assess the physiological processes of the kidneys. And although the examination of urine dates to perhaps many years before the advent of written history, in earlier times little was known about the other body fluids as valuable clinical specimens nor was it written about in ancient documents.

Review Questions

1. Name the three basic types of examinations performed during the evaluation of body fluids.
2. Discuss uses of a urine analysis for the evaluation of a patient
3. What are the visible characteristics examined for with the macroscopic examination of urine and other body fluids?
4. Why is a urine such a valuable and effective means of discovering diseases involving body organs and systems?
5. What are some similarities of urine relative to body fluids other than whole blood?

Answers Found in Appendix C

Quality Assurance and Laboratory Regulation

2

Objective(s)

Understand quality assurance and the components comprising a QA program

Compare quality control and quality assurance, providing similarities and differences

Discuss the role of quality control (QC) in the performance of laboratory procedures

Compare quality control functions and that of proficiency testing

List the areas that are monitored and evaluated in an effective quality assurance program

Contrast reliability, accuracy, precision and variance as components of a QA program

2.1   Quality Assurance or Quality Management and Regulation of Laboratory Practice

Several agencies provide guidelines for programs designed to ensure that specimen collection, handling, testing and reporting are handled in a systematic manner that limits errors in both testing and the handling and use of results. The program is one of continuous implementation and monitoring of the program to prevent both technical and procedural errors that would negatively impact the quality of care afforded the patient. Quality assurance provides for an on-going evaluative process that is implemented, monitored, and evaluated on a regular basis to insure quality results as it applies to the clinical laboratory. There are several elements of this program that are practiced at least daily or for each work shift in the medical laboratory.

A set of processes called *Quality Control* (QC) is part of the evaluative process and is the most prominent element of quality assurance programs for the clinical laboratory, where commercially prepared sets of samples are processed along with patient samples. These samples are used to insure reproducibility of quality control specimens on a regular basis. They will signal problems with the *analytical* portion of the

© Springer International Publishing AG, part of Springer Nature 2018
J. W. Ridley, *Fundamentals of the Study of Urine and Body Fluids*,
https://doi.org/10.1007/978-3-319-78417-5_2

procedure (pre- and post-analytical elements are equally important and are discussed later in this textbook). Quality control is not the only component of a quality assurance program found in the laboratory, but it is the most visible and effective means for insuring quality results for laboratory values obtained by clinical testing. Quality assurance for the lab consists chiefly of quality control measures for evluating accuracy in test performance. Quality assurance for the laboratory is a part of the quality assurance program for the entire facility and are interrelated. Discussions found in this textbook will generally refer specifically to the study of urine and other body fluids.

Both *internal quality control* and *external quality control* is employed in the quality control program of most health care facilities. The major differences in these two types of quality control samples lie in the source of the samples used for testing. External quality control programs utilize samples that are purchased from a commercial provider. These controls will contain several levels of results, from low to high levels for the constituents tested for in each procedure. Control samples may be either assayed or unassayed, meaning that expected results are provided with assayed samples, while unassayed samples are normally used only after the facility performs sufficient numbers of procedures which would allow the laboratory to calculate its own range of acceptable values. Internal controls may be obtained from patient specimens that are pooled and are preserved for up to several months and are performed at intervals during the day. Significant deviations that develop indicate that some sort of malfunction of equipment may be the cause. Another area that may cause deviations from expected quality control values occurs when testing supplies or controls may have deteriorated when the samples are improperly stored or handled.

Besides quality control procedures, the *quality assurance* program involving other areas of the facility includes evaluation, communication and monitoring the activities that include coordination with the facility, other laboratory departments and the clinical staff including the physicians and designated care providers such as physician's assistants and nurse practitioners. Failure to pay heed to all three areas may present a barrier to effectively providing timely and accurate results to facilitate adequate patient care. Regardless of the clinical setting where laboratory procedures including tests on urine and other body fluids are performed, there are basic requirements to insure quality of work that must be followed. Other settings besides hospital laboratories (Fig. 2.1) that are mandated to employ quality assurance programs range from reference laboratories, physician office laboratories (POLs), multi-physician clinics, rehabilitation and long-term care facilities.

Both voluntary accreditation agencies and governmental agency requirements play a role in the use of a quality assurance plan. The laboratories in all the settings previously listed must first be governed by internal standards established by managers of the facility itself. In addition, the program must comply with the requirements of a quality assurance program that will be required by a professional accreditation agency. For hospitals and clinics, voluntary accreditation bodies such as the *Joint Commission* and the College of American Pathologists (CAP) inspect sites for compliance with their established standards for laboratory practice. In addition, categorical accreditation agencies for areas of the laboratory exist for specialty areas including blood banking (*immunohematology*) and microbiology, among others.

Points to Remember
Steps must be made daily to insure valid results through laboratory testing. A quality assurance program is necessary in any type of laboratory, ranging from physician office labs to specialized medical center laboratories. Quality control programs are an essential part of insuring that test results can be trusted in the diagnosis and treatment of disease.

Fig. 2.1 Hospital laboratory

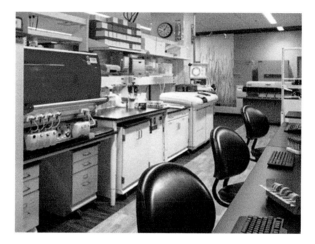

2.2   Regulations That Govern Laboratory Testing

The federal government began the regulation of laboratories somewhat simultaneously with the advent of Medicare in 1965. The result was legislation that became effective under the *Clinical Laboratory Improvement Amendments of 1967* (CLIA '67). This legislation originally included only hospital, independent and reference laboratories which engaged in interstate commerce where these labs accepted test samples that crossed state lines. This regulation was made necessary in a series of highly publicized cases where erroneous laboratory results were provided by both hospital and reference laboratories. The initial federal regulation of laboratories provided for inspections and accreditation of hospital and independent laboratories that performed tests on Medicare patients and billed the federal government for these tests.

In October of 1988, Congress began even more stringent regulation of laboratories through the *Clinical Laboratory Improvement Amendments* (CLIA '88) which replaced the CLIA '67 act as well as all previous regulations mandated by *Medicare* and *Medicaid*. The CLIA '88 requirements are funded by the Health Care Financing Administration (HCFA), a division of the US Department of Health and Human Services (HHS). These new regulations were met with a storm of comments, some in protest of the increased regulation of certain laboratories, and particularly those from physician office laboratories (POL's). These CLIA regulations divided laboratory tests into *waived, moderately and highly complex* procedures based on difficulty and those that required interpretation of results. The laboratories themselves are categorized into one of these divisions, and the category to which the lab is assigned is based on the types of tests that may be performed by each and specifies the level of training required of employees that perform the complexity levels of tests.

Terminology was utilized under CLIA '88 that sought to include all laboratories, by describing laboratories as diagnostic facilities that were established for testing biological, biochemical, serological, microbiological, immunohematological, hematological, biophysical, *cytological*, and *pathological* specimens. Some other examinations of materials from the human body to be tested were also regulated based on the level of treatment diagnosis and prevention or treatment of any medical condition afflicting human beings. Laboratories which performed only minimal procedures of low complexity such as those by physician office laboratories (POLs) were required to apply for a certificate of waiver as a response to complaints from some of these offices.

Those performing moderately complex and highly complex procedures were required to obtain a registration certificate. In January of 1993, an addition to the regulations allowed physicians to perform six different microscopic examinations on his or her patients with no official oversight by an external agency, either local or federal. Some components of a urinalysis are waived, but the microscopic examination is a moderately complex test, and is not performed as a *waived test* procedure. Not all regulations pertaining to the clinical laboratory are established on the federal level. Some individual states and in some cases local governmental agencies have regulations that are equal to or more stringent than those of the federal government. For example, most of the states require state licensure of laboratory professionals and other practices that contain requirements that exceed those established on the federal level.

2.2.1 Other Regulatory Agencies

Accreditation by voluntary agencies is sought by many laboratories to enhance their public images and to provide for continuing education and professional activities by their members. But along with CLIA, many states require facility and/or personnel licensure as well as compliance with other non-voluntary regulatory requirements of clinical laboratories. In addition, medical education programs are also regulated by state governments as well as by voluntary agencies. Some of the states have established strict personnel standards that are enforced before an individual may work in any capacity where medical laboratory procedures are performed and where results are produced that are used in diagnosing and treating patients. There are some additional regulatory offices (Table 2.1) that have at least minimal oversight of medical laboratories, both voluntary and non-voluntary.

> **Points to Remember**
> Some agencies exist for the sole purpose of setting and enforcing standards that lead to overall quality of a laboratory's operations. Some of these are governmental and require licensure and verification that minimum standards for the facility and its personnel are met. Other agencies called professional accreditation bodies have similar goals to those of governmental agencies. Membership in these organizations is voluntary and requires the meeting of standards for the accredited facility as well as its members. The main goal of professional organizations is to advance the public image of the profession, while insuring that educational standards are met.

Table 2.1 Regulatory offices with oversight of medical laboratories

OSHA	Occupational Safety and Health Administration
EPA	Environmental Protection Agency
COLA/HCFA/CLIA[a]	Commission on Office Laboratory Accreditation for physician office laboratories (COLA), and Health Care Finance Administration (HCFA) considered equivalent to standards by Clinical Laboratory Improvement Act (CLIA) regulations
The Joint Commission	Formerly the Joint Commission on Accreditation of Healthcare Organizations (JCAHO)
NCCLS	National Committee for Clinical Laboratory Standards (NCCLS) provides educational standards for both national and international educational and training programs for laboratory professionals
ASCP	American Society of Clinical Pathologists (ASCP) provide for credentialing of laboratory professionals, including pathologists (MDs) who are in addition licensed by their respective states in which they practice

[a]Equivalent regulatory requirements in these agencies

2.3   Elements of an Effective Quality Assurance Program

A quality assurance program is an ongoing and continuous process that encompasses all the areas of operation. The program is designed to improve the quality and efficiency of the laboratory, although in a medical facility, the quality assurance program is not confined to the laboratory, but to the entire facility. In the laboratory, where test results are vitally important in the diagnosis and treatment of the patient, a commitment by all personnel is paramount to comply with the quality assurance program to be effective. When records are complete, and accuracy has been assured and problem areas are resolved, the employees will be fulfilled and will become more self-confident and more likely to continue to adhere to the protocol established.

Essentially, the quality assurance program will monitor the procedure for requesting procedures, proper identification of the patient, accurate specimen procurement, identification of samples and the transporting of samples to the laboratory. Required processing of the samples and distribution of the samples to the appropriate laboratory department or section is one step in an outlined sequence that is called the *preanalytical* portion of the performance of the procedure. The actual performance of the procedure is the analytical step, and includes laboratory personnel performance, instrumentation, reagents and the technical or *analytical* step. *Postanalytical* concerns involve insuring that a reasonable result based on the clinical data available was achieved and transmitted to the appropriate person or department, that acceptable turnaround times for completion and distribution of the results occurred, and maintenance of the sample as required by the standards in the event a procedure must be repeated for confirmation (Table 2.2). Components of a quality assurance program for a clinical laboratory or department within the laboratory include, but not limited to:

Points to Remember
A quality assurance program incorporates all elements of a facility that may affect the appropriateness of services rendered. In the laboratory, personnel qualifications and the effectiveness of the quality control policies are the main components of the quality assurance program as it addresses laboratory testing.

Table 2.2 Components of laboratory quality assurance program

Quality control protocol and records of results and corrective actions
Procedure manuals outlining all aspects of the performance and reporting of test results
Actions to take to remedy out-of-control results for quality control specimens
Management of the collection, distribution and testing of patient samples
Specimen collection, transport and processing
Determining adequate turnaround time for specimen collection to reporting results
Comparison of test results
Proficiency sample testing
Test results and the correlation with clinical information for each patient
Evaluation of quality control results on a scheduled basis
Follow up in complaint resolutions
Technical competence through assessment of personnel qualifications and practice
Provision of continuing education and opportunity for personal improvement
Routine personnel evaluations to identify concerns, weaknesses and strengths
Maintenance of quality assurance records
Scheduled review of quality assurance program and results with staff
Improvement of the physical location and organization of the laboratory site
Access to library sources and professional journals and articles
Review of proficiency test results for improvement, recognizing outstanding performance
Elimination of safety hazards through training and adherence to safe practices

2.3.1   Quality Control, a Component of a Quality Assurance Program

Quality control as a component of the quality assurance program is a means by which the laboratory ensures that results obtained from testing are valid. Quality control records are a vital component in the inspection of the laboratory by both voluntary accreditation agencies as well as by offices of the state and federal governments. In the final CLIA regulation of 1988, it is stressed that the laboratory must establish and adhere to a written quality control plan that includes each procedure performed. The purpose of the written quality control standards is intended to monitor and evaluate the effectiveness of the testing methods used to assure accuracy and reliability of patient test results.

Several terms relating to the description of reliability, which simply means "can the results be trusted" are used by inspectors of the laboratory. But some medical laboratory professionals are unsure of the distinction between *precision* and *accuracy* (Fig. 2.2). The term 'precision' refers to the reproducibility or repeatability of a result for a given control sample or samples and should not vary significantly for different days or during a 24 period. In a quality control program, there should be very little variance between the results obtained from the control samples for each 'run' or batch of tests performed. It should be remembered that control samples are included in each batch of tests for each procedure performed, even during the same day.

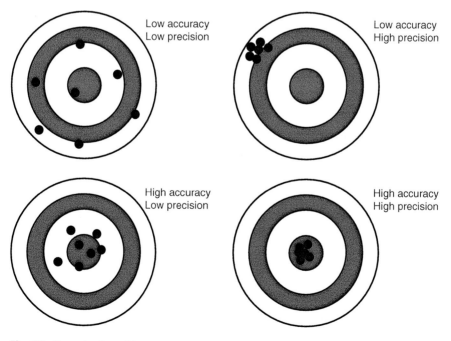

Fig. 2.2 Example of precision versus accuracy

Therefore, reproducibility or precision does not refer to accuracy, although some laboratorians equate precision with accuracy. The term 'accuracy' is used for results that are close to the absolute or true value of the analyte (test component) that is being measured. So, it can be deduced that precision can be present while accuracy may fall short of reflecting the true value of the product being tested for. Several variables are related to but are not limited to the work environment. These include heat and humidity among other physical conditions, the age and condition of the instrument components, the operator, and variations in the electrical supply may be minimal as some small variations in the day-to-day performance in a laboratory are inevitable.

Accuracy is best achieved by using standardized procedures to minimize as many of the variables associated with the testing procedure as possible. When procedures are modified, or new methods are adopted, valid comparisons must be performed which assess the correlation of the two procedures while using the same set of standards and controls for both methods. Another valuable component of assessing accuracy is found in the use of *proficiency testing* programs, in which prepared samples are provided to the laboratory. The results transmitted to the provider are compared with other similar laboratories using similar methodology. Standardized reports enable the laboratory staff to assess their performance for each procedure and to take remedial steps for values outside the acceptable ranges. Unacceptable performance on proficiency samples used to assess accuracy may result in punitive action by regulatory agencies that inspect a medical lab.

Precision is best assessed by including standards, reference samples or control materials in each set of procedures. Statistical determinations of variances from the mean average signal that either technical or other problems may exist. Quality control charts may be manually prepared or are often provided by the more automated instruments used to perform the tests. Statistically significant deviations from the expected results require a systematic approach for troubleshooting the methodology. The error(s) may occur with the control materials themselves, the reagents used for testing, malfunctions of the analytical equipment, poor specimen handling, or poor technical performance by the operators (laboratory personnel). Day-to-day control samples, between a run (a set of samples) processed in the same day, or by incorporating blind samples to assess reproducibility from a previous run are commonly utilized to assess precision.

Points to Remember
Precision and accuracy are related but are separate entities. Accuracy without precision, or reproducibility, would be pointless. Precision is accomplished through the periodic use of control samples, and accuracy is achieved by analyzing samples sent by a provider of programs that include all departmental testing in the laboratory.

2.3.1.1 Statistical Variance

Statistical variance exists for all testing, whether using patient samples, control samples or proficiency specimens. It is impossible to obtain the exact same measurements each day due to a variety of variables that may affect the procedure. Environmental factors such as humidity, temperature, equipment fatigue, slight differences in dilutions of reagents and control samples all can play a part in any variances. An *acceptable* level of variance is determined after repetitious testing over an established length of time. Assayed values of controls from the manufacturer of the samples are used initially, until the facility develops its own values, which are often more stringent than those provided by the manufacturer. This spread of data is determined by calculating the standard deviation, or spread of data, from repeat testing of the same control materials over an agreed time span. Remember that many labs at this point develop their own control samples from pooled specimens that are stored and used for a considerable length of time, often for a year's time.

A quality assurance program also serves to establish the technical competence of the professional staff, and this is affected by the level of education, training and due diligence exercised by each individual working in the laboratory. CLIA regulations regarding the practice of quality control are complicated and address the complexity of testing using waived tests, and medium and high complexity tests and agree to *pre-approved* procedures to be performed in a laboratory. Appropriate controls of urine or other body fluids must be adequate for all constituents tested for in the laboratory.

Some controls are semi-quantitative and are thusly named as they do not provide a numerical level, ie. 100 mg/dL such as is found in a plasma glucose determination. Controls will be provided for testing the chemical components of the urine sample where a dipstick is utilized with color-reactive chemically-impregnated pads. This is a semi-quantitative type of method, with results reported as trace, small amount, moderate amount, or large amount whereby no specific numerical value is obtained that is documented on a Levy-Jennings or other chart. Confirmatory tests must be performed on some positive results measured by the dipstick, since there are many interfering substances and conditions that will yield false positive and false negative results. The microscopic portion of the urinalysis procedure provides a more *quantitative* result where an actual narrow range of solid components such as blood cells, crystals and microorganisms are enumerated.

Results for control samples that exceed the allowable range are rejected and patient results cannot be released until certain remedial actions take place in which the samples are retested. In general, two control specimens, usually a normal and an abnormal level must be utilized at a minimum. Many control samples come in a set of three, where one will give results in a low abnormal range, the second will provide normal level results, and the third will often provide results in an abnormally high range. The quality control program to assess the reliability of laboratory results must contain documentation of results and must monitor the following areas that might impact the quality control and test results (Table 2.3):

Table 2.3 Factors impacting test results	Facility conditions (air quality, temperature, lighting, etc.)
	Condition of test reagents, supplies and materials
	Education and training of technical personnel
	Protocol for specimen collection, maintenance, preservation and transport
	Regular updating of procedure manuals
	Methodology suitable for all types of testing
	Required maintenance of equipment records
	Calibration records for each instrument
	Schedule of quality control testing (control processes)
	Remedial actions plan for out-of-range results
	All quality control records of results for a required length of time

Levy-Jennings QC Chart
Control X Constituent

	1	2	3	4	5	6	7	8	9	10	11	12	13	14	15
3 SD															X
2 SD			X									X			
1 SD	X					X	X						X		
Mean		X			X				X		X				
-1SD				X						X				X	
-2SD						X									
-3SD															
Day	1	2	3	4	5	6	7	8	9	10	11	12	13	14	15

Fig. 2.3 Sample Levy Jennings Chart used for recording quality control values

Statistical variances are sometimes shown by a Levy-Jennings chart (Fig. 2.3) and is sometimes displayed graphically. But the results of individual "runs" where various levels of control samples are included in the set of patient data produced and must be stored for required periods of time. With computer storage widely available, QC results are automatically saved by components of many of the major analytical instruments when sample are run as an automated procedure. Major errors may cause faulty results when testing body fluids such as urine for accurate clinical data. These errors most frequently occur when medical laboratory professionals deviate from established principles outlined in the procedure manual and when violations of quality assurance standards occur.

Examples of some of these departures from good, standard practice are:

1. Using urine or other fluid samples that were left at room temperature for a length of time
2. Collecting samples in dirty of inadequate containers
3. Reagent strip bottles have been exposed to moisture and heat
4. Tablet reagents have become moist
5. Failure to follow procedures provided by package inserts or the procedure manual
6. Inadequate mixing or failure to mix the sample causing poor distribution of solid components in the body fluid
7. Failure to observe interfering substances such as medications
8. Clerical errors, a postanalytical process resulting in faulty or misdirected results
9. Failure to repeat procedures on new samples with extremely unusual or confusing results
10. Failure to recognize an abnormal specimen or result
11. Focus on a single test without comparing results with clinical data and other test results

2.4 Reporting Patient Results

There are two types of controls, quantitative and qualitative. Qualitative merely provide a result of *positive* or *negative* and the quality control records are quite simple, where the two controls are performed with each *run* or set of samples to be tested. The quantitative tests provide an actual value that is reported, for example, 35 mg of a certain chemical as established quantitative volumes that correlate with the test. The quantitative procedures may have as many as three different levels of results, and the data must be documented. These documents are examined by accrediting and licensure agencies when their representatives make an official visit to a laboratory. In the complete urinalysis procedure, the dipstick chemical results are semi-quantitative, where results may be graded as positive, small amount, negative or high level. Some of the components of other body fluids are performed as quantitative procedures where the glucose for a cerebrospinal fluid, for instance, may yield a value of 49 mg/dl (100 ml). The quantitative procedures and the units in which they are reported are covered thoroughly in clinical chemistry textbooks.

A system for evaluating quality control results to determine if patient results are valid and can be reported to the physician or other clinician frequently utilizes a set of standards called Westgard's Rules. Control results must fall within a certain predetermined range each time a given procedure is performed. The control results must be within a range established by a statistical measurement called the standard deviation. In most cases, the control results must be within two standard deviations before reporting patient results as valid.

1. Warning Rule–It is broken when one control measurement exceeds the ±2 SD guideline. Other rules must now be tested by examining other control values in the run (within run) and in previous runs (across runs) before deciding on the acceptability of the patient's results. If any of the remaining rules are violated, the laboratory professional must thoroughly examine the test's analytical procedure, perform troubleshooting measures, and perform maintenance or other established measures before making any decision about releasing the results or re-running the test.

2. Within-run Only Rule–Detects random error but may also point to systematic error. The run is considered out-of-control when one control value exceeds the ±3 SD limits

3. Systematic Error–This rule detects systematic error and can be applied within and across runs. It is violated when two consecutive control values exceed the same ±2 SD limit.

4. Range Rule–applied within run only to detect random error. It is violated when the SD difference between two consecutive control values exceeds 4 SD.

5. Systematic Error Within and Across Runs–This rule detects systematic error and is applied within and across runs. It is violated within the control material when the last four control values of the same level exceed the same ±SD limit. A violation occurs across control materials when the last four consecutive controls for different levels exceed the same ±1 SD.

6. Systematic Error Both Within and Across Runs–This rule detects systematic error and is applied both within and across runs. It is violated within the control material when the last ten values for the same control level are all on the same side of the mean. If violated across control materials when the last ten consecutive values, regardless of control level, are the same side of the mean. The number of values considered can be decreased if three or more levels of control are run

2.5   Selection of Assayed or Unassayed Control Materials

For quantitative methods, laboratories can use either "assayed" or "unassayed" control materials. Assayed controls are controls for which the manufacturer of the materials has established the acceptable limits or range for the control test results. Generally, the limits represent a two to three standard deviation (SD) range. When control results fall outside the limits, the laboratory must take corrective action. Unassayed controls are controls which the laboratory tests initially along with assayed controls. The laboratory will establish confidence levels for the unassayed controls and then will cease using assayed controls and will use its own statistical analyses to establish an acceptable range for control values. Most laboratories will eventually establish a narrower range or limits of 2 SDs after operations have been in place for a given length of time, and this indicates improvement in the functions of the laboratory.

Most quality control rules will detect either random or systematic error. There is actually an acceptable level of random errors, but these are usually so minimal in number and clinical significance that patients are not harmed in most instances.

There are some built-in safeguards for various pieces of laboratory equipment that will alert the operator that a result should be repeated or confirmed. Effective quality control procedures require sensitivity to both types of error and an acceptably low false rejection rate. Improved sensitivity to both random and systematic error can be achieved by combining quality control rules. Quality control procedures using a combination of rules are called "multirule control procedures" or multirule procedures. Multirule procedures define both the rules and the order in which the rules are applied to the control data. According to the CLIA requirements, when control results are outside established criteria for acceptability, the laboratory must take and document remedial action to correct the problem. The control results must be acceptable prior to reporting patient results and if the corrective action taken indicates that the patient test results could be affected, the laboratory must retest patient specimens. The laboratory's quality control procedure for corrective action will most often include the following guidelines in the sequence provided.

1. Repeat testing using the same control or calibrator material.
2. Repeat testing with a new vial of control or calibrator material.
3. Verify all reagent lot numbers and expiration dates in use.
4. Look for obvious variations or instrument failures.
5. Repeat testing using a new lot of control or calibrator material, if available.
6. Perform basic preventive maintenance.
7. Recalibrate, if appropriate, and repeat control testing.
8. Open new reagent, calibrate and repeat testing, if appropriate.
9. Call service.
10. Notify supervisor.
11. Document all corrective action.

   All corrective actions and records or repeat testing or confirmation of results must be retained as items that will be examined by an inspector of a licensure or accreditation body. In summary, a "quality" control program that ensures that steps and documentation are taken ultimately ensures that the laboratory is reporting accurate and reliable patient test results. Note that patient results cannot be reported in the following cases (Box 2.1). The "run" should be rejected if:

Box 2.1: Conditions Where Results Are Not Reported
1. One control exceeds the mean by ±3 SD
2. One control exceeds the mean by 2 SD in the same direction (±) two consecutive times for two controls in the same run or two controls in the same run
3. Two controls in same run differ by 4 SD (ie., one +2 SD while second is −2 SD)
4. Four consecutive controls exceed the mean by 1 SD or more in the same direction
5. Ten consecutive values fall on the same side of the mean

Points to Remember
In order to report patient results that will be used in the diagnosis and treatment of patients, statistical means are used to insure that a "run" or batch of samples can be insured of being reasonably accurate. Consistent rules are followed and when deviations from the expected range of results of control values, occurs the patient values cannot be reported until remedial action is taken.

2.6   Summary

A quality assurance program is a complex plan that incorporates a large number of entities that may affect determination of the accuracy of results and their proper reporting. While it is the most involved of the components of a quality assurance system, quality control for control samples is not the only area which may make it necessary to troubleshoot the steps leading to the completion of a procedure. Quality assurance plans and in particular quality control results and calculations are required by a number of licensing and accreditation bodies, and must be available for examination during an inspection of the facilities. The precision and accuracy of laboratory procedures are verified through the practices required by an effective quality assurance program. This entails concurrent running of control samples with each set of procedures, and compiling the data to insure precision. Proficiency testing programs are run as regularly scheduled to insure accuracy when compared with values from other laboratories with a similar menu of tests and methodology.

Review Questions

1. What is the importance of quality assurance?
2. Quality assessment would be best described as:
3. What is meant by quality control? Describe key elements of a quality control program.
4. When a new procedure is adopted, what would be an initial responsibility of the clinical staff of the laboratory?
5. The primary goal of an effective quality assurance program is:

Answers Found in Appendix C

Safety Practices in Testing Areas

3

Objective(s)

Understand the importance of safety regulations for laboratory personnel

List potentially hazardous conditions in the clinical laboratory

Explain why biohazardous wastes should be separated from basic wastes in the medical laboratory

Discuss the need for an infection control plan

Explain how laboratory wastes are discarded

Understand precautions necessary to avoid exposure to hazardous conditions in the laboratory

Describe personal responsibility of the worker for maintaining a safe environment

List a number of physical hazards associated with the workplace

List some sources of bodily specimens with the potential for transmitting infectious diseases

Understand the role of the medical facility in protecting the medical workers and the patients

List examples of work practice controls

List examples of engineered controls in the typical medical care facility

List pre-exposure procedures (don't forget education and training components)

Discuss processes involved in post-exposure activities

3.1 General Description of Safety in the Laboratory

An overall and integrated plan for safety is a management level responsibility. All departments and offices of a modern health care facility formulate a plan specific to each department, which is then integrated into a facility-wide plan. Safety should be foremost in the minds of all employers and employees providing health care. Training is provided on a regular basis in order to maintain a valid program which includes patient safety, employee safety and facility safety. In addition to workers

© Springer International Publishing AG, part of Springer Nature 2018
J. W. Ridley, *Fundamentals of the Study of Urine and Body Fluids*,
https://doi.org/10.1007/978-3-319-78417-5_3

and patients, safety of visitors and others who enter the facility, even for business purposes, must be considered. After adoption of a safety plan, the program is implemented, maintained, and regularly evaluated for any needed revisions as to effectiveness. During facility surveys from accreditation and licensing agencies both for single departments and those including the entire facility, safety plans are evaluated. The extensive safety programs include *biohazards*, toxic hazards from materials dangerous to humans and even use of certain medications. Proper maintenance and use of equipment in order to avoid injuries due to defective equipment, maintenance and design of the physical plant itself are vital components of a safety program. Any accidents or accidental exposures to toxic or biohazardous materials must be reported to the appropriate officials.

> **Points to Remember**
> Safety is a responsibility of the facility as well as of ALL employees. There are legal implications and economic reasons for providing safety for employees, patients and visitors in a medical facility.

3.1.1   Clinical Laboratory Safety Standards

Standards for safety of laboratory workers is designated by federal, state and sometimes local governmental authorities, agencies and committees. These standards are intended not only for protecting workers in the laboratory, but other healthcare personnel, patients under treatment and visitors who enter the grounds or the facility. The Occupational Safety and Health Administration (OSHA) in 1970 promulgated a system of regulations stipulating certain safeguards in buildings, grounds and within departments to ensure safe and healthful working conditions. OSHA, operating under the U.S. Department of Labor, regulates any business with one or more employees, and is interpreted to mean ALL businesses. OSHA standards, at a minimum, require appropriate warning labels and signs to alert workers of potential danger, and require PPE or personal protective equipment, procedures for exposure control and documentation of training and educational programs. In 1991, the advent of a newly discovered infection called HIV 1 forced adoption of two new standards, one for bloodborne pathogens and the other for hazard communications.

Hazards in the medical laboratory are manifold. Chemical, electrical, fire and explosion risks are present in many of the tasks performed in the lab. Biological hazards, based on handling of body fluids, and cultures of bacterial organisms are addressed in an Infection Control document that is also known as the Exposure Control program. Barrier devices for personal protection requires masks, face shields, gloves, and proper biohazardous discard containers for disposal of contaminated wastes are placed conspicuously in work areas. This facilitate quick disposal of these materials and ease of pickup by housekeeping for approved disposal at designated waste disposal sites in a systematic manner.

3.1.2   First Aid in the Clinical Laboratory

Since the employee's safety is paramount from an efficiency and economic standpoint as well as from a legal view, first aid is required as part of the clinical laboratory student's education. Of course, first aid is only the primary treatment to save lives and further damage before more definitive care can be rendered. Both educational programs and medical facilities must have effective safety plans as required by accreditation agencies. Medical facilities must offer annual courses on first aid as a part of their safety plan. This training may be considered as an integral component of the continuing education requirements for all personnel and documentation of training is open to inspecting agencies. Significant numbers of potential hazards exist in a clinical laboratory and each facility will establish its own protocol to follow in the event of an accident or "near accident." It is necessary to evaluate near accidents, in order to prevent repeat occurrences of an unsafe act.

Providing first aid is only a temporary stop-gap effort intended to reduce the effects of an accident or illness until a more advanced level of medical treatment is available, and means for the rescuer to provide for his or her own safety must be included. Basic steps in first aid training plans include the topics of stopping bleeding, preventing shock, restoring heartbeat and breathing. Additional measures to increase the victim's comfort and to avoid further complications of the illness or injury should be stressed.

3.1.3   Facility Safety Plan

Although the facility's safety plan addresses the entire institution, laboratory accreditation teams who perform a site visit in the medical laboratory also inspect safety programs pertinent only to the laboratory. Often joint overlap exists between agencies looking for similar violations of safety rules. Commonly a medical laboratory safety and exposure plan is adopted with input from a facility-wide *Safety Committee* in the hospital setting. The *Infection Control Committee* or *Exposure Control Committee* will have also have input into the policies and procedures specific to each department. Exposure or infection control committees are highly formal in nature and are an integral part of the administrative team involved in fulfilling the regulations imposed by state, federal and accrediting organizations.

Safety issues are most often managed by a committee that is separate from the infection or exposure control committees, although many of the functions overlap and there is a great deal of cooperation between these major committees. Both committees monitor activities that are facility wide, since biohazardous materials are found throughout many areas of the hospital. The safety committee monitors occupational risks that extend to patients and visitors as well as risks found on the grounds and the environment surrounding the facility. Where biohazardous materials or toxic chemicals are stored or used, these areas are clearly identified by signs (Figs. 3.1 and 3.2) warning of the presence of these materials. Material Safety Data Sheets are also provided in areas where certain materials are found that pose the potential to harm those who come in contact exists.

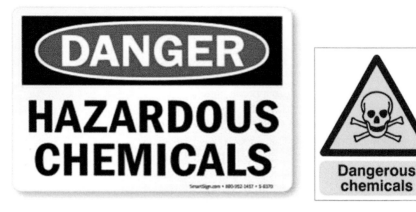

Fig. 3.1 Symbols and signs warning of chemical hazards

Fig. 3.2 Biohazard sign

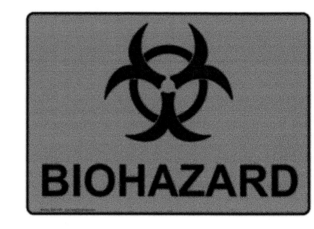

3.2 Potentially Hazardous Situations in the Laboratory

The clinical laboratory contains a number of safety hazards, and certain precautions must be taken by those working with patients and patient samples to avoid becoming infected with a serious microorganism. In order to maintain safety of its employees and students, the medical laboratory training programs are required to expend considerable time and effort toward educating workers and students of laboratory science regarding the multitude of possibilities for injury and infection. Primarily, those performing tasks within the laboratory environment must be informed of hazards that are present as a "right to know." Basic precautions associated with each of these hazards and how to use common sense and training for continuous safety requires orientation and training for each worker. Oftentimes, exposure leading to the contraction of a disease occurs when a laboratory staff member becomes complacent regarding associated risks or violates certain safety policies.

It bears repeating that potential hazards exist in all medical laboratories. Biological, chemical and physical components follow this order of precedence and are major threats to safety in a laboratory environment. The use of toxic chemicals, some with the risk of promoting respiratory problems or even death if inhaled require the use of a properly installed and maintained fume hood. Students and workers who handle both biohazardous chemicals and certain microorganisms that are highly contagious should be trained in the use of this protective device. Some hoods are specifically designed for microorganisms such as virulent bacteria, viruses, and fungi, yeasts and molds only. Different types of hoods are used when working with toxic chemicals which are opened and poured under a hood, preventing vapors from being breathed by the workers. A number of safety components for physical hazards are mandated by building codes, and certain safety equipment is required by state and local law for certain tasks. These regulations have greatly decreased the number of accidents and *exposure incidents,* and no doubt death for some.

> **Safety Alert**
> Safety in a medical facility is more complex than that of other types of industrial plants. There is a potential for likely exposure to infectious organisms and toxic chemicals on a regular basis, and to electrical hazards and other environmental hazards. Any personal involvement with the medical facility, regardless of category of occupation or as a visitor, is subject to being exposed to these potentially hazardous conditions and materials.

3.2.1   Biological Hazards

An understanding of the methods by which biohazards (microorganisms) are spread is graphically depicted by the *Chain of Infection* (Fig. 3.3). Hazardous materials and conditions are separate components of a plan for insuring safety of all who work in or otherwise come in contact with the typical health care environment. The health care facility has a responsibility to protect its employees, the patients it treats, and its visitors, vendors and any contract workers who may be exposed to hazardous conditions or materials. Many governmental and private regulatory agencies and organizations contribute to efforts to set standards and policies with a goal of achieving safety for everyone who has any relationship with a health care facility. The overriding goal of hospitals or other health care facilities is to provide quality care while assuring its employees and patients are safe by providing a healthful and safe environment.

There must be a link between the source of an infection, the mode of transmission, and a host that is susceptible to becoming infected in order for an infectious disease to be communicated. Breaking this chain of infection is a requirement for avoiding or halting the spread of biohazards. In some cases, an immunocompromised person may be more susceptible for contracting an infectious disease than one with an intact immune system. However, a healthy individual with a good

Fig. 3.3 Chain of infection

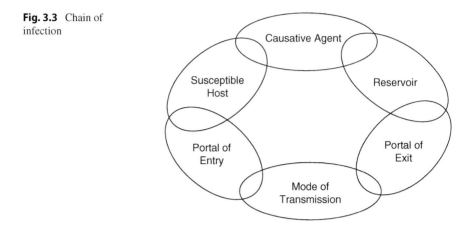

immune status and with no breaks in the skin may also become infected. Susceptibility is often increased in a hospital setting via the administration of certain medications, debilitating illnesses, and even those with a genetic predisposition for becoming infected. It is called *direct contact* when accidental infection occurs through direct contact with an infected patient. Indirect contact transmission occurs where no direct human-to-human contact has occurred. This type of transmission occurs from a reservoir of organisms on a contaminated surface or object. A less common mode of indirect contact occurs when vectors such as mosquitoes, flies, mites, fleas, ticks, rodents or dogs transmit an infectious agent to the health care employee or patient.

Infection Control Flash

The symbolic unraveling or breaking of any link in the Chain of Infection may expose a number of persons to the potential for harm due to a biohazardous material. The spread of disease to others in a short time may lead to a widespread outbreak when conditions are suitable. An exposure may spread a disease beyond the walls of the medical facility when employees and visitors leave the building(s), leading to a local epidemic.

3.2.2 Exposure to Non-biological Hazardous Materials

OSHA's Hazard Communication Standard (HCS) requires that information will be provided by the employer to all workers that may be exposed to hazardous chemicals in all industrial enterprises. This standard is based on the assertion that employees have both a need and a right to know the hazards and the identities of the chemicals they are exposed to in their individual workplaces. They are also mandated to be provided with information and equipment that afford protective measures to limit exposure to dangerous materials. Steps to take to minimize and prevent potential adverse effects from occurring are required through training and must be provided regarding any hazardous material, either biohazardous or otherwise, capable of presenting risks to the health of the employee.

It is estimated that more than 30 million workers are potentially exposed to one or more chemical hazards through their work at any given time. There is a growing arsenal of both naturally occurring and person-made chemicals that is currently estimated at more than 650,000 different compounds. Many of these cause serious side effects upon exposure and present employers with the challenge of assuring adequate transmission of knowledge to each employee through education and training. Any job changes require that an employee be provided additional training to meet new challenges.

The HCS requires information regarding physical hazards such as flammability or possibility of explosions, and health hazards that include acute effects, some of which may result in life-long medical conditions. Through the HCS requirement, information must be available to both employers and employees regarding potential hazards for the mammoth list of chemicals used for industrial purposes. Published recommendations of training for precautions leading to proper use of certain materials should reduce the number of illnesses and injuries caused by chemical exposure.

Fortunately, many chemicals used in the medical laboratories and health care facilities have been engineered to be less caustic or dangerous as methodologies change. Employers are provided the information they need from product inserts that may be used to design an appropriate training program for employees and any operational changes requiring additional training. It should be noted that when employees change positions, they will be immediately oriented as to the risks of any new materials with which they will have contact. With proper knowledge, employees are more willing to participate in these programs effectively when they understand the hazards involved, and understand measures necessary to protect themselves. Together, joint actions and responsibilities of the employer and the employee actions will prevent the occurrence of adverse effects caused by exposure to chemicals in the workplace.

The HCS establishes uniform requirements to make sure that the hazards of all chemicals imported into, produced, or used in U.S. workplaces are evaluated and that this hazard information is provided to employers and employees who may be exposed to hazardous materials. Chemical manufacturers and importers are required to publish the hazard information they learn from their evaluations to employers who use the materials. Containers must be labeled with standard labels as to their contents, and material safety data sheets (MSDS's) are transmitted to the companies using the products. In addition, all covered employers must have a hazard communication program to inform their employees as to the meaning of labels and warning signs where certain products are used. Material safety data sheets are required to be filed in the work areas for emergency treatment (see Appendix B, Sample Material Safety Data Sheet).

Safety Alert
The employees of the institution must be informed of and trained for the appropriate measures designed to prevent exposure to hazardous and toxic materials. These practices are mandated by a federal agency and are often incorporated into the standards published by accreditation agencies. Again, avoiding exposure and potential injury to the employee, the patient and the visitor is a joint responsibility of the employer and each individual.

All workplaces where employees are exposed to hazardous chemicals must have a written plan which describes how the standard will be implemented in that facility. The work operations which do not have to comply with the written plan requirements are those where employees only handle chemicals in sealed containers. But any broken container that is leaking must be reported immediately. The written program must reflect the duties each employee performs in a particular workplace. For example, the written plan must list the chemicals present at the site, indicate who is responsible for the various aspects of the program in that facility and where written materials will be made available to employees. In addition, the written program must describe how the requirements for labels and other forms of warning, material safety data sheets, and employee information and training are going to be met in the facility.

3.2.3   The Effect of Federal Law on State Right-To-Know Laws

The HCS requirements supersede all state laws in states without OSHA-approved job safety and health programs or any local laws which relate to issues handled by HCS. This exemption is without regard as to whether a state law conflicts with, complements, or supplements the federal standard, and without regard to whether the state law appears to be as effective as HCS federal standards. The only state worker right-to-know laws that are authorized would be those established in some 26 states and jurisdictions that have OSHA-approved state programs. Federal workers that work under the hazard communication standard are covered by executive order.

3.2.4   Internal Sources for Providing a Safe Workplace

Health care facilities will have a more thorough understanding of risks inherent to the enterprise that will external agencies providing inspections and surveillance. This responsibility of the facility in providing for the safety of employees, patients and visitors is an extremely important function. Regulations and guidelines are provided by a number of licensure and accrediting agencies. The biological component of safety known as *biohazards* and the chemical and physical components of safety are sometimes handled by two separate committees, although the duties may overlap and are sometimes handled by a single committee. These committees are comprised of individuals appointed from all of the major areas of the health care facility. Committees are responsible for initiating policies regarding safety and procedures designed to prevent contraction of disease through exposure to all categories of hazards in the workplace. These committees were previously discussed and may be called by various names but the number of committees and the scope of their responsibilities are provided for in the organizational structure of the facility. Remember, there may be one all-inclusive committee with overlapping duties and responsibilities, or there may be separate Infection Control, Exposure Control and Safety Committees.

The laboratory department is often used as a vital adjunct to either or both infection and exposure control committees. Environmental sampling may be done on a periodic basis to determine if *decontamination* and general cleaning of the equipment and the physical building itself is adequate (Fig. 3.4). Environmental surveillance in general where the facility had bacterial cultures taken from work surfaces, drinking fountains, equipment and other areas was at one time more prevalent than currently but may no longer required by accrediting agencies. However, surveillance may be performed on select surfaces and equipment and efforts may be expanded if the numbers of certain bacterial infections increase dramatically to determine the source of the infections.

Outbreaks of *nosocomial* infections, described as those that are hospital acquired, are investigated by the laboratory for the infection control committee. A common term for a hospital-acquired disease that occurs as a result of providing medical care during medical procedures such as surgery or chemotherapy is that of *iatrogenesis*. The medical staff, headed by the chief of staff, receives antibiotic usage of data compiled by the laboratory as to the effective use of antibiotics. Reports from housekeeping, the dietary department, and other areas pertaining to unsafe or biohazardous conditions are reported to the infection control committee which may utilize the laboratory's expertise in addressing problem areas.

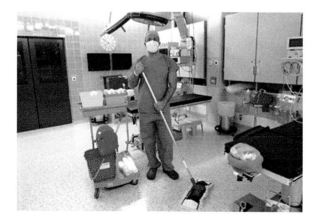

Fig. 3.4 General housekeeping

Most often there is a representative on the infection control committee from the medical laboratory. Infection control, exposure control and safety are difficult to separate from each other, and although there may be three separate committees, they demand a cooperative and combined effort from all areas of the facility in order to be totally effective. But the laboratory is a key component in completing surveillance to determine if indeed a problem exists and in providing a solution to many of the problems related to infection for all three committees.

Not all patients who are harboring an infectious disease are readily identifiable, and some show no symptoms or signs of disease. These persons may be termed 'carriers' but are often difficult to identify. Therefore, all patients and specimens from them should be handled with caution. It is a good practice to avoid direct contact with patients and their specimens in general. This is possible through care in handling of patient samples and by using barrier devices, called Personal Protective Equipment or PPE to avoid coming in direct contact with materials and persons who may expose the worker to the risk of contracting an infection (Fig. 3.5). Due to the nature of medically related work, and the persons with whom the workers are in contact, the risk to workers and

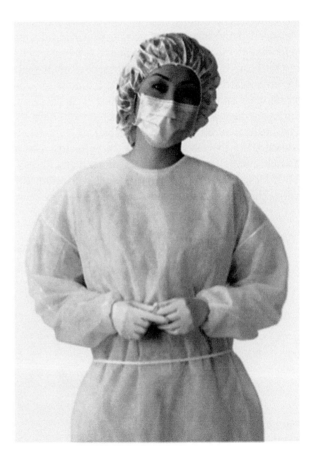

Fig. 3.5 Wearing PPE

patients of becoming injured or infected is amplified. It is also wise to include visitors to the facility when discussing means of preventing injuries and illnesses.

Health care workers should seek to provide superior patient care while insuring the environment for both patients and workers is conducive to maintaining physical and emotional health. Safety issues are more than just a responsibility to one's coworkers, self, and the patients. It is a volatile legal issue as manifested by suits brought by both patients and workers who have been harmed by injuries and by the contraction of preventable infections. In the late 1970s a focus on safety was spurred by the arrival of the *human immunodeficiency virus* or *HIV* that causes the dread acquired immuno-deficiency syndrome called AIDS. The advent of this serious infection contributed greatly to the strengthening of policies and procedures to prevent contraction of this disease, and by extension aided in avoiding other types of infections as well.

Two types of controls are provided for health care employees to protect their patients, their coworkers and themselves. *Work practice controls* include training and forethought by preplanning the work before initiating a procedure. This includes components such as good housekeeping practice scrupulous personal hygiene to reduce the exposure to all sorts of hazardous materials through common sense and application of knowledge. A good example of work practice controls is that of correctly performing handwashing both before and following medical procedures (Table 3.1). *Engineered controls* in a medical facility is an OSHA term indicating the use of manufactured devices for self-protection, such as hypodermic needles that contain a self-sheathing mechanism to prevent accidental skin punctures with a used needle or filters that clean the air to avoid the exposure of employees and patients to potentially harmful environmental hazards.

> **Points to Remember**
> All departments work together in a medical facility to provide a safe environment for all individuals connected with the institution. Committees are established to promulgate policies that are used in creating procedures that incorporate safety into the practices by the employees. The facility should be constructed with safety in mind, to prevent injury to individuals, and will include engineered controls for ease of safe practices. All personnel will receive appropriate safety training pertinent to their occupations, and training is updated on an annual basis and when job responsibilities change.

Table 3.1 Effective handwashing technique

Effective handwashing technique
1. Using warm but not *very* warm or cold water, wet the hands and wrists
2. Apply soap from dispenser that should be available at all handwashing facilities
3. Lather hands and between fingers well; massage soap into nails and nail beds using the fingers
4. Knead the hands together briskly, producing friction, for at least 20 s
5. Rinse thoroughly with warm water; dry completely with absorbent towel or air stream device
6. If the sink is not equipped with foot or knee controls, turn off faucet with dry paper towel

3.2.5 External Sources for Providing a Safe Workplace

Federal and state laws and agencies have been adopted and organized to protect workers and patients against contracting disease from biohazardous materials, as well as exposure control laws regarding toxic and hazardous chemicals. The hazards, chemical and biohazardous, that are experienced in a clinical laboratory are numerous. However, many of the chemicals used for laboratory procedures are now less toxic than previously, when carcinogenic materials such as benzene were widely used in chemistry reagents. Internet resources abound where the laboratory employee can gain information regarding the toxicity of chemicals and materials found in the laboratory. The Occupational Safety and Health Act adopted by the U.S. Congress in 1970 mandates appropriate training for employees by their employers. The training is dependent upon the procedures and degree of exposure they may potentially experience on a routine basis. As a "right to know," a worker must be made aware of the potential for harm from any material with which he or she is likely to come in contact in the workplace. HAZMAT, an acronym derived from hazardous materials, is required training that provides information for employees of health care facilities who come in contact with hazardous wastes and hazardous materials.

Each state also has its own laws requiring this training which complies with individual states and their OSHA and DOT training requirements. OSHA is the agency of the US government that has the power to force employers to comply with safety issues and criminal charges may be brought for violation of laws enacted to protect the worker in almost all industries. A rule promulgated by OSHA in 1983 was expanded in 1987 and it required employers to provide safety training, maintaining a safe work environment, and provision of personal protective gear (PPE) such as gowns, jackets, gloves, boots, etc., when working in certain areas. This is especially true in hospitals where multitudes of work areas require protection from explosive gases, blood and other body fluids and tissues, electrical hazards, and any other common potential sites for accidents from falls and being cut with broken glass and other devices.

Other agencies that require and monitor practices within the clinical laboratory contain provisions for the safety of employees as a part of their standards for accreditation. These groups include the voluntary accrediting agencies including the *Joint Commission* [formerly the Joint Commission for the Accreditation of Healthcare Organizations (JCAHO)], the *College of American Pathologists* (CAP), and categorical departmental agencies such as the *American Association of Blood Banks* (AABB) provide safety requirements as a part of the accreditation process. Non-voluntary federal agencies such as the *Centers for Disease Control and Prevention* (CDCP) and the Food and Drug Administration (FDA) also mandate and regulate laboratory practices and safety requirements. And in most states, strict regulations are imposed by Medicaid laws, public health and environmental laws are in effect, particularly in those states where laboratories and in some cases personnel are licensed by individual states (Table 3.2). Some state and local regulations may even be more stringent than those endorsed by either voluntary or non-voluntary agencies.

Table 3.2 Timelines for federal guidelines and laws going into effect concerning biological safety

1970 CDC published "isolation techniques for use in hospitals"
1975 CDC revised "isolation techniques" to include category-specific precautions and prohibition of recapping needles
1983 CDC issued nonbinding guidelines for isolation precautions in hospitals, designating seven isolation categories
1985 CDC introduced universal blood and body fluid precautions (universal precautions known as UP), primarily in response to HIV/AIDS epidemic
1987 CDC issued body substance isolation guidelines
1988 U.S. congress enacted clinical laboratory improvement amendments of 1988 (CLIA '88)
1991 OSHA issued bloodborne pathogens (BBP) standard, which mandated the use of UP
1996 CDC issued standard precautions, synthesizing UP and body substance isolation
2000 U.S. congress enacted needle stick safety and prevention act
2001 OSHA revised BBP standard in response to needlestick safety and prevention act

The possibility of exposure to bloodborne *pathogens* for medical workers led to additional guidelines and regulations by the Centers for Disease Control and Prevention (CDCP) and the Occupational Safety and Health Administration (OSHA) intended to prevent the exposure to bloodborne pathogens. CDCs version of Universal Precautions was initiated in 1987 where all patients are considered as potential carriers of bloodborne pathogens, which allowed for protection of the workers only. These precautions excluded urine and body fluids not visibly contaminated with blood. A modification of Universal Precautions included *body substance isolation* (BSI) which effectively eliminated concern about certain specimens that may not meet the criteria of containing visible blood, by considering all body fluids and moist body substances to be potentially infectious.

In 1996, the guidelines for *Universal Precautions* and for BSI were incorporated, resulting in a new set of guidelines called *Standard Precautions*. It should be noted that while Universal Precautions were generally intended to protect the health care employee, provisions in Standard Precautions serve to protect the patient as well as the health care provider. Even though these guidelines are basically addressed for direct patient care, the principles address the handling of patient specimens in the laboratory. Standard Precautions are as follows:

Infection Control Flash
Over a period of several decades, federal guidelines designed to protect health care workers have evolved. The guidelines were originally designed to protect only the worker, but eventually focused on both the health care provider and the patient. Most of these guidelines have been combined in Standard Precautions, along with needlestick guidelines issued by the US Congress and revised the following year.

3.3   Key Components of Standard Precautions

Certain elements of standard precautions are employed during almost all medical activities and procedures. The list provided here is an amended list that is presented in a sequence in which the most common applications of these precautions are listed first and early in the list.

- Handwashing
  Handwashing is one of the most basic but effective measures to be employed against contracting an infectious disease and is performed basically every time a procedure is performed. Where policy permits a waterless antiseptic may be used, and this practice is growing in acceptance as being as or more effective in preventing infections than mere handwashing. Handwashing is required before donning gloves, after touching blood, body fluids, secretions, excretions and contaminated items, and immediately after removing gloves. When moving from one patient to another, handwashing is also required to prevent cross-contamination. An associated use of antiseptic agents is that of cleansing the skin or mucous membrane prior to surgery, cleaning wounds, or cleaning the hands with an alcohol-based antiseptic product where a sink and soap are unavailable.
- Gloves
  Although gloves are a barrier device, they are used in practically all medical procedures and therefore are treated separately from the other barrier devices. Consider every person (patient or staff) as potentially infectious and susceptible to infection. Washing the hands before gloving and upon removing the gloves following a medical procedure is the most important procedure for preventing cross-contamination (person to person or contaminated object to person) between patients and from patient to employee. Wear gloves on both hands before touching anything that is moist such as broken skin, mucous membranes, blood or other body fluids, soiled instruments or contaminated waste materials. Any time an invasive procedure is performed, the wearing of gloves is extremely important.
- Barrier Devices
  Barrier devices include equipment called Personal Protective Equipment (PPE) that is required by OSHA for those who have a potential for exposure to infectious materials. Gloves are worn for contact with blood, body fluids, secretions and contaminated items, mucous membranes and non-intact (cut, chafed or abraded) skin. These devices when appropriately worn serve to protect the skin from blood or body fluid contact. Gowns and sometimes aprons that are impermeable to fluids should be worn to prevent the soiling of normal clothing during procedures that may involve contact with blood or body fluids. This protective equipment serves to protect the mucous membranes of eyes, nose and mouth when there is potential contact with blood and body fluids through the use of face masks and goggles. A face mask must be replaced if it becomes damp from respirations and the mask is usually not effective for more than 30 min of use.
  Physical barriers such as protective goggles, face masks and aprons should always be used when there is a likelihood of splashing and spilling of any body

fluids (secretions and excretions) while cleaning or repairing instruments and other items. When a face shield is used to prevent contact with aerosols and splatter of body fluids, a face mask is also required to be worn under the shield. For infectious diseases that are respiratory in nature, including in particular tuberculosis, a specially fitted respirator must be provided for each employee who comes in contact with a patient who is suspected of having the disease. Patient resuscitation requires the use of mouthpieces, resuscitation bags or other ventilation devices to avoid mouth-to-mouth resuscitation. These devices are intended to protect the employee providing resuscitation and these items should be discarded as biohazardous wastes as they have come in contact with mucus membranes.

- Linen and Patient Care Equipment
  Proper handling of soiled linen to prevent touching skin or mucous membranes is required. Linen is also transported for one area of the building to another in a carrier with impermeable sides to prevent spread of organisms from the linen. Soiled linens in patient care areas should never be pre-rinsed in a patient area prior to being transported to a laundry facility. Handling of soiled equipment in a way that prevents contact with skin or mucous membranes in order to avoid contamination of clothing and surrounding work areas. Reusable equipment should always be decontaminated prior to reuse or prior to transport to a repair facility or for storage. Single-use pieces of equipment are common in hospital and in the laboratory, and are disposed of properly as medical waste, depending upon the exposure to potential pathogens.
- Environmental Cleaning
  Routine care, cleaning of and disinfecting of equipment and furnishings in patient care areas is required upon discharge or transfer of a patient with an infectious disease. Procedures are required for the routine care, cleaning and disinfecting of areas that are frequently touched by patients, visitors and employees of the hospital. Patient rooms require disinfecting of beds, bedrails, bedside equipment and supplies. Some equipment must be sterilized or cleaned by use of high-level disinfecting processes. Work surfaces of laboratories are routinely and regularly disinfected, often with a 10% sodium hypochlorite solution, prepared fresh daily (effective for 1 month if stored in an area protected from light and extreme temperatures). When cleaning work areas and for cleaning areas where spills have occurred, the solution is applied to the surface and allowed to air dry.
- Patient Assignment
  House patients who may contaminate the environment or cannot maintain appropriate hygiene are assigned to private rooms. Isolation rooms with an anteroom for personnel decontamination and disposal of infectious materials are required for a number of infectious diseases. In addition, patients with weak or immuno-compromised systems are placed in isolation rooms in order to protect them from hazards associated with being confined to a health care facility. These specially-designed rooms have largely replaced the need for tuberculosis and similar sanitariums for those patients who pose a great risk to those with which they come in contact, such as tuberculosis and leprosy.

- Sharps Precautions
  Place all used "*sharps*" such as needles and scalpels in puncture-resistant containers to prevent injury and infection of those handling these wastes. Avoid recapping of used needles or removing used needles from disposable syringes as well as bending, breaking and otherwise manually manipulating used needles. Puncture proof and rigid containers are required in all areas where sharp supplies such as needles, scalpels, glass slides, etc., are used. The laboratory operations produce a large number of sharps in both phlebotomy procedures as well as some routine work.

- Waste Disposal
  Safely dispose of infectious waste materials to protect those who handle them and prevent injury or spread of infection to the community. Except for urine samples, all biological wastes must be placed in appropriately labeled and designed containers with a biohazard symbol attached. Urine samples may be poured into a laboratory sink, and flushed thoroughly with water for disposal. The sink used for disposal should be cleaned by a 10% bleach solution on a regular basis. Empty urine containers may be disposed of into standard waste containers along with routine non-biological hazardous wastes. Biohazardous wastes must be collected properly and stored in areas where they are sequestered from traffic, and the areas must be labeled as such. Commercial providers collect the wastes and charge by the pound for transporting and disposing of the materials, most often by burning in high-temperature incinerators.

3.4 Urine Samples and Body Fluids as Potential Biohazards

The body fluid, urine, is not considered under federal guidelines as posing a significant hazard to the health of the employees who perform tests on the material. However, if blood is present in the urine sample, as often occurs in some medical conditions and disease processes, there is at least the potential for being exposed to *bloodborne pathogens* when the sample is not handled properly. Although exposure to body fluids other than blood are less likely to transmit infectious organisms, they are nevertheless responsible for transmitting viruses, bacteria and other pathogens such as fungal elements and even certain parasites. Therefore, it must be kept in mind that a number of other body fluids are capable of transmitting infectious diseases and require the same respect for handling that blood and blood products do.

Medical procedures in which aerosols are produced such as in cauterization or when bronchial aspirations are performed require complete personal protective equipment for optimum safety.

The body fluids and materials that are known to be capable of transmitting disease agents are semen, vaginal fluids, cerebrospinal fluid, synovial fluid, peritoneal fluid (*transudate*), amniotic fluid, and bronchial washings. The laboratory professional may be required to perform a variety of laboratory procedures on any of these fluids. In addition, the handling of urine, feces, nasal secretions, saliva, sweat, sputum, tears or vomitus are not directly implicated in the spread of disease, but if they are tinged with blood, transmission of microorganisms through these types of specimens is possible.

Fluids from *exudates* or wounds where discharges and transudates which are fluids that ooze from membranes, are all capable of enabling the transmission of pathogens, usually in the form of bacteria, from one person or object to another. It should also be noted that while sputum is not ordinarily considered as a hazardous material, it can be the source of transmitting tuberculosis (TB) and will often be blood tinged when the respiratory disease of TB is present.

Safety standards that regulate the safety of workers in clinical laboratories are designed to protect the health care worker from a variety of hazards. Those who are trained adequately will have an understanding of the potential for becoming infected or harmed by exposure to toxic materials or of becoming injured through unsafe practices. The aforementioned safety plan and standards and procedures promulgated by the infection control and exposure control committees are all-inclusive and should address physical, biological and toxic sources of danger. The safety program is required of all clinical laboratories and the identification of potential hazards of all categories is an integral part of the program. Accidents involving the contraction of diseases through carelessness or accidents should be eliminated with proper adherence to safety protocol.

Since blood is the source for harboring most likely the most hazardous organisms, an infection control plan that focuses on the handling of blood, regardless of source, is managed in most cases by the Infection Control Committee. Although often used synonymously with the Exposure Control Committee plan, the exposure control focuses on eliminating or minimizing employee occupational exposure to blood, many other body fluids, and defines *other potentially infectious materials (OPIM)*. Most body fluids are formed as *ultrafiltrates* of the blood plasma, so they are therefore capable of transmitting blood borne pathogens such as the Human Immunodeficiency Virus (HIV) and *Hepatitis B* and *C* (HBV and HBC), although other organisms are also spread through the exchange of body fluids. CDC has recommended safety precautions when handling all body fluids, with the exception of sweat, tears and urine, through its standards available to all facilities.

These Standard Precautions are designed to protect the health care worker who is handling blood and bloody materials. It should be noted that the term "Standard Precautions," designed to protect the patient in a health care facility for acquiring and infectious disease while undergoing medical treatment, is now used in health care facilities. The current regulations called Standard Precautions include the elements included in both Universal Precautions and Standard Precautions. These policies are based on the fact that different specimens inherently carry different risk levels and differing types of exposure is presumed to carry varying degrees of risk.

3.5   Physical Hazards in the Health Care Facility

Although physical hazards are not intrinsically linked to the study of urine and body fluids samples, certain environmental hazards must be avoided. In the health care environments, slipping on spills as well as tripping and falling are common, for both hospital employees and patients. During a recent 10-year period, injuries as a result of falls comprised the second-highest means by which injuries occurred in health care facilities. In the areas of laboratories where body fluids are examined, centrifuges are often employed for various procedures, particularly for concentrating certain elements of the fluid into a sediment "button."

Centrifuges rotate at extremely high revolutions, and are capable of causing breakage of tubes, and the spreading of aerosols. Most modern models of centrifuges have a safety features which prevent opening the instrument until the spinning movement has stopped. But removing broken glass and plastic from the centrifuge, and the aerosols generated by the process of spinning, can result in the spread of *pathogens* (organisms that cause disease). Most local governments require inspections by fire marshals that inspect facilities for safety features as well as for the risk of fire and explosions.

As added risks to the health of the laboratory employee, noise levels in certain areas of the department are considerable. Some levels may be so extreme that hearing loss may occur over a period of time. However, newer models of equipment often yield lower levels of operating noise or are enclosed inside shielded barriers that provide a quieter environment. Chemical hazards still exist but have been greatly minimized through the development of newer and safer chemicals used for laboratory tests. Some of the older methodology utilized quite toxic and even carcinogen (cancer-causing) materials that have been greatly eliminated over the years. Faulty equipment and conditions that employees consider a health risk should be reported to the appropriate parties.

3.5.1 Waste Disposal and "Sharps"

Policies must be provided for the proper disposal of both biohazardous wastes as well as toxic chemicals. Training for healthcare employees is required for effectively preparing and removing wastes and toxins. All biohazardous wastes must be disposed of according to state, local and federal regulations. These regulations can vary from one location to another and will change due to research or changing policies by safety committees and even government agencies. Most hospitals now procure the services of a commercial waste disposal firm that provides for the safe collection and storage of biohazardous materials, prior to the pickup of biohazardous wastes for transport to a facility where the materials are incinerated at an extremely high temperature.

In the past, facilities were allowed to burn their own wastes, but this is no longer done. However, the collecting facility is ultimately responsible for the wastes until it arrives at the disposal site, even when transport is by commercial facilities. Smoke from some of these materials is toxic so the smokestacks are often built to a height of more than a 100 ft, and a distillation process may also be employed to capture and recycle some of these wastes produced by burning the materials. No less hazardous than smoke and exposure to hazardous waste is that of the disposal of hardware that is capable of causing injury when mishandled. The term "sharps" refers to broken glass, needles, scalpels, and metal devices with sharp edges or corners that must be safely disposed of (Fig. 3.6) in specially designed, rigid and marked to warn handlers of the possibility of danger.

Toxic chemicals although not nearly as prevalent in the medical laboratory as they have been in past years, regulations for proper disposal of used chemicals or chemicals that should be discarded are to be followed in each facility. Some chemicals may be poured into the sewer system if highly diluted with water. But most, especially those containing azides, copper, chromium, lead or mercury require special handling by trained toxic waste disposal personnel. Eyewash stations (Fig. 3.7) are to be situated in areas where chemicals or biohazardous materials may splash into the eyes.

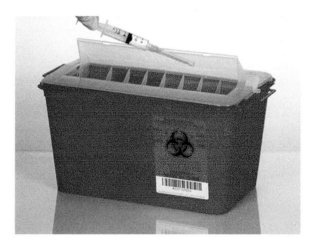

Fig. 3.6 Basic sharps container

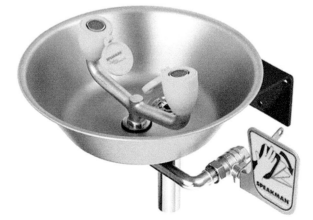

Fig. 3.7 Eyewash station for emergency incidents with biohazards, toxic chemicals

3.6   Disposal of Biological and Contaminated Waste Materials

Some bodily fluids such as feces and urine are not considered as dangerous materials but if they contain visible blood they should be treated as potentially dangerous. Solid wastes that are contaminated with blood or other body fluids should be placed in a red bag affixed with a red Biohazard symbol. These bags are strong and impervious to fluid leakage from the contained items. The bag is sealed with a twist tie or tape and placed into a box with a Hazardous Medical Waste sign. Soaked items such as chemical wipes, gauze sponges and paper towels where blood or other fluids can be squeezed from it or where blood may flake from the item, are considered regulated medical waste.

Sharp items, most frequently referred to as simply "sharps" include needles, broken tubes, and disposable items may that may cause injury if carelessly handled. When these items are contaminated with patient blood or other bodily fluids, a secondary danger lies in the potential for these items to transmit infectious diseases if improperly handled. When the skin is no longer intact as a barrier against microorganisms through cuts, chafing and burns, infection might easily occur. As a precaution, used needles should never be recapped, bent or broken in preparation for disposal. Syringes, needles, broken glass, and other sharp items should be placed in the appropriate container strategically located in work areas, on a work counter and in any sterilization area (see Fig. 3.8).

Disposable items that may contain body fluids of patients, but are not subject to medical waste regulations if not soaked with blood or tissue, such as gloves, paper towels from basic handwashing and absorbent paper for use on laboratory counters, should be placed in a lined trash receptacle. Red bags should _not_ be used for non-regulated waste. Some containers for Biohazardous Wastes will have a foot-operated lever for opening the lid to protect the person discarding the wastes by avoiding unnecessary handling (see Fig. 3.9). To place unregulated wastes into a red biohazard bag such as gloves that have no significant blood on them would involve a great deal of expense borne by the health care facility which has in paying for the disposal of non-biohazardous wastes.

Infection Control Flash
The disposable of contaminated wastes are subject to strict regulation. The collection, storage and transportation are documented as they are collected and transported for final disposal, generally by a commercial waste disposal company, through incineration by a certified method.

Critical Thinking Scenario
An accident involving a truck responsible for collecting biohazardous wastes and toxic materials from medical laboratories is involved in an accident enroute to the disposal site. Although the owner of the disposal service calls in biohazardous crews to clean up the spill, who is ultimately responsible for the proper recovery and disposal of the wastes?

Fig. 3.8 Containers for disposal of contaminated sharps

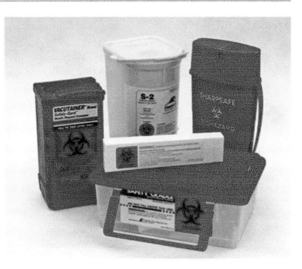

Fig. 3.9 Foot-operated biohazardous waste container

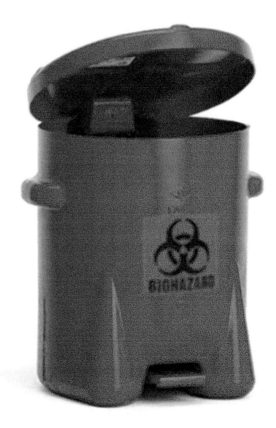

3.7   Summary

An integrated plan to provide for the safety of health care professionals, patients, and visitors to a medical facility must be provided. One or more committees is or are formed to provide guidance to the facility and to interpret regulations and requirements of accrediting and licensing bodies. These committees develop policies from which procedures are in agreement with the policies and which are adopted by the administration of the health care facility.

Potentially hazardous materials must be properly handled, collected, and stored in order to create a safe environment for everyone who is associated in any fashion with a health care facility, including even the casual visitor or contract worker. It is economically advisable for the hospital to protect its workers and patients, to avoid unwarranted absences and medical expenses. In addition, patients and families may file a lawsuit if injured or harmed while in the facility. The students of health care programs and those working in a medical facility should become aware of the measures to be taken to protect themselves and their patients.

Review Questions

1. Name three specimen types that are not included in the list of samples that are significant sources of infection in medical laboratory employees.
2. The two bloodborne pathogens which require training as mandated by the federal agencies are:
3. The most common disinfectant used for cleaning work surfaces in the laboratory is:
4. The agency that requires a medical facility to provide adequate protective equipment which includes gloves is:_____
5. When washing the hands, which of the following activities is not a requirement?
   a. Using a paper towel to turn on the faucet after completing a medical procedure
   b. Rubbing the lathered hands to provide friction
   c. Scrubbing the nail beds against the palms of the hands
   d. Using warm water when available
   e. Hands should be washed with the fingers pointed in an upward position
6. Centrifuging a specimen is likely to create:_____
7. Which of the following legislative regulations led to the standards required of ALL medical laboratories?
   a. Healthcare Finance Administration
   b. Occupational Safety and Health Administration
   c. Clinical Laboratory Improvement Amendments of 1988
   d. Centers for Disease Control and Prevention
8. Name the three categories of laboratory tests that were established by CLIA '88.

Answers Found in Appendix C

Metabolic Origins of Urine and Other Body Fluids

4

Objectives

Discuss the evolution of urine as a material used for diagnosis of disease, to modern day testing.

Describe the functional units of the kidney and the genitourinary system.

Explain how urine and body fluids are formed.

Discuss some ways in which body fluids can be related to a particular disease process.

List the major functions of the kidney to include filtration of waste products, reabsorption, and secretion.

Provide the chemical components of urine.

Demonstrate an understand of changes that occur in improperly collected and stored urine specimens.

4.1   Formation of Body Fluids

Urine is a sterile liquid by-product derived from metabolic processes of the body and is secreted by the kidneys via a process that may be called micturition, urination or voiding. After secretions, reabsorptions and other processes often governed by hormones, the remaining urine consisting mostly of water is excreted through the urethra. Cellular metabolism generates a number of toxic waste by-products of which many are rich in nitrogen, and are filtered from the bloodstream and into the bladder for elimination from the circulatory system. Both chemicals and formed elements may be found in the urine and are detected by a set of procedures called a urine analysis, combined into the term 'urinalysis.' A closely related fluid is that of amniotic fluid found in the uterus of pregnant females that also serves to aid in eliminating wastes from the body of the fetus.

Urine is continuously formed by the kidneys in varying amounts depending on physical activity, the time of day, and the activity of hormones such as *antidiuretic*

© Springer International Publishing AG, part of Springer Nature 2018
J. W. Ridley, *Fundamentals of the Study of Urine and Body Fluids*,
https://doi.org/10.1007/978-3-319-78417-5_4

hormone (ADH). While not formed by the kidneys, *amniotic fluid*, cerebrospinal and other fluids are closely related to *urine,* and many of the analytical procedures are the same, and will be further discussed in the chapters devoted to each of these body fluids. All body fluids are similar in the sense they are all actually ultrafiltrates of blood plasma except arguably that of cerebrospinal fluid. Some body fluids are richer in certain constituents derived from the blood and surrounding tissues than others. In the kidneys, some materials including glucose, *amino acids,* water, and other substances essential to body metabolism are normally reabsorbed but this is not always true in certain disease processes. Physiological processes occur by which approximately 170 L of filtered plasma is converted to the average daily urine output of 1.2–1.5 L of urine, although average normal ranges may cause considerable variations from these amounts. Certain factors as discussed in the next section will cause variations from these normal volumes.

> **Infection Control Flash**
> Urine is not considered as capable of transmitting infectious organisms in the same manner as blood and other body fluids. Urine may be disposed of in the sewer systems, and the containers may be disposed of in regular trash.

4.1.1   Daily Volume of Urine

Daily urine volume is greatly dependent upon a number of factors, but generally equals the amount of intake of water and watery fluids such as beverages. Ingestion of water occurs chiefly through the drinking of water and other beverages, but is also influenced by foods that contain water. The volume of urine excreted per day is dependent upon the amount of water that is actually excreted through the kidneys, but water can be lost through conditions other than the amount that is voided from the bladder. Water is a major constituent of urine so the amount excreted is usually determined by the body's state of hydration, or amount of water present in the vascular system and in the tissues of the body. Extreme losses of water from the tissues results in *dehydration,* or the absence of water in the body organs, as the blood system will extract fluids from the tissues in order to maintain adequate blood flow to the tissues, a function called perfusion.

Factors that influence urine volume include fluid intake, fluid loss from non-renal sources, variations in the secretion of antidiuretic hormone, and the necessity to excrete increased amounts of dissolved solids, such as glucose or salts. Taking these factors into consideration, it can be seen that although the average daily urine output is 1200–1500 mL, a range of 600–2000 mL may be considered normal. Remaining well-hydrated during illness, especially if the illness is accompanied by a fever, is a concern of the nursing personnel.

Oliguria, a decrease in the normal daily urine volume, may occur when the body enters a state of dehydration due to excessive water loss through vomiting, diarrhea, perspiration, or severe burns and other miscellaneous causes. Oliguria may lead to anuria, a complete cessation of urine flow, and often results from shock or a serious level of damage to the kidneys or from a decrease due to a diminished flow of blood to the kidneys. Two or three times more urine is excreted during the day than during the night. This increase in the nocturnal excretion of urine is termed nocturia and occurs through action of a hormone called ADH, or anti-iduretic hormone. Polyuria, an increase in daily volume, results in an increase in daily urine volume, and is frequently associated with *diabetes mellitus* and *diabetes insipidus*. However, an artificially increased output may be the result of the use of (*diuretics*, caffeine, or alcohol, which suppress secretion of antidiuretic hormone. It should be noted that beverages containing high levels of caffeine and alcohol tend to induce dehydration and are a poor choice of beverage when working in hot and/or dry environments.

Diabetes mellitus and diabetes insipidus produce polyuria for different reasons, and analysis of the urine is an important step in the differential diagnosis. Diabetes mellitus is caused by a defect either in the production of insulin by the pancreas or in the function of insulin, resulting in an increased body glucose concentration. The excess glucose is not reabsorbed by the kidneys, necessitating the excretion of increased amounts of water to remove the circulating glucose from the body. Although appearing to be dilute, a urine specimen from a patient with diabetes mellitus will have a high specific gravity because of the increased glucose content. Diabetes insipidus results from a decrease in the production or function of antidiuretic hormone and occurs in a process where water required for necessary body hydration is not reabsorbed from the plasma filtrate of the kidney. In this condition, urine will be quite dilute and will reveal a low *specific gravity*, indicating a higher level of water with fewer dissolved substances. Fluid loss in both diseases is characterized by excess ingestion of water, resulting in even greater volume of urine output. Polyuria and increased fluid intake may be the first symptom of the two types of diabetes.

Points to Remember
Urine results from the ingestion of fluids and is controlled by the needs of the body based partly on environmental conditions. The volume of urine excreted is controlled by hormonal influence as well as the amount of fluids entering the body and the amount of water that is consumed through breathing, perspiring, and bowel elimination. The volume of urine excreted is controlled by the amount of fluids available, while other body fluids are regulated by the physical constraints of the bodily cavities, and the purposes for which they are produced.

4.2   Anatomy of the Urinary System

The urinary system is comprised of two kidneys, their associated glands and *ureters* leading from each kidney to the bladder where urine collects for excretion. Urine is excreted from the body through the urethra that leads from the bladder where muscles called sphincters enable the urethra to open and release the urine into the environment. The pair of organs called the kidneys is bean-shaped, and each is roughly the size of an adult's fist. They are located near the middle of the back in an area called the retroperitoneal region, which is the area behind the peritoneum, a serous membrane-lined cavity of the abdominal cavity.

When viewed from the exterior of the body, kidneys are located just below the rib cage with kidneys normally found on each side of the spine but in rare cases, three kidneys may occur. The kidneys are sophisticated reprocessing organs that are able to filter massive amounts of blood each day. It is estimated that up to 25% of the body's blood volume that is pumped through the heart is received by the kidney at all times (Fig. 4.1). Every day, a person's kidneys process of up to 200 L (a L or liter is slightly more than a quart of blood) slightly more than a quart of blood, sifting out about 2 L of waste products and extra water. The wastes and extra water become urine and flow to the bladder through tubes called ureters. The bladder stores urine before releasing it from the body by urination.

The kidneys require a rich supply of blood which provides oxygen and nutrients to the organs as well as being intrinsically involved in the filtration process of removing toxins and metabolites while reabsorbing essential chemical constituents.

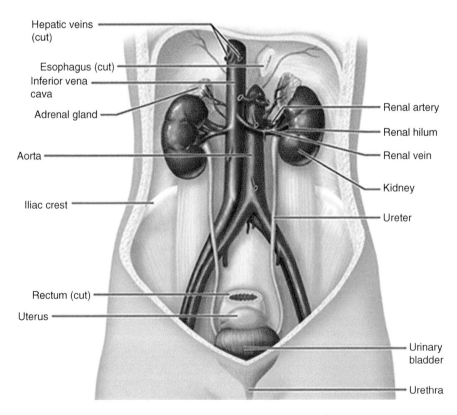

Fig. 4.1 Position in Human of Generalized Structures of the Urinary System

The renal artery carries the blood to the kidney, where the artery branches into smaller and smaller units, eventually becoming afferent (transporting toward) arterioles that enter the glomeruli leaves the glomeruli through efferent (transported away from) arterioles.

The renal tubules of the nephrons are directly in contact with the efferent arterioles and it is here that reabsorption of essential chemicals and secretions between the blood and the filtrate of the glomeruli take place. The actual removal of wastes occurs in tiny units inside the kidneys called *nephrons*. Each kidney has about a million to 1.5 million nephrons. In the nephron, a *glomerulus* consisting of a tuft of tiny blood vessels called capillaries, intertwines with a tiny urine-collecting tube known as the tubule, a structure that is a long and narrow tube. Selective excretion and reabsorption of various chemical compounds occurs in different areas of the tubule, ie. proximal, medial and distal portions of the Loop of Henle.

The glomeruli (plural form of glomerulus) act as filtering units, or sieves, and retain normal constituents of the vascular system, while allowing excess fluid and water to be excreted. These materials are reabsorbed by the three areas of the tubules, the proximal, medial and distal areas in the Loop of Henle, and are returned to the blood where they are diffused by the blood throughout the body. In this manner the kidneys return certain chemicals, the most common of which are chemicals called electrolytes that include sodium, potassium, chloride and phosphorus the blood to return to the body while allowing wastes to pass through. A complicated chemical exchange takes place as waste materials and water leave the blood and enter the urinary system following reabsorption of essential products.

As one of the most complex and important organ systems of the body, the kidneys through release and retention of certain ions, contribute to the overall pH of the body, which remains in a slightly alkaline state, and may require significant attention. The tubules receive a combination of waste materials but also chemicals that the body requires for metabolic functions. In addition, the kidneys, through selective excretion or reabsorption, help to regulate the body's level of substances such as hydrogen ions and bicarbonate ions in order to manage any alkalinity or acidity of the blood. It is critical that the kidneys operate correctly to maintain the correct chemical balance that is necessary for life.

4.2.1 Functions of the Kidneys

In summing up the functions of the kidneys and indeed the entire urinary system, the system is perhaps the most important system, performing vital functions in order to maintain life and health. They monitor the metabolism of the body day and night, and perform their functions well unless illness interdicts. This is done through complex functions which occur throughout the day and the night to keep the body in a state of equilibrium called homeostasis. The kidneys remove wastes and excess water from the blood to form urine while reabsorbing needed chemicals for insuring homeostasis or normal conditions of the body. Urine flows from the kidneys to the bladder through the ureters. Wastes in the blood come from the normal breakdown of active tissues, such as muscles, and from food. The body uses food for energy and self-repairs. After the body has taken what it needs from food, wastes are sent to the blood. If the kidneys did not remove them, these wastes would build up in the blood and damage the body when the blood became toxic.

Points to Remember
Although urine primarily functions in releasing waste products from the body, many other vital functions involved with the health of the individual are provided by the kidneys. Retention of vital components of the blood through reabsorption as needed provides for an optimum concentration of certain chemicals necessary for carrying on a normal metabolism of the body.

4.2.2 Renal Physiology

In summary, and to repeat some of the functions provided earlier, the physiology of the kidneys relate simply to the functions of filtration, reabsorption and secretion. The remaining components of the urinary system basically serve to collect, store and release the urine following these three functions. Of course kidneys are complex and are responsible for a variety of functions. It should also be noted here that the kidneys are composed of two distinct anatomical areas called the cortex and the medulla. The *cortex* is the outer layer of the kidney and includes the glomerular portion of the nephrons as well as the *proximal tubule* (tubule closest to the glomerulus). The *medulla* includes the *Loop of Henle*, a structure which lies between the proximal and the *distal convoluted tubules* and which lead into the collecting ducts where the fluid enters the ureters leading to the bladder. The *medial tubule* lies intermediate to the proximal tubule and the Loop of Henle (Fig. 4.2). These structures are all vitally involved in the excretion and reabsorption of chemical elements necessary for the metabolism of the entire human body.

4.3 Major Physiological Functions of the Kidney

1. Waste products are removed as the primary function of the kidneys, which include mostly nitrogenous wastes from protein metabolism. These wastes called kidney function tests are measured in panels of blood chemistry tests and the levels are increased in diseases where the kidneys have been damaged.
2. Water and electrolyte balance is a major function of the kidneys, where excess water is excreted, and when dietary consumption of water is insufficient, the kidneys function to slow excretion until sufficient water is maintained in the body. Excess electrolytes (sodium, potassium and other elements) are excreted until a normal level is achieved in the blood.

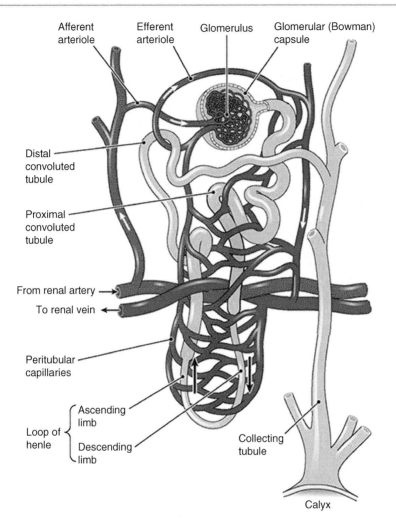

Fig. 4.2 Nephron, functional unit of kidneys and associated structures

3. Retention of glucose and proteins through reabsorption into the bloodstream enables the body to maintain adequate levels of these vital nutrients.
4. Acid-base balance is essential to maintaining the pH (acidity or alkalinity) of the blood within a limited range. Many of the vital functions of the body would be impossible if the pH falls or rises to an abnormal level. Adjustment by the body of the pH level when necessary is achieved by excreting hydrogen ions if the blood becomes abnormally acid, and excreting bicarbonate ions when the blood is too alkaline.

4.3.1 Hormonal Influences of the Kidneys

In addition to removing wastes, the kidneys are responsible for forming and releasing three important hormones important to the proper functioning of the body.

- *Erythropoietin* or EPO, a hormone produced by the kidneys, stimulates the bone marrow to produce red blood cells. This hormone is often decreased in certain disease states affecting the kidneys and leads to *anemia*, a decrease in the level of red blood cells.
- *Rennin* is a hormone which is produced by the kidneys. Rennin splits angiotensin I to angiotensin II, which stimulates vasoconstriction and secretion of *aldosterone*. Along with other factors, rennin helps to regulate the blood pressure of the body.
- *Calcitriol*, the active form of vitamin D, serves to help maintain calcium for bones and for the normal chemical balance of calcium in the body, an ion important to muscular function. This hormone form of vitamin D promotes absorption of both phosphate and calcium in the intestines and decreases calcium excretion through the kidneys, working in conjunction with *parathormone* produced by the parathyroid glands.
- Aldosterone is produced by the adrenal cortex of the kidneys and is an extremely active *mineralocorticoid* hormone. This hormone serves to regulate reabsorption of sodium by the kidneys, which in turn affects indirectly the retention or excretion of potassium, chloride, and bicarbonate. Other effects of this hormone are that of the regulation of blood pH, blood volume and blood pressure.

4.4   Composition of Urine

Blood is a valuable contributor to the process of excretion of certain wastes and in the maintenance of other levels of nutrients and chemicals. In general, urine consists of *urea* (the chief nitrogenous waste) and other organic materials and chemicals dissolved in water. Considerable variations in the concentrations of these substances can occur due to the influence of factors such as dietary intake, physical activity, body metabolism, endocrine function, and even body position. Urea, a metabolic waste product produced in the liver from the breakdown of protein and *amino acids*, accounts for nearly half of the total dissolved solids in urine. Other substances include primarily creatinine and *uric acid*. Major inorganic solids that are dissolved in urine are chloride, followed by sodium and potassium. Small or trace amounts of many additional inorganic chemicals are also present in urine.

Although not part of the original plasma filtrate, the urine may also contain formed elements such as cells, casts, crystals, mucus, and bacteria. Increased amounts of these formed elements are often indicative of disease. Should it be necessary to determine whether a particular fluid is actually urine, the specimen can be tested for its urea and creatinine content. Inasmuch as both of these substances are present in much higher concentrations in urine than in other body fluids, the demonstration of a high urea and creatinine content can be used to identify a fluid as that of urine.

This is sometimes an important consideration when fluids have leaked from the body and must be differentiated as to the source of the formation of the fluid. In addition, when a urine sample must be collected for drug studies, some creative persons may attempt to dilute their urine with water or will submit a sample of water from the toilet, so testing the fluid would be vital in these instances.

4.4.1 Water Balance and Reabsorption

Maintenance of the body's water balance is primarily by regulation of the *osmolality* of the body's fluids. The loss of hypotonic fluid by the lungs (mostly water) and the skin tends to increase the osmolality and the intake of fluids by mouth tends to reduce osmolality. The osmotic pressure of the extracellular fluid is predominantly maintained at a constant level primarily by regulation of water excretion by the kidneys. The hypertonic or concentrated interstitial fluid surrounding the tubules of the kidneys provides a high osmotic pressure for the removal of water. Since water flows into a more concentrated solution such as the interstitial fluid, a passive process requiring no energy, fluid is lost as needed through the urine. Also, transmembrane channels in the plasma membranes of capillaries that are made of a protein called *aquaporin,* increases the permeability to water, allowing water to flow into and from the tubules into the blood vessels.

The antidiuretic hormone *(ADH),* is also known as *vasopressin*) and is produced by the posterior pituitary (neurohypophysis) of the brain, the release of which is regulated by the osmotic pressure (concentration) of the blood. ADH then stimulates the rising of another hormone called cAMP within the cells which initiates a series of reactions that increases the number of aquaporin channels. A negative-feedback reflex mechanism regulates the osmotic concentration of the extracellular fluid surrounding the tubules by controlling the secretion of ADH.

An increase in secretion of ADH is accomplished through a rise in ECF (extracellular fluid) osmotic concentration. The sensors or osmoreceptors are located in the anterior hypothalamus near the neurons that produce ADH. The receptors react to changes in the intracellular volume or osmotic concentration caused by changes in the osmotic concentration of the fluid surrounding them. Axons of these receptors appear to be on the secretory neurons and impulses are transmitted from the receptors to the secretory neuron endings in the posterior pituitary. The ADH, which is increased during sleep, causes increased water reabsorption and results in the retention of water, with some edema (swelling) with increased tissue water observable upon waking with tightening of the skin and puffiness around the eyes. Along with continued dissolved solids excretion, there is a reduction in the osmotic concentration of extracellular fluid, resulting in biofeedback to the osmoreceptors. This stimulates a fall in levels of ADH production and release when the body returns to normal activity.

Another vital factor in the regulation of water and solute levels was discovered only within the past 2 decades. The *atrial natriuretic peptide (ANP)* is an *atrio-peptin* (protein polypeptide) hormone that is a powerful vasodilator. Other names used for ANP include that of *atrial natriuretic factor (ANF)* or the *atrial natriuretic hormone (ANH)*. This hormone is involved in homeostasis where control of water, sodium, potassium and fat which is known as adipose tissue are balanced. Produced by secretion from the muscle cells in the atria of the heart in response to high blood pressure, the hormone reduces the water, sodium and adipose loads in the circulatory system, serving to reduce blood pressure.

Activities and medical conditions may contribute to the dehydration of the body, to include such reactions as perspiring heavily, vomiting excessively, or prolonged diarrhea. A lengthy bout of high fever also leads to an extreme loss of fluids, mostly water, from the body. This loss of water increases the osmotic pressure of the blood and turns on the production of ADH which in turn prevents further loss of water that would lead to a more serious medical condition. It is of vital concern when episodes of vomiting, diarrhea and sweating, especially in the very young and the very old, rapidly turn into a full blown medical emergency, even progressing to a life-threatening state. The feedback mechanisms that stimulate increases or decreases in the ADH concentration by increased production are quite sensitive and only a 1% change in the plasma oncotic concentration may cause swelling of the tissues, resulting in a change in plasma ADH concentration that alters the osmolality of both plasma and urine quite rapidly.

The normal threshold level for the concentration of plasma ADH ranges from 280 to 295 mOsm/kg of water. Small changes in plasma ADH concentration of only approximately 15 mOsm/kg is sufficient to stimulate changes in the glomerular flow rate (GFR) of the kidneys. This small variation in plasma osmolality may cause the urine osmotic flow rate and concentration to vary by 20 L/day. When the osmotic concentrations of ADH fall below 280 mOsm/kg H_2O, the level of ADH in plasma remains relatively constant at about 0.5 pg/mL (10^{-12} g/mL).

Therefore results in the plasma osmotic concentration is maintained at a normal level. The significant sensitivity of this feedback mechanism is so reactive that a change of 1% in the plasma osmotic concentration (approximately 3 mOsm/kg H_2O) may possibly result in a change in the plasma concentration of ADH by 1 pg/mL. This amount is sufficient to alter osmolality of a urine sample by roughly 250 mOsm/kg H_2O. In an individual weighing approximately 150 pounds, this change can be produced by merely drinking 400–450 mL or 14 fluid ounces of water.

4.5 The Artificial Kidney

The human kidney is also an endocrine gland which performs some of its functions by secreting two hormones as listed earlier. These hormones are erythropoietin and calcitriol (Vitamin D_3), the active form of vitamin D and accompanied by the enzyme called rennin. The operation is technically quite easy for placing a donor kidney into a patient with failing kidneys, but there are major problems associated with obtaining and maintaining an acceptable human kidney from a donor. There are two types of dialysis, one of which involves using an artificial kidney and is called *hemodialysis*. The other method is for those with less serious kidney malfunction and is called *peritoneal dialysis*. Neither of these methods are perfect, as the artificial device requires blood transfusions along with the procedure on a regular basis of perhaps three times per week, and the dialysis machine does not provide the hormones that are a function of the natural kidneys.

An artificial kidney uses the principle of artificial dialysis similar to that of the kidneys to remove toxins from the blood where one's own kidneys are no longer functional. In this method, a patient's blood is treated by removing small molecules including primarily urea from the blood. These particles freely diffuse between the blood and the bath fluid of the dialysis unit. It is necessary for large molecules including plasma proteins and blood cells to remain in the patient's blood. The bath fluid has essential salts found in the blood of the patient that are added to avoid loss from the blood of these ions called electrolytes. Anticoagulant must be added to the blood to prevent clotting while passing through the instrument. The anticoagulant must then be neutralized as the blood returns to the patient's circulation to stave off dangerous hemorrhage that would occur.

Artificial kidneys greatly benefit patients with acute kidney malfunction but are only a temporary solution until the patient's own kidneys again begin to function or a kidney for transplant is available. These devices have enabled people suffering from chronic kidney failure to remain alive, but at great expense of time, money and emotional issues for the patient. Dialysis is effective in removing wastes but cannot perform the functions of a natural kidney. The natural kidneys provide hormones including erythropoietin (EPO) demanded by the body for blood production. The inability to monitor the blood and provide homeostatic control of sodium and glucose the body requires, along with essential hormones other than EPO is problematic. So without constant monitoring and treatment of the inherent difficulties of continuous transfusions, the dialysis patient will become anemic without being provided synthetic erythropoietin.

4.5.1 Completely Artificial Kidney

To alleviate the problem of a shortage of donor kidneys accompanied by the dangers of rejection of the foreign tissue and transmission of infectious diseases, development of improved artificial kidneys is currently being widely pursued. Rejection of a donor kidney frequently occurs, even when the donor and the recipient are generally genetically compatible. Even absent of immediate and severe rejection of the donor organ, the organ recipient must be placed on anti-rejection drugs for life to prevent the problem of graft rejection. The recipient's immune system, unless both donor and recipient are identical twins, will recognize the donated tissue as "foreign." Ongoing research is attempting to develop a dialysis instrument that will "pick up" the essential hormones, molecules and ions and reintroduce them into the patient's blood.

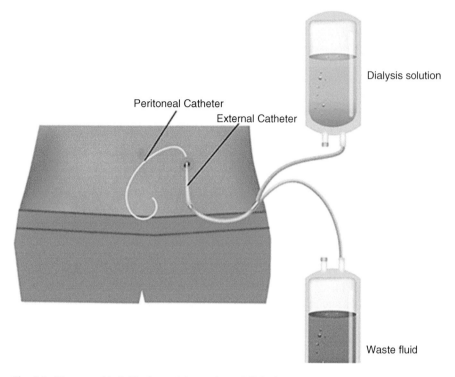

Dialysis solution

Peritoneal Catheter

External Catheter

Waste fluid

Fig. 4.3 Diagram of individual practicing peritoneal dialysis

Peritoneal dialysis is the second method of dialysis that can be performed by the patient at home but only for less severe kidney disease. The patient must be physically and mentally able to perform self-dialysis. For this treatment, a soft catheter is implanted into the abdominal or peritoneal cavity with a port that has been installed permanently. The abdominal cavity is filled through the inserted tube with a special cleansing solution. The walls of the abdominal lining or peritoneum is rich with small blood vessels called capillaries which have a rich blood flow. The peritoneum and the capillary walls filter the blood in a similar manner as do the filtering units of the kidneys. The solution usually remains in the abdominal cavity for prescribed lengths of time, a period of typically up to 6 h. The solution contains dextrose, a sugar in solution that is capable of receiving wastes from the blood. Residual fluid remains in the abdominal cavity. The peritoneal cavity is filled and after the prescribed length of time is drained back into the original bag containing the dialyzing solution. This process may require perhaps four exchanges per day, depending upon the patient's needs and requirements (Fig. 4.3). An additional form of peritoneal dialysis is available and used by some, whereby a machine called a cycler fills and drains the abdominal cavity, most often while the patient sleeps.

Points to Remember
While artificial kidneys function well in removing toxins from the blood, they are at this point unable to provide through biological feedback the hormones necessary for regulating excretion, and those required for stimulating the formation of red blood cells. Reabsorption of needed constituents that are initially excreted may also be problematic.

4.6 Laboratory Tests to Assess Filtration

For certain specific needs based on the patient's medical condition, it is necessary to evaluate the functions of the kidneys as to the efficiency of the kidneys in the concentration of and excretion of urine. There are basically two separate tests to attain this information. A procedure known as the clearance test may measure either creatinine or inulin, both metabolic products that are not readily reabsorbed to any appreciable extent. Clearance tests measure the volume in mL's per minute of urine passing out of the tubules by using laboratory data to complete a somewhat complex calculation for obtaining diagnostic data.

4.6.1 Osmolality

Sometimes a procedure mentioned earlier and known by the term osmolarity is used, and slight differences exist between osmolality and osmolarity. The osmolality test measures the concentration of minute particles in urine per kilogram of water. One liter of pure water weighs exactly 1000 g, and a kilogram would change with the concentration of solutes or solids dissolved in the solution. Osmolality or particles in a kilogram of water and osmolarity, measuring particles in a liter of solution may be confusing. However, for dilute fluids such as urine, they are essentially the same. Both osmolality and osmolarity are performed on urine, plasma and serum samples. There are, however, significant differences between tests for plasma versus serum. Since plasma contains a protein called fibrinogen used in the clotting of blood, and serum would contain no fibrinogen since clotting had already occurred and would be enmeshed in the clot. Normal values for osmolality (Box 4.1) of the urine are as follows.

Box 4.1: Normal Osmolality Values
- Normal Random specimen: 50–1200 mOsm/kg
- With 12–14-h fluid restriction: Greater than 850 mOsm/kg

Note: The normal value for osmolality determinations as well as for most other procedures will vary somewhat among laboratories where different instruments and reagents, as well as testing personnel produce differing results.

The sensation of thirst is produced due to an increased concentration of ionic particles dissolved in a solution such as plasma of the human body, and decreased concentration will prompt a lower intake or ingestion of fluids. Therefore, manipulation of fluid intake may be used by medical personnel when determining osmolarity or osmolality of plasma. Freezing and boiling points of liquids are called physical characteristics of the liquid. Dissolved materials will affect the boiling and freezing points of a solution. The physical characteristics of a patient sample to be used for determining osmolality is measured by a process called the freezing point depression. As an example, an iceberg consisting of water from rain or snow, floats in the ocean which is composed of salt water. Sea water has more particles or particulate matter in it than does the frozen liquid of the iceberg. Therefore, the sea water with more dissolved particles will require a significantly lower temperature in order to freeze. Since urine has electrolytes along with other dissolved particles, and when compared with pure water, will require a lower temperature is order for the sample to freeze the sample. From these differences, the concentration of the sample is determined based on the differing temperature for it to freeze when compared with pure water.

4.6.2 Creatinine Clearance

Creatinine is a waste product produced by a compound called creatine as an energy source by the muscles. Therefore, the clearance test is somewhat affected by the muscle mass of the patient. A creatinine clearance test is used to aid in evaluating the rate and efficiency of the kidney to filter blood plasma and measures the amount of urine passing from the nephrons of the kidney, most of which are reabsorbed into circulation (Table 4.1). The normal value for one with no kidney disease should have a

Table 4.1 Calculation for Creatinine Clearance

Clinical information for calculation	24-h total urine volume
	Creatinine value for *plasma* sample
	Creatinine value for *urine* sample
	Minutes in a day (1440)
Equation	$$\frac{\text{Value for urine sample}\left(\text{mg}/\text{dL}\right)\times\text{Volume of urine}\left(\text{mL}\right)}{\text{Value for plasma sample}\left(\text{mg}/\text{dL}\right)\times1440\,\text{min}/\text{day}}$$
Sample calculation	Urine volume = 850 mL
	Urine Creatinine = 225 mg/dL
	Plasma Creatinine = 1.2 mg/dL
	Minutes in day = 1440
Determination of results	$$\frac{225\dfrac{\text{mg}}{\text{dL}}\times850\,\text{mL}}{1.2\dfrac{\text{mg}}{\text{dL}}\times1440\,\text{min}}=\frac{191250\,\text{mL}}{1728\,\text{min}}=110.7\text{mL}/\text{min}$$

creatinine clearance value of approximately 120 mL/min. This value is used to help detect and diagnose kidney dysfunction where a decreased blood flow to the kidneys exists. In patients with known chronic kidney disease or congestive heart failure (CHF), where there may be a decreased blood flow rate, a creatinine clearance test may be necessary for monitoring progress of the disease (prognosis) and to evaluate the extent of any glomerular damage. The values obtained may also be used to determine the need for kidney particular type of dialysis or organ transplant.

4.7   Summary

Urine and other body fluids are formed from the liquid portion of blood, called plasma, and may have similar constituents including chemicals and cells, but the normal levels vary depending upon the fluid being tested. As is presented in this chapter, the kidneys are much more than just filtering devices that remove wastes from the body that are produced through metabolic processes.

Mechanisms exist for dictating the amount of the various body fluids, and disruptions in the production of and flow of the fluids may occur in a disease process. Urine is one of if not the most often tested body fluid, other than blood. The kidneys help to control the volume of water being excreted or retained and the amount of certain chemicals such as electrolytes being retained or excreted. The body is finely tuned to monitor through biofeedback the levels and concentrations of urine as well as other body fluids.

Some of the functions of either retaining or excreting electrolytes through the urine is accomplished by the action of hormones, which are also involved in influencing the production of blood cells and the levels of calcium and phosphates found in the bones. Other vital functions of the kidneys include control of the blood pressure and sensory impulses indicating a need for water when the concentration of the filtrates in the kidneys becomes more concentrated. Laboratory tests based on the filtration and concentrative abilities of the kidneys may be used to determine blood flow to the kidneys, congestive heart failure and the renal flow per minute through the nephrons of the urine.

Review Questions

1. Blood flow through a nephron of the kidney follows which of the following paths?
   a. Efferent arteriole, peritubular capillaries, afferent arteriole
   b. Afferent arteriole, ureters, efferent arteriole
   c. Efferent arteriole, afferent arteriole, peritubular capillaries
   d. Afferent arteriole, peritubular glomerular capillaries, efferent arteriole
2. The electrolyte affected by rennin-angiotensin-aldosterone hormone is:
   a. Magnesium
   b. Potassium
   c. Chloride
   d. Sodium

3. The daily volume of urine excreted depends would be affected by:
   a. Water intake
   b. Dehydration
   c. Congestive heart failure
   d. All of the above
4. Why is an adequate flow of blood, or perfusion, important to the kidneys?
5. Which of the following would not be a function of the renal system?
   a. Filtration
   b. Reabsorption
   c. Formation of blood cells
   d. Secretion
6. The hormone most responsible for the regulation of sodium in the blood is:
   a. Calcitriol
   b. Erythropoietin
   c. Aldosterone
   d. Antidiuretic hormone
7. The test used to determine the concentrating ability of the kidneys is:
   a. Macroscopic evaluation
   b. Creatinine clearance
   c. Osmolality
   d. Measurement of daily volume
8. The three methods of determining the specific gravity of a urine sample include all the following except:
   a. Refractometric measurement
   b. Measurement by urinometer
   c. Weighing a given urine sample
   d. Chemical measurement of ions

Answers Found in Appendix C

Microscopic Components Common to Body Fluids

5

Objectives

Explain how and where urine and body fluids are formed.

List ways in which body fluids can be related to a particular disease process.

Describe the major functions of the kidney to include filtration of waste products, reabsorption, and secretion.

List the solid components (cells, crystals) of body fluids.

Provide the chemical components of urine.

Demonstrate an understanding of changes that occur in improperly collected and stored urine specimens.

5.1 Microscopic Components of Body Fluids

In the previous chapter, the formation of urine as a body fluid was discussed. The constituents found in urine which is formed by a single system as a group of organs called the urogenital system. These organs are treated separately from that of the formation of body fluids found in other bodily cavities that are associated with the functions of tissues and organs. Some of the microscopic and chemical elements found in urine may also be found in other body fluids of the human, but at different levels and numbers based on the body site where the various fluids are formed. Therefore, a discussion of the formation of body fluids other than urine is presented in this section along with microscopic features of the major fluids of the human body. "Formed elements" include a variety of forms, from living cells to crystals formed from chemicals in the body fluid, to artifacts that have no clinical significance.

© Springer International Publishing AG, part of Springer Nature 2018
J. W. Ridley, *Fundamentals of the Study of Urine and Body Fluids*,
https://doi.org/10.1007/978-3-319-78417-5_5

5.2   Body Fluid Formation

Other body fluids arguably with the possible exception of cerebrospinal fluid are also formed as ultrafiltrates of blood as is urine but are not found in the large volumes that urine is. Fluids other than urine and blood will be discussed more fully in the following chapters devoted to each of these. Some disagreement exists between medical professionals and researchers as to the extent blood plasma plays in the formation of cerebrospinal fluid. It should be noted that the volume of body fluids other than urine and blood are not controlled by hormones to the extent of urine, although some hormonal controls may contribute to fluid retention, particularly in the hormonal fluctuations in women.

These fluids also do not function in the same way that urine does particularly with respect to the filtration of fluids for excretion as they basically serve to nourish the tissues of the regions of the body where they are found. The fluids found in the cerebrospinal region of the body serve to protect and nourish the central nervous system, as well as to regulate pressure within the *intracranial* region and to circulate nutrients and remove waste products. Fluids associated with joints such as legs and arms in particular are *synovial* fluids, and are found in the spaces surrounding the articular cartilage. They provide lubrication to prevent friction between the cartilaginous coverings of the bones and supply nutrients to the cartilage itself. *Serous fluids* include those found in the *pleural* (chest) region, *pericardial* (surrounding the heart) and *peritoneal* (*abdominopelvic* region) of the body. Levels of chemical constituents of each of these types of fluids vary due to the physiological needs and functions of the body regions associated with them, but many of the components of the associated fluids that are normally tested regardless of body site where found are similar.

5.2.1   The Formation, Distribution and Excretion of Body Fluid

As an ultrafiltrate of blood, body fluids normally seep into and out of the blood vessels through the blood capillaries. These fluids primarily perform both nourishing and lubricating functions and originate as components of blood. The consistency of these fluids and the levels of components found in them vary by the body sites where they are found. Since the origin of all body fluids is the liquid portion of blood, the constituents for which body fluids are tested may contain some of the same materials that are found in blood. Although the levels of most components will not be the same in both blood and other body fluids, blood levels do serve to somewhat affect the levels in body fluids.

A possible exception to the use of an ultrafiltrate of blood forming all body fluids is that of cerebrospinal fluid (CSF). Only relatively recently it was generally believed that the choroid plexuses were the major source of the cerebrospinal fluid. But considerable current data now indicate that substantial additions to CSF are made at extrachoroidal regions outside the choroid plexuses. Studies of the formation of CSF in rhesus monkeys support the theory that at least some extrachoroidal CSF formation is probable. The exact mechanisms for the formation of CSF are still unknown at the present time but some sort of ultrafiltration is probably involved as in the other major body fluids.

The term 'body fluids' is a collective term for all liquids that are normally found in the human body, with similar fluids found in other mammals. Body fluids are composed of two types. *Intracellular* fluids are found within the cells of the body while *extracellular* fluid is found in the cavities of the body. Laboratory testing of any of these fluids will almost exclusively be extracellular fluids. Other fluids are in minor proportion to that of extracellular fluids, and are distributed to the surface and pores of the body for moisturizing the skin, hair, muscles, eyes, nose and mouth but are seldom tested in the laboratory. Major fluids in the hollow internal organs, marrow, brain and spinal cord all have the function of nourishing the organs surrounded by body fluids. For the study of body fluids other than blood and urine, this section is devoted to the formation of these body fluids and determination of the presence of various constituents in the fluids.

Body fluids originate in the blood and osmoses into the appropriate body spaces, and originates with ingested food and water, where water is often a major component of various beverages. Water is also formed during digestion in the stomach before becoming a component in the formation of blood in the bone marrow. When blood circulates throughout the body, the liquid portion is then filtered into the various body cavities where it is maintained in a form containing essential nutrients for a specific organ or system it surrounds. Key organs maintaining the balance of water in the body involve the lungs, spleen and liver as vital components of body fluids. Transportation and distribution of body fluids are accomplished greatly by the lungs due to their mechanical effects in the *thorax*, and by the kidney with the major role it plays in regulating water metabolism. Transportation of the body fluids involve the heart and the entire vascular system in the distribution of body fluids and are responsible for the circulation of oxygenated blood to the tissues of the body, all the while contributing to the formation and storage of body fluids in the correct spaces.

> **Points to Remember**
> All body fluids, arguably with the exception of cerebrospinal fluid, are ultrafiltrates of the blood plasma. In addition to the regulation of fluids of the blood and the various body cavities, the lungs, spleen and liver also play a major role in the regulation of water balance.

5.2.2 The Body Fluid Compartments

The two main body fluid divisions or compartments are both intracellular and extracellular. But it should be noted that the majority of laboratory tests performed on body fluids are of the extracellular variety. Only a few very esoteric tests would ever involve intracellular fluid. However, there are times when cells are destroyed in

Table 5.1 Reservoirs for Extracellular Body Fluids

Blood plasma	Extracellular fluid found in the blood vessels and from which the tissues derive their water and other nutrients
Interstitial fluids	Chiefly extracellular fluid outside the blood vessels that is separated from plasma by the walls of the capillaries
Transcellular fluids	The term 'transcellular' means fluids that are found between cells as fluids with specialized functions. The transcellular fluids are separated from the plasma by a cellular membrane such as those that line body cavity walls and organs, contributing to their shape and formation, along with the capillary walls. Examples of this type of fluid include synovial fluid (cushions and lubricates joints), cerebrospinal fluid which nourishes and protects the brain from trauma, and the aqueous humor and the vitreous body of the eyes (which maintain the shape of the eyeball and supports the alignment of structures such as the retinas that are found within the eyeballs)

order to obtain intracellular fluid. The extracellular compartments are found in the following table (Table 5.1).

5.3   Major Body Cavities

In addition to the divisions of the body fluids into either intra- and extracellular compartments, the entire body is further divided into body cavities that are further divided into planes. Vital body organs are confined to these body spaces, and fluids are identified by the body cavity where they are found. Two major divisions of these cavities include those called the ventral or frontal and the dorsal or posterior cavities (Fig. 5.1). The ventral cavities are larger than the dorsal cavities which are those found in the spinal region of the body of a mammal. The dorsal cavity is further divided into the cranial and spinal cavities, and the dorsal cavity also contains a region called the retroperitoneal cavity containing the kidneys and associated structures such as the adrenal glands. The ventral cavity is subdivided into the thoracic cavity that houses the lungs and heart, then the abdominal and pelvic cavities, most often combined as the abdominopelvic cavity. The digestive organs and the reproductive organs are found in the abdominopelvic region.

5.4   Volume of Body Fluids

The volumes of the compartments containing body fluids are regulated in part by the intake of fluids in the body along with any losses from metabolic functions and disruptions due to illness resulting from an elevated temperature. The body has a number of feedback mechanisms that aid in the removing, retaining or gaining of water in order to maintain homeostasis, the balance of life within the living organism. In addition to obtaining water from drinking fluids and from the water found in foods, some water is derived from metabolic processes such as oxidation of the simple sugar called glucose, which is derived from food, as shown (Table 5.2) below. When the body experiences a certain pathological condition, water may be retained or lost at a great rate, resulting in edema or swelling when too much is retained, or becomes

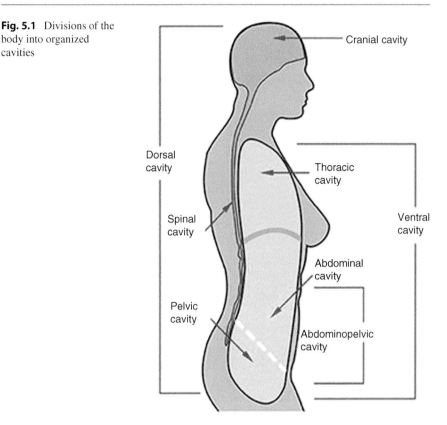

Fig. 5.1 Divisions of the body into organized cavities

Table 5.2 Metabolically-derived Water From Glucose Oxidation

$C_6H_{12}O_6$	+	$6\,O_2$	→	$6\,CO_2$	+	$6\,H_2O$
Glucose		Oxygen from respiration		Carbon dioxide		Water

dehydrated when too much water is lost. The concentration of electrolytes (elements that carry a charge) and in particular the sodium ions in the extracellular fluid greatly influence the volume of body fluids in various areas of the body in a significant number of ways. There are also many other solutes whose concentration in the body fluids that are kept within necessary limits by a variety of mechanisms that serve to adjust the retention or loss of these solutes, mostly by the kidneys. In a healthy individual, a human would have roughly twice the amount of intracellular fluids as that of the extracellular fluids, which may include plasma, *interstitial* and transcellular fluids.

5.4.1 Solutes Within the Fluids

The solutes in the body fluid vary in concentration and type between the partitions outlining the compartments of the body (Table 5.3). The cellular membranes between extracellular fluid and intracellular fluid, capillary walls between plasma

Table 5.3 Differences between intra- and extracellular fluids

	Extracellular (mmol/L)	Intracellular
Sodium (Na⁺)	142	↓ than extracellular concentration
Potassium (K⁺)	3.5–5.0	↑ than intracellular concentration[a]
Chloride (Cl⁻)	110	No reference values
Bicarbonate (HCO⁻₃)	25	No reference values

[a]Chiefly a result of hemolysis of RBCs

and interstitial fluid, and cellular layers between interstitial fluid and transcellular fluid are semi-permeable, where water can move in and out readily. This enables water to move into and out the body through the osmotic concentrations of the solutes in the different compartments due to differences in osmotic concentration. This process is known as a *passive transfer* and does not require energy for the transfer of water from one side of the barrier to the other. Where the osmotic concentration is the same on either side of the membrane, water will not move through the barriers when this condition is achieved. There is a major difference in the concentration of ions between intracellular and extracellular fluid, enabling a constant exchange from one side of the membrane barrier based on the needs of the body under certain conditions (Table 5.3).

5.4.2   Regulation of Water Exchanges Between Compartments

A continual exchange between plasma and extracellular fluid of water and solutes takes place between the body fluid compartments through the walls of the capillaries, which are the smallest of the blood vessels and where most ionic changes take place. This movement occurs as a result of two forces, the hydrostatic pressure within the capillaries, pushing water and solutes out, and due to an osmotic gradient relative to the plasma proteins in the capillaries, water is drawn into the capillary veins. The capillary walls are permeable to a number of solutes but in general are not permeable to most plasma proteins.

A protein fraction called albumin is the chief contributor to the *oncotic* pressure found in the blood. This concentration of protein results in a marked pressure difference between plasma and interstitial fluid. Any excess of fluid volume where fluid leaving the capillaries slightly exceeds the fluid re-entering the cells, results in the accumulation of excess extracellular fluid, and is referred to as "swelling." This excess interstitial fluid is taken up by the lymph vessels and is returned to the vascular system at the base of the cervical neck where the main lymph vessel, the thoracic duct, joins the venous system.

5.4.3   Regulation of Volume and Osmolality

How are the volumes of the various body fluids regulated? For intracellular fluid, the volume of fluids that are maintained is a somewhat simple process. Cell membranes are permeable to water, therefore water will cross the membranes into and out of the cell if there are differences in solute concentration (osmolality) that will result in differences in osmotic pressure between the two sides of the cell membranes. Individual cells can thus regulate their volume by adjusting their membrane transport processes to increase or decrease their solute content; this will lead to corresponding increases or decreases in volume as water osmotically follows the solute. In addition, if excess water is incorporated into the cell, the membranes of the cell may rupture (lyse).

For extracellular fluid, volume regulation is more complicated than that for urine because of the limited capacity of some of the compartments compared with the urinary system. And because the extracellular fluid solute concentration (osmolality) is kept constant, the water content will depend on the solute content. The regulation of body fluid volume is intrinsically linked with regulation of the concentration of sodium ions in the extracellular fluid. There are numerous other solutes whose concentration in the body fluids are kept within necessary limits by a variety of mechanisms which eventually adjust their retention or loss, mostly in the kidneys. For example, an increase in the amount of sodium (Na^+) in the body through ingestion of salty foods prompts a sensation of thirst so more water is drunk to bring the Na^+ to the correct concentration. This results in an increased volume of blood. Because sodium (Na^+) and its associated negative ions such as chloride are the main solutes of the extracellular fluid, the volume is regulated indirectly by controlling the Na^+ content of the body.

Sensors in the circulatory system detect the blood pressure and the amount of blood returning to the heart from the rest of the body. Both of these measures tend to increase if the extracellular fluid volume increases, and nerve signals from the sensors, relayed to the brain, ultimately lead to changes in the concentrations in the blood of hormones that regulate Na^+ excretion by the kidneys. The main hormones controlling the retention of sodium come from *angiotensin* II and aldosterone. Both of these act to retain Na^+ (and consequently water) so their secretion is inhibited when extracellular fluid volume increases. An increase of volume also has more direct effect by diminishing secretion of the water-regulating hormone, vasopressin (antidiuretic hormone or ADH), the action of which is to promote retention of water in the kidneys. The water is then returned to the blood and the tissues of the body.

5.5   Incidental Physical Constituents of Body Fluids

Body fluids, depending upon the type represented, vary greatly. Descriptions of cells that are often found in body fluid specimens but that may be incidental to the collection of the sample or for other reasons may be found in body fluids. For instance, cells may be found based on the source of the body fluid, such as those found in both normal and abnormal cerebrospinal fluids (CSFs). CSF samples may include cells from the lining of the ventricles (ventricles or cavities of the brain), *choroid plexus* or ependymal cells (cells of the central nervous system that line the ventricles) in both normal and abnormal specimens. Blood cells, particularly red blood cells, may be found due to the trauma of having a body compartment pierced by a needle and fluid withdrawn. Some of the red cells may come from the skin and the lining of the cavity where capillaries abound. Bacteria from the skin may also be found in various samples of body fluids, and careful attention to testing is required to rule out an infection by using the correct protocols for the procedure.

5.5.1   Significant Morphologic Characteristics of Cells in Body Fluids

Blood cells found in body fluids usually retain the physical features exhibited in hematology procedures, where studies of the morphology and physiology of blood is accomplished. Multiple varieties of cells found in the hematologic or myeloid (blood cell) lineage, those of the lymphoid system (stems from immune cells) and even muscle cells) will not be discussed here as would occur in a hematology text. These cells may be implicated in the diagnosis of a number of conditions that cause clinically significant changes or are evidenced in body fluids other than urine and blood.

5.5.1.1 Peripheral Blood Cells
Many of these cells will appear as easily recognizable cells from the bloodstream but it is possible that some of the physical characteristics may be different from the cytologic representations found in hematological procedures. This may be due to alterations during collection and the processing of the fluids using a specialized *centrifuge* that may alter some of the cellular features (Fig. 5.2). Early white cells called blasts are particularly sensitive to cellular distortion during centrifugation.

Blood cells that may be a result of contamination or of allergic processes are:

Erythrocytes Red blood cells (RBCs) in body fluids may be a result of contamination during collection, but may be present when trauma has occurred, especially the finding of RBCs in CSF.

Eosinophils Eosinophils possess a characteristic set of coarse red-pink granules and are found in abundance in some allergic conditions (Fig. 5.3). A thin smear of nasal fluid that is stained with a hematological stain will enable differentiation between an allergic rhinitis (nasal inflammation) and that of a bacterial infection.

5.5.1.2 Phagocytic or Mononuclear Cells
Phagocytes are specialized white blood cells (leukocytes) that are called *mononuclear cells* as they have a single, non-lobular and intact nucleus. They are capable of phagocytosis which means in a literal sense that a condition of eating cells exists. These cells are called macrophages and are very large monocytes which have a large nucleus. They are characterized by the material they have ingested as a unique diagnostic characteristic (Fig. 5.4). These cells are actually monocytes that have grown too large to pass through the capillaries of the vascular system which have passed from the blood vessels into the surrounding tissue. Ironically, monocytes that transition to macrophages have a lifespan that is quite long, but those which remain in the blood vessels

Fig. 5.2 Centrifuge used
for general laboratory
purposes

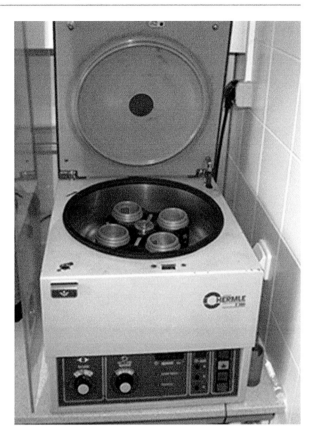

Fig. 5.3 White blood cells
called eosinophils

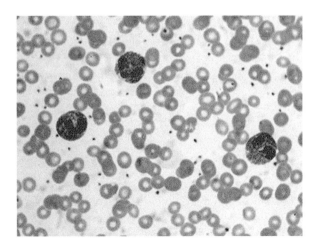

Fig. 5.4 Large monocyte

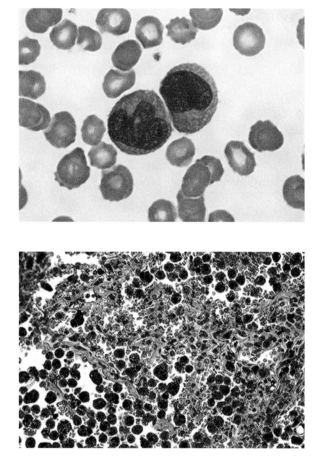

Fig. 5.5 Alveolar
macrophage

only survive for a matter of days. Some autoimmune diseases, where a body's defenses react against its own tissues, may reveal phagocytic cells that have ingested other cells of the body. Any pigmented material observed in a macrophage should be differentiated from yeasts and bacteria which have a recognizable shape and are physical elements that many white blood cells are capable of ingesting.

There are as many as five different phagocytes that are classified based on the location in which they are found and the ingested materials. They are:

Alveolar macrophages
Alveolar macrophages (Fig. 5.5) are found in bronchial washings, a procedure called bronchial lavage, and sometimes sputum from patients with respiratory illnesses such as asthma. These cells are also called dust cells as they are known to ingest both pathogens and environmental particles such as smoke and air pollutants, including dust.

Kupffer cells
Kupffer cells are specialized macrophages (Fig. 5.6) located in the liver and lining the walls of the sinusoids that form part of the reticuloendothelial system (RES) where blood cells are also formed.

Fig. 5.6 Kupffer cell

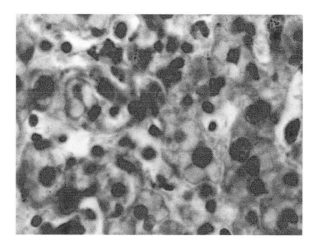

Siderophages

The prefix sidero- refers to iron. Siderophages ingest red blood cells (RBCs) and the iron from the hemoglobin of the RBCs. These iron granules (hemosiderin) stain brown to black when stained with Prussian Blue and are found in cerebrospinal fluid (CSF) where a cerebral hemorrhage leaks blood into the CSF. The presence of hemosiderin granules in the siderophage indicates that a true hemorrhage has occurred rather than the finding of RBCs related to the needle aspiration from the spine.

Lipophages

The prefix lipo- refers to the presence of fat. Lipophages are macrophages that ingest fatty materials from extracellular (outside the cell) following a variety of medical procedures such as a cerebral infarction (death of tissues of the brain). When significant tissue destruction has occurred in the pleural (chest) region, these cells may be found.

Neutrophages

When the leukocyte called a neutrophage (a type of white blood cell) that contains a segmented nucleus rather than the round or oval shape of the mononuclear cells, is ingested by the neutrophage, the lobes of the nucleus become separated and are small round remnants or become pyknotic (nucleus becomes compacted).

Points to Remember

Specialized cells that are specific to certain organs of the body exist for the purpose of maintaining cells of the organs and removal of organisms, cellular debris and environmental materials from a particular region of the body. These large and specialized types of cells are called macrophages, or "big eaters" and are generally characterized as white blood cells. Several different types of white blood cells are capable of ingesting undesirable components to be removed from the body, and these cells exhibit some of the characteristics of the cell line to which they belong.

5.5.1.3 Cells from Linings of Body Cavities

Somewhat characteristic cell types are found in the linings of the large cavities of the body, including the thoracic, *pericardial* (surrounding the heart) and *abdomino-pelvic* regions. These linings are mucoid and are designed to prevent friction between the space or organ lined by a protective lining and the organs that come in contact with them. Cells found in these regions are somewhat incidental and may be a result of inflammation but provide no specific diagnostic data.

Mesothelial cells

Mesothelial cells may be increased in chronic conditions where an effusion (collection of liquid) may be found. Mesothelial cells are capable of becoming phagocytes and transformation into macrophages.

Cells lining bronchii

Bronchial linings are found in the bronchi of the respiratory system. These cells are ciliated (contain hair-like projections) around the periphery of the cell (Fig. 5.7). These cells can be confused with ciliated protozoal (one-celled parasites) as they are quite active and motile when obtained from bronchial sputum or from bronchial lavage.

Synoviocytes

Synovial membranes line all spaces around articular surfaces of joints of the body. Inflammation of synovial membranes occur in conditions including rheumatoid arthritis or traumatic joint injury may require aspiration of synovial fluid which might contain synoviocytes.

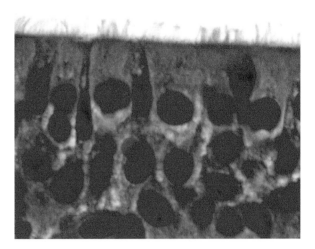

Fig. 5.7 Ciliated bronchial cells

Ependymal (choroid) cells
These cells form an epithelial lining of the ventricles of the brain and the central canal of the spinal cord as a single and continuous cell layer. Motile cilia may be found on the outer surface of this lining.

Points to Remember
Normal cells line the cavities of the body and are important in maintaining the fluid where articulation between tissues is found and are named after the organs or tissues where they are found. These cells are most often more prevalent in inflammatory conditions but are not indicative of any particular pathologic finding.

5.5.1.4 Miscellaneous Cell Types
Most of the miscellaneous cells found in body fluids are included in the fluid during collection, as a needle is usually the means for collecting these fluids and some of the cells are dislodged as they are pierced.

Squamous epithelial cells
These cells are most often found in cerebrospinal fluid due to the piercing of the epithelium during collection of the sample. However, squamous carcinoma (cancer) cells may be found in the sample and must be differentiated from normal skin cells. This is accomplished by the presence of atypical nuclei of cancer cells as opposed to a simple and typical appearance in normal squamous epithelial cells (Fig. 5.8).

Lupus erythematosus (LE) cells
An autoimmune disease commonly called lupus is characterized by the presence of neutrophils called LE cells (Fig. 5.9) that contain large and smooth pink inclusions which are from phagocytized nuclear material from other cells. They may appear in both pleural and synovial fluids but the disease is diagnosed most commonly by the presence of antinuclear antibodies and not from the cells that exhibit the phenomenon described here.

Chondrocytes
The term 'chondrocytes' refers to cells found where cartilage is found in particular areas where cushioning fluids of the synovial joints are found. Those with osteoarthritis (bone) and injuries to the joints and long bones of the body are present.

Cells found in malignancies
A variety of cells indicating cancer may be found in any of the body fluids. Metastases of cancer reveal cells that may be found in the CSF in malignancies

Fig. 5.8 Squamous
epithelial Cells

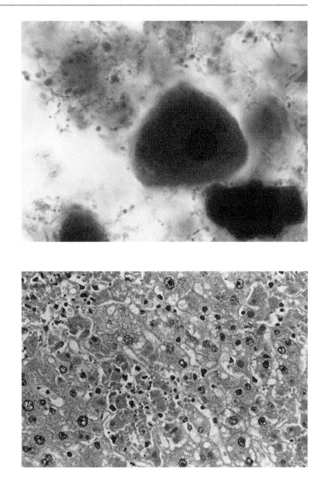

Fig. 5.9 LE cells

of the central nervous system (CNS). It is not common to find malignant cells in the synovial fluid. Diagnosis is made by a pathologist or a cytologist who makes special preparations of the cells on glass slides that are stained and studied microscopically.

Microorganisms

It is possible to identify a number of infectious microorganisms that are found in body fluids, and that might contribute to a disease. Yeasts and bacteria are commonly found and these organisms may require staining in order to visualize morphologic characteristics for identification or differentiation from cellular debris. Parasites and their eggs may be found in body fluids that may lead to the identification of a number of species of parasites. An experienced parasitologist or microbiologist is required for diagnosing many of these diseases. Bacteria may require incubation on a nutrient media using a Petri dish before definitive identification can be made (Fig. 5.10).

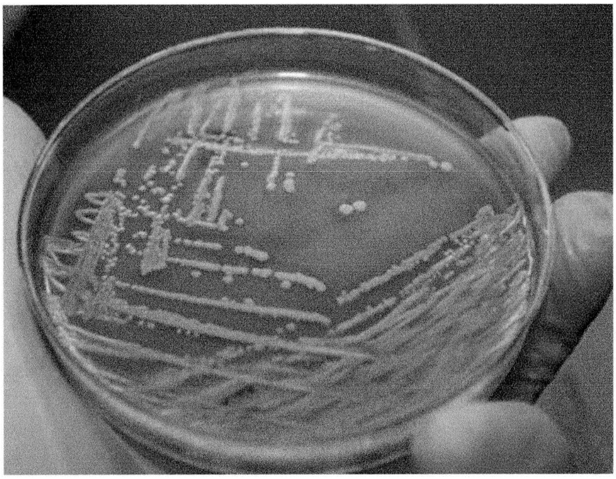

Fig. 5.10 Petri dish with
bacterial growth

Crystals
A variety of crystals related to synovial fluids may appear in the aspirated material.
A condition called gout may reveal the presence of monosodium urate crystals in
fluid from the affected joint. Hematin crystals from ingestion of RBC's may be
found in macrophages of the CSF following CNS hemorrhage.

Points to Remember
Some cells, organisms, and formed materials such as crystals are found where
disease processes are occurring. Abnormal cells may be found in malignancies and in autoimmune diseases such as lupus erythematosus. When organisms such as parasites and bacteria invade the tissues, the result may be an
increase in fluids or changes in the normal concentration of certain constituents of the fluids.

5.6   Chemical Analytes

Since electrolytes in body fluids are an essential means for maintaining fluid balance in body spaces, it is not common but studies of body fluids other than blood
may be required in specific instances. Chemical constituents of body fluids also
function in a protective role, reducing the impact of trauma on particularly the brain
and the large joints of the body. As a source of nutrients, the body fluids often contain glucose and other chemical constituents for nourishing the tissues of the body
site. The most common chemical analyses performed on a variety of body fluids are
those of glucose and the various fractions of the protein of the fluids which that
originate in the blood plasma. The concentration of total proteins may change in
response to disease processes, and is sometimes used to differentiate between

certain medical conditions, including the various fractions of the total protein. These analyses are often used to differentiate between viral and bacterial infections in the areas from which the fluid is obtained.

5.7   Other Miscellaneous Artifacts

Artifacts are not a significant problem when examining body fluids but are frequently found in urine samples. However, most solid and visible particles known as artifacts are harmless and are only incidental to the collection of the various samples of body fluids. Starch granules may be present due to contamination by body powders. Products of coagulation from the blood plasma may form small fibrin strands that might confuse the inexperienced microscopist. The identification of some foreign materials from implanted prosthetic devices made of silicone or polyester may challenge the professional examining the fluid.

A simple procedure called a *wet mount* in which a sample is placed on a slide with a cover slip and examined microscopically may provide valuable clues to the presence of a number of constituents that may be useful in indicating the need for further testing. In some cases, the finding of artifacts that may have imparted a cloudy appearance may enable a quicker completion of the evaluation of a body fluid sample. A quick survey for the approximate number of white and red blood cells, epithelial cells, crystals, and sometimes parasitic organisms and yeast will be helpful to the laboratory professional. An example of one of these findings is indicated where epithelial cells from a vaginal specimen may be coated with a certain species of bacteria which are called "clue cells" (Fig. 5.11), indicating the presence of vaginosis.

5.8   Summary

Body fluids include the most commonly tested fluids of blood and urine, but there are a number of body fluids in addition to these two types of fluids that provide critical clues as to certain medical conditions of the body. Although all body fluids originate as blood plasma with the arguable exception of cerebrospinal fluid (CSF), the constituents and the concentrations of each depend upon the body site form which the fluid is obtained, and disease processes occurring in the body. Analysis of a body fluid specimen requires correct and careful collection, transport, handling and testing of the material. The appearance and condition of the specimen may be affected drastically by faulty collection, preservation and transport. Faulty collection may reveal the presence of blood and other contaminants which might lead to an erroneous diagnosis even when sufficient knowledge of the clinical value of the specimen and when adequate procedural steps are followed.

A variety of disease conditions may be determined through the physical and chemical analysis of body fluids. The fluids are observed and tested for the presence of infectious processes, as evidenced by the presence of cellular presence among

Fig. 5.11 Vaginal epithelial cells called clue cells, are coated with bacteria

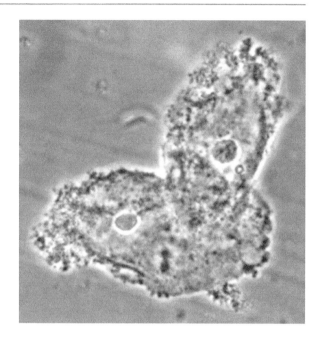

other clinical findings. It may even be possible to visualize a number of causative and infectious organisms by quick and simple procedures that may require further analysis by certain professionals for confirmation and diagnosis. Even crystals that might form during a disease process may lead to physical damage to articular joints such those found in gout.

A body fluids specimen must be sequentially evaluated for appearance and physical characteristics, as well as a microscopic evaluation. The presence of certain blood cells may provide clues for the diagnosis of a number of pathological conditions, including malignancies that might have metastasized throughout the body. Sometimes the presence of body fluids in certain anatomical regions of the body will require testing to even determine the source of the fluids, particularly following an injury. When examining body fluids, the same safety precautions are necessary that pertain to the performance of procedures involving blood, since infectious organisms may be present. The importance for analyzing any body fluids should never be underestimated.

Urine and other common body fluids derive from the same origin, that of blood plasma, although the concentration of the various fluids differ. Dissolved chemicals in urine as well as the other body fluids include electrolytes, glucose and protein. The other common elements found in major body fluids in certain disease states involve the presence of formed elements. Blood cells are the most common of the clinically significant formed elements, but in some cases, such as crystals, both normal and abnormal, that may be found in joint fluids (synovial fluids), are included in formed elements. Both peripheral blood cells and tissue cells are important in maintaining the health of the individual or in reacting to pathological conditions.

Body fluids may be either intracellular (inside the cell membranes) or extracellular and that are found chiefly in the cavities or body compartments of the body. A third, transcellular fluids, refers to fluids found between cells and tissues and have specialized functions. They usually line the body cavities and are separated from the plasma by a cellular membrane. Examples of this type of fluid are that of the synovial fluid, CSF and the aqueous humor and vitreous body of the eye. The fluids are consistent with the needs of the tissues of these various cavities and provide for protection and nourishment of the areas in which they are found. Some organs such as the lungs, spleen and liver are instrumental in maintaining the volume and fluid balance of the various liquids, of which water is a major component of the fluids. The transport and distribution of the fluids are a function of the spleen and by the mechanical functions of the lungs which affect the contraction and expansion of the thorax. The kidneys are vital in maintaining a critical water balance and certain hormones of the kidneys and even the heart effective in this vital role of regulating the retention and evacuation of fluids of the body.

The volume of the fluids is regulated by the intake of fluid and the feedback mechanisms which cause a transfer of fluids to other compartments and to the excretory organs. Certain illnesses serve to disrupt this exchange and transmission of fluids resulting in an extreme loss of fluids or gains in fluids resulting in congestion, edema and swelling. The volume of fluids and the exchange of the fluids will cause a variation of concentration of fluids as a passive movement from one side of a membrane to another, based on concentrations of solutes such as electrolytes. The fluids in some cases contain small numbers of specific cell types, but increases of certain cells are present in infectious diseases and where tissue damage has occurred. Bleeding into the compartments based on trauma may also reveal the presence of red blood cells which will not occur in any of the cavities of the body under normal circumstances.

Phagocytic cells are found throughout the body in both the blood and in some organs where they provide vital functions to maintain the health of the body. Other specialized cells are found as linings of particular body cavities and are involved in both protection and functional aspects of the associated organ or tissue found in the cavity. Chemical analytes such as electrolytes, glucose and protein found in the body's cavities and compartments correlate with the needs of the organs or cavities where the body fluids are found. In some cases, extraneous and often harmless formed elements that may be either organic or inorganic are found in the body fluids, and may or may not signal a medical condition requiring medical attention.

Case Study

A 65-year-old man was doing some repairs on the rails of his deck when an entire side of the deck collapsed and he was thrown to the ground. He was initially unconscious due to striking his head on a brick wall near the deck. When he regained consciousness, he summoned his wife and was taken to the local emergency room by ambulance. During the first hour, after a routine X-ray of the head showed no skull fracture, he began to suffer from severe headaches and blurred vision. As his condition deteriorated, the physician decided to perform a lumbar puncture, for an examination of the CSF.

Three tubes were used for apportioning the CSF sample, and a small amount of blood was observed macroscopically in each of the three tubes. The samples were sent to the laboratory for examination. Chemistry tests for protein and glucose were performed along with cell counts and a Gram stain. Using a special stain, the technologist also found black-colored coarse granules in some of the large white blood cells of the sample.

1. What type of stain did the laboratory technologist most likely use for this test?
2. What are the cells called that contained the granules?
3. What would be the likely condition from which the accident victim is suffering?

Review Questions

1. How are body fluids other than urine and blood formed?
   a. As an ultrafiltrate of blood plasma
   b. By specialized cells that produce fluids in some systems
   c. By the bone marrow of the body
   d. a & b
2. Elements found in the examination of urine that have no clinical significance are:
   a. Formed elements
   b. Artifacts
   c. Cells of tissues and organs
   d. Any chemical component
3. Body fluids include all of the following except:
   a. Synovial fluid
   b. Cerebrospinal fluid
   c. Urine
   d. Blood
   e. All the above are body fluids
4. Intracellular fluid is contained:
   a. Inside body cavities
   b. Outside cell walls
   c. Inside cell walls
   d. Only inside the nuclei of cells
5. Most of the fluids in the body are derived from:
   a. Other organisms
   b. Formation of fluids by body chemistry
   c. Foods and water
   d. Formed in body cavities and absorbed
6. Organs and tissues that play a major role in water balance include all except:
   a. Spleen
   b. Kidneys
   c. Liver
   d. Lungs
   e. All of the above organs

7. The term commonly used for the body fluid compartments of the human body are:
   a. Blood and urine
   b. Intra- and extracellular fluids
   c. Interstitial, transcellular
   d. Serous and plasma fluids

8. The concentration of greatly influence the volume of body fluids found in various areas of the body?
   a. Tissue cells
   b. Concentration of electrolytes
   c. Infectious organisms
   d. None of the above

9. The term "osmolality" is best related to:
   a. Concentration of dissolved materials
   b. Volume of fluids in the body
   c. Water balance
   d. Bone density

10. The term "phagocytosis" refers to:
    a. Production of certain white cells
    b. Displacement of red blood cells
    c. A specific autoimmune disease
    d. Eating of the body's cells

11. The disease called gout is based on the presence of:
    a. Large numbers of white cells
    b. Blood found in the urine specimen
    c. High levels of electrolytes
    d. Presence of monosodium urate crystals

Answers Found in Appendix C

Specimen Collection of Body Fluids

6

6.1 Collection and Handling of Body Fluid Specimens

It is essential to handle any laboratory specimen in the proper manner. Issues of proper collection, transport and identification of the samples, and storage when the samples are not immediately tested, must be addressed routinely. Improper collection of samples will distort and delay the results and are useless as diagnostic tools in the treatment of the patient, causing undue discomfort to the patient in some instances, and even extra costs for recollection.

6.1.1 Specimen Collection and Handling of Urine Specimens

The collection and preservation of urine samples for the various types of analytic testing must follow a strict protocol in order to ensure valid results. The handling of urine specimens requires that Standard Precautions be observed, although urine is not normally considered as a prime source for transmitting infectious diseases to others. The specimen should be collected in a clean dry container and a sterile container is required when the specimen is tested by bacterial culture. The specimen must be properly labeled and delivered to the laboratory promptly, as physical and chemical changes will occur if the sample sits at room temperature for more than a few minutes. Urine samples that are collected for a culture to determine the presence of bacteria require more care in order to avoid a contaminated specimen that will yield confusing results. A sterile container that is tightly capped upon collection and is promptly transported to the laboratory or stored in the refrigerator for transport to a laboratory at another location is paramount in importance. When a *catheterized specimen*, as the preferred method of collection, is inconvenient or impossible, steps must be taken to cleanse the external genitalia of women through the use of antiseptic towels. Care must be taken not to contaminate the urine specimen with the bactericidal agent used on the towel, as this would prevent bacterial

© Springer International Publishing AG, part of Springer Nature 2018
J. W. Ridley, *Fundamentals of the Study of Urine and Body Fluids*,
https://doi.org/10.1007/978-3-319-78417-5_6

growth when cultured. A midstream specimen, where the initial flow is discarded after interrupting urination, then the next portion, or midstream urine, is collected.

Some changes occur even if the sample is refrigerated for a considerable period of time. Urine has been known as an indicator for measuring health and well-being of humans and other mammals for thousands of years, and remains as an important tool in the diagnosis of many illnesses. Abnormalities discovered during the examination of the constituents and characteristics of a urine specimen are not confined to diseases of the genitourinary system, but may indicate medical conditions of other organs and tissues of the body. The clinical findings obtained from the examination of a urine specimen are favorably influenced by proper collection methods that include timing, handling, preservation and storage. A wide range of collection and transport containers for urine specimens are available from a variety of medical supply companies. The urine collection method employed and the container chosen will depend on the type of laboratory procedure requested by the medical professional.

Points to Remember
It is important to understand that an improperly collected and/or handled specimen is useless even when testing procedures are carefully conducted. Erroneous medical information is more dangerous than no information at all, in some cases. An old adage, "No test result is any better than the specimen that was collected," is appropriate.

6.1.2   Urine Specimen Handling Guidelines

General considerations for the collection of urine samples and proper handling of the samples during collection, transport and testing require that certain elements of care be observed. Some are mandatory and are imposed by both federal and state accrediting and licensing agencies. Others may be promulgated by voluntary accreditation agencies and must be adopted by the medical facility as a requirement for maintaining the integrity of the sample and professional accreditation. These points will be emphasized in all areas of this text where applicable.

6.1.2.1 Labels
Affix an identification label for the patient that may include name as well as other identifying data such as patient account number or barcode. Insure the information on the label and the requisition form and report forms match. If the collection container undergoes transport to another area of the facility, the label should be placed on the collection container and not on the top, as the lid could be removed and then placed on another patient's container. All labels should be firmly affixed to the container and will remain on the container when refrigerated.

6.1.2.2 Volume

A minimum volume is required for many laboratory examinations and should be insured prior to transporting the specimen to the testing area or site. In addition, under filling or overfilling of collection containers with preservative may alter the specimen-to-additive ratio and could result in altering results, either on the lower or higher spectrum. Patients who have difficulty voiding or are dehydrated often have difficulty in providing an adequate sample, sometimes resulting in a contaminated specimen. So collection might need to be delayed when practical in order to rehydrate the patient and to collect a valid sample.

6.1.2.3 Collection Date and Time

Always include the collection time and date on the specimen label, many of which provide for this information. This will confirm that collection was done properly. For timed specimens, verify the starting and stopping points (beginning and ending times) of collection. Documentation should include the time at which the specimen was received in the laboratory for verification of proper handling and transport after collection. Some facilities provide a standardized label that contains much of the necessary information needed to insure a properly identified specimen and that the proper procedure is being performed.

6.1.2.4 Collection Method

The method of collection should be checked when the specimen is received in the laboratory to ensure the type of specimen submitted meets the criteria required for the test requested. An example of an optimum specimen and test match includes a first morning specimen for complete urinalysis and microscopic examination.

6.1.2.5 Proper Preservation

Check to determine if a chemical preservative is present or if the specimen has not been refrigerated for a period of >2 h post collection. After accepting the test request, ensure that the method of preservation used is appropriate for the selected test or tests. If the proper preservative was not used, the test cannot be conducted and the sample should be recollected.

6.1.2.6 Light Protection

Verify that specimens submitted for testing for constituents of the sample that might be light-sensitive analytes are collected in containers that protect the sample from light, particularly sunlight or fluorescent lights. Failure to protect the sample from light for certain metabolic constituents may lead to erroneous results, and subject the patient to unnecessary treatment or no treatment as all. Although the collection of urine samples appears to be a simple process on the surface, the specimens must be collected in adherence with certain standards or may not produce valid results.

The menu of tests that can be performed on urine samples is significant and of utmost clinical importance. Therefore, it is critical to be able to adequately evaluate the entire process from steps in collection through transport and testing. These steps are just as important as those of actually producing valid test results by conscientious practice, and in troubleshooting any problems encountered during the entire sequence. An increasing number of tests that are available for home use where urine is the sample of choice may lead to erroneous results for the untrained practitioner producing test results.

6.1.2.7 Preservation of Urine

The most routine method for preserving urine samples is refrigeration when the sample cannot be tested immediately. Increase of specific gravity and precipitation of *amorphous phosphates* (found in alkaline urine samples) and *amorphous urates* (found in acid urine samples) will occur after a few hours in a refrigerated environment, and measures must be taken to return the sample to room temperature before testing is initiated. When *preservatives* are required, bacterial growth must be inhibited, and formed elements must be preserved, without interfering with the chemical constituents. Some urine specimens require an acidifying agent such as hydrogen chloride to prevent changes in chemical elements that would occur if the specimen was not preserved.

A number of changes in unpreserved urine specimens where testing procedures are delayed. Both chemical and physical changes occur, ranging from the disappearance of some elements, to the formation of others. In the best scenario, urine samples should be tested soon after collection to prevent changes from occurring that might lead to erroneous diagnosis or treatment (Table 6.1).

6.2   Types of Urine Specimen Collection

Laboratory urine specimens are classified by the method of collection employed to obtain the specimen. Basic types of collection methods are established for the purpose of obtaining a suitable sample, and to insure that testing will either be performed as soon as practicable or can be stored or preserved in a manner that will prompt testing at the first opportunity after delaying the procedure. The basic

Table 6.1 Changes in urine samples following collection

Increased *pH* from breakdown of urea to *ammonia*
Decreased glucose due to *glycolysis* (destruction of glucose) with bacterial utilization of glucose
Decreased ketones
Decreased *bilirubin* from exposure to sunlight or ultraviolet light
Decreased urobilinogen (changes to urobilin)
Increased *nitrite* content due to bacterial reduction of *nitrate*
Increased bacterial growth
Increased turbidity by bacteria or *amorphous sediment* (particularly in refrigerated samples)
Disintegration of RBC's and casts; may occur within minutes as *casts* cannot be preserved
Changes in color due to oxidation or reduction of metabolites

methods of collection that are tailored to the procedure to be performed are outlined in the following category of collection techniques (Figs. 6.1 and 6.2).

6.2.1   Random Specimen

This is the specimen most commonly sent to the laboratory for analysis, primarily because it is the easiest of all collection methods to obtain and is almost always readily available. This specimen is usually submitted for a complete urinalysis and microscopic analysis, although it is not the specimen of choice for either of these tests. Random specimens can sometimes give an inaccurate view of a patient's health due to the patient's amount of fluid intake causing dilution of constituents of the urine. If the specimen is too dilute, analyte values may be artificially lowered, providing an erroneous picture of the patient's health. Pediatric specimens that routinely undergo chemistry and microscopic analysis are generally collected as a random specimen. As the name implies, the random specimen can be collected at any time of a 24-h day for testing. Although there are no specific guidelines for how collections should be conducted, especially avoiding the introduction of

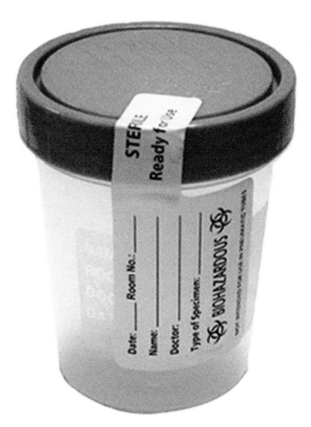

Fig. 6.1 Capped and sterile clean-catch urine containers

Fig. 6.2 Use of transport bag for safety

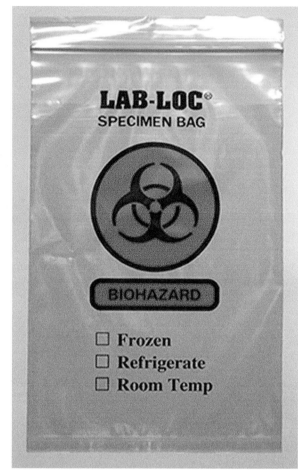

contaminants into the specimen. Utilizing the clean catch method while using a sterile or clean container is always advantageous for this purpose and requires explicit instructions to patients so they do not touch the inside of the cup or cup lid during the process of voiding.

6.2.2 Early or First Morning Specimen

This is the specimen of choice for urinalysis and microscopic analysis for the urine will generally be more concentrated by the urine having remained in the bladder for a considerable length of time. Therefore the specimen will contain a relatively higher level of both cellular elements and chemical analytes such as protein, if any are present. The first morning specimen is also called an 8-h specimen and is collected when the patient first awakes and has not emptied the bladder since going to sleep. While the urine sample can be collected over any 8-h period, the collection time must be practical for patients who may have an atypical work and sleep schedule. Proper collection practices accompanied by accurate recording of the collection time are important criteria for a first morning specimen. For an 8-h collection, any urine voided during the 8-h collection period should be pooled and refrigerated to insure that a true 8-h specimen is obtained.

6.2.3   Fasting (Second Specimen of the Morning)

The general practice for a 24-h collection is to discard the first morning sample but retaining the second specimen. This avoids any test bias in collection since the first urine passed in the morning represents collection of concentrated urine from the bladder during the previous night. Also, a representative sample is collected when a glucose tolerance test is being performed to determine a diabetic condition. When glucose is found in the urine of a patient, this fact does not establish that the blood glucose is elevated as there is up to a 2 h delay when the plasma glucose is elevated to obtaining a positive glucose in the urine sample. An elevated blood glucose level may have returned to normal at the time of collecting the urine sample and would represent a blood glucose value from one to 2 h earlier.

6.2.4   Glucose Tolerance Sequence of Collections

Some years ago, the 5-h *glucose tolerance test* (GTT) was performed to establish a diabetic condition, but is rarely prescribed today. Most often, a fasting specimen (see previous description) of urine and a blood sample are collected and tested for glucose. A measured amount of glucose based on the body size is administered at certain intervals, such as after a fasting state. This test measures the body's ability to utilize carbohydrates by measuring the plasma glucose level at stated intervals after ingestion or intravenous injection of a large quantity of glucose. Then most commonly, 1 h following the administration of the glucose, the blood is again collected along with a urine sample and is tested for the presence of glucose.

6.2.5   Two-Hour Post Prandial

A 2-h post prandial urine sample is collected when indicated following the ingestion of a meal or drinking a beverage containing a measured amount of glucose or carbohydrates before being tested for glucose. This is a screening test for diabetes, and is often sufficient for diagnosing Type II diabetes. A blood sample is collected at the same time and the results are correlated with the patient's response to the glucose or carbohydrate "load." Diet and exercise are often sufficient to successfully treat this medical condition.

6.2.6 Twenty-four Hour or Timed Collection

Timed collection of urine specimens is required for a number of analytic procedures for diagnosing various medical conditions. A 24-h sample indicates the
excretion of a particular analyte over a period of time where variations may occur
for various reasons, such as heavy ingestion of fluids. Among the most commonly
performed tests requiring timed specimens are those measuring *creatinine*, urine
urea nitrogen, glucose, sodium, potassium, or analytes such as catecholamines
and 17-hydroxysteroids that are affected by diurnal variations. A 24 h collection
is also commonly used for patients who show higher than normal levels of protein
in their urine as established by the complete urinalysis procedure.

Although the 24-hour specimen is most common, a timed specimen is collected
to measure the concentration of these substances in urine may range over a specified
length of time from 8 to 24 h. In this collection method, the bladder is emptied by
initially voiding prior to beginning the timed collection. Then, for the remainder of
the designated time period, all the urine voided is collected and pooled into one collection container, with the final collection taking place at the end of the specified
period. The specimen is normally refrigerated during the collection period, but for
some procedures a preservative such as boric acid is added to prevent the deterioration of certain components found in the urine. Accurate timing and strict adherence
to instructions is critical in order to properly calculate the results to determine concentrations of constituents of interest for individual patients. Interpretations that are
reached based on faulty calculations may result in an improper diagnosis that can
negatively affect the medical treatment rendered.

6.2.7 Midstream Clean Catch Specimen

This is the preferred type of specimen for bacterial culture and sensitivity testing in order
to reduce the likelihood of cellular and bacterial contamination. Patients are required to
first cleanse the urethral area with an antiseptic wipe containing castile soap or other
antiseptic. The patient is instructed to void the initial portion of the urine stream into the
toilet. These first steps significantly reduce the opportunities for preventing the release
of skin contaminants into the urine stream prior to collection. The urine stream is then
directed into a clean dry container and any remaining urine is voided into the toilet. This
method of collection can be conducted at either day or night.

6.2.8 Catheterized Specimen

This procedure is conducted when a patient is bedridden or cannot urinate independently. The healthcare professional inserts the outside end of an indwelling Foley
catheter (Fig. 6.3) that was previously implanted. The terminal end of the catheter is
inserted into a container but care must be exercised not to contaminate the sterile
collection container by the end of the catheter. A simple "in and out" catheter may

Fig. 6.3 Indwelling Foley catheter for male patient

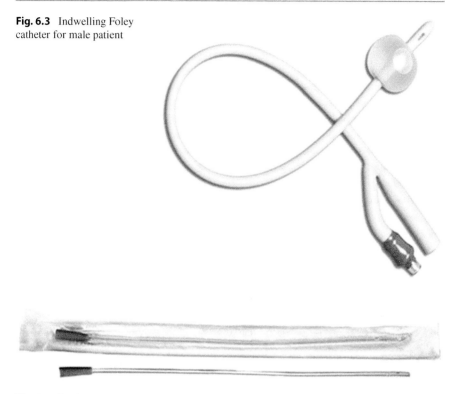

Fig. 6.4 Straight "in and out" urinary catheter

be inserted through the urethra and into the bladder to collect a urine specimen from patients who do not require an indwelling catheter for long-term use (Fig. 6.4).

6.2.9 Suprapubic Aspiration Specimen

This method may be necessary in some cases when a bedridden patient cannot be catheterized and obtaining a required sterile specimen would be difficult. Patients with some degree of paralysis may be unable to void normally so this type of procedure may be the only manner in which a sterile sample can be obtained. The urine specimen is collected by inserting a needle through the abdominal wall and directly into the bladder by using a syringe to draw the sample from the bladder. In this procedure, careful cleansing of the puncture site and care following the process may be necessary for the patient's safety

6.2.10 Specimen for Prostatic Evaluation

Since the prostate glands of the male patient often affect and even diminish the flow of urine. Inflammation or enlargement of the prostate glands are a common occurrence as males age, making it difficult to produce a strong urine stream. When inflammation or cancer is present, careful study of the urine of patients with *prostatitis*, the term for inflammation of the prostate, is important. When a routine urine sample from a male includes the presence of microscopic *spermatozoa* is also common and warrants further study. Urine samples collected following prostatic massage by the physician or other health care professional may require microscopic examination as well as bacterial cultures to determine if a causative agent is present. But in most instances of chronic prostatitis, negative bacterial cultures may be obtained. Men with chronic prostatitis may suffer sporadically from elevated temperature and periods of *pyuria*, a term indicating the presence of white blood cells in the urine. This condition may be confused by other conditions such as cystitis, *urethritis*, testicular condition called *orchitis*, or a venereal disease.

6.2.11 Pediatric Specimen

Collecting a urine sample from the very young patient presents a challenge to the pediatric nurse and others responsible for such collections. In addition, the laboratory tests often prescribe a volume of at least 10 mL for a complete urinalysis, although a smaller volume may yield some useful information. However, scanty samples pose a problem as they may be contaminated and the results may be inconclusive. For infants and small children, a special pediatric urine collection bag or PUC is attached adhesively to the skin surrounding the urethral area. When the collection is complete, the urine sample is poured into a collection cup. If the sample is small, it may be poured directly into a quantitative urinalysis tube or transferred by pipette to the tube. Urine collected from a diaper is not acceptable as a sample in that it will not provide accurate laboratory test results. Remnants of fibers from the diaper may result in contamination of the sample, contributing material that will likely affect the test results (Fig. 6.5).

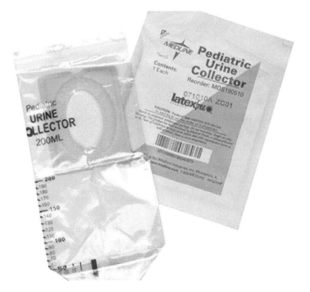

Fig. 6.5 Pediatric urine collection device

6.3   Verification that Urine Specimen Has Been Properly Collected

Many legally required samples and even some that are required for specific diagnostic purposes may be altered or attempts made to alter the sample by the patient for a number of reasons. Patients may attempt to avoid prosecution or even to please the physician by adulterating their urine with water to dilute the urine or to cover an accidental loss of part of a sample or failure to collect all of the sample during a 24-h collection. A creatinine level can be performed to insure that the sample is indeed urine. Creatinine is a waste product of muscle metabolism that is excreted by the kidneys and a negative result or a very low creatinine level may signify an incomplete urine sample.

6.4   Urine Collection Products

Multiple manufacturers provide urine collection containers in an extremely large variety of sizes and shapes. Information regarding the proper use and needs for a specific product must be evaluated when selecting a particular brand or type of urine container. Routine urinalysis systems offer collection containers and assorted tubes and pipettes are used to standardize the volume of urine tested, insuring an adequate performance of the complete urinalysis coupled with efficiency, accuracy and consistency of results. Urine collection containers such as cups for routine urinalysis and larger containers for timed collections used in collection and transport are readily available in institutional settings such as hospitals. Urine collection container cups come in various shapes and sizes, some with screw-on caps and others with snap-on lids to minimize leakage during transport. Containers are designed to protect healthcare personnel from exposure to contents of the containers and prevent exposure of the specimen to contaminating bacteria and other objects. Most specimens are now collected and transported in containers with effective leak-resistant covers. Containers to be used in transporting the samples to specialty labs which meet the requirements of state and federal agencies are also available.

6.4.1   Urine Collection Containers (24-h Collection)

Urine collection containers for timed specimens, including high capacity 24-h specimens are available in a variety of shapes and colors. Color and an opaque color are necessary to protect samples from light, which would invalidate the sample. Many are of 3 L capacity to insure sufficient capacity for individual variations in the volume excreted is allowed. Containers that are amber in color to protect light-sensitive constituents such as porphyrins and urobilinogen from being destroyed by exposure to light. Not only sunlight, but fluorescent lights also have a deleterious effect on sample results.

Warning labels and complete patient identification must be placed on the container (Fig. 6.6). If more than one preservative is acceptable, the least toxic or hazardous

Fig. 6.6 24-h urine
collection container

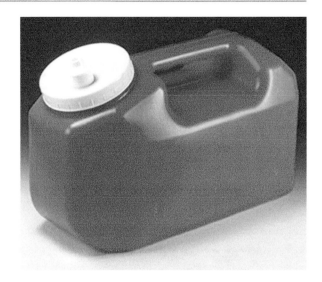

chemical should be used if there is a choice. Material Safety Data Sheet or important excerpts from the MSDS form should be given to the patient along with an explanation of the risks involved when coming into contact with any preservative, and actions to be taken if accidental exposure to the preservative or sample occurs. Preservatives selected are based on the specific procedure to be performed, and commonly include boric acid, hydrogen chloride which is a strong acid, acetic acid and toluene.

6.4.2   Urinalysis Specimen Tubes

Urine specimens are poured directly into urinalysis tubes that are sometimes equipped with screw-on or snap-on caps. Evacuated tubes similar to tubes may be used in some systems for performing urinalysis procedures, similar to those sued for blood collections. Urinalysis tubes come in a variety of shapes with either a conical bottom, round bottom, or flat bottom. The most commonly used type is that of the conical bottomed tube (Fig. 6.7) which provides a good collection method for microscopic analysis of formed elements of the urine. Some tubes that are designed for use with a pipetter that is matched to the tube in diameter allows for standardized sampling by extracting a standard and consistent volume. Sufficient strength in the walls of the tubes selected should be able to withstand forces exerted on them during centrifugation. Volumes required for the urinalysis tubes will differ in range for total volume, and methodology is designed to provide accurate estimates of the contents of the centrifuged sample.

6.4.3   Preservatives for Urinalysis

Clinical and Laboratory Standards Institute (CLSI) was formerly known as the National Committee for Clinical Laboratory Standards (NCCLS) and publishes recommended guidelines for the use of preservatives used in urine samples. CLSI

Fig. 6.7 Urinalysis
centrifuge tubes with
pipettes for charging slides

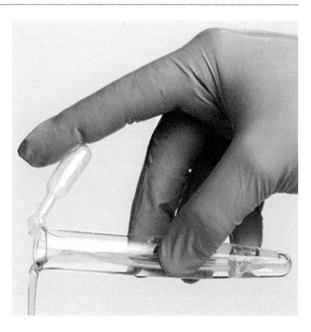

recommends as a general practice that all urine samples be tested within 2 h of collection. However, refrigeration or chemical preservation of urine specimens may be useful when testing or refrigeration of the sample(s) is delayed for more than 2 h. A variety of urine preservatives most commonly used to include acids such tartaric and boric acids, are readily available from commercial laboratory supply vendors. With an acid pH of the sample due to the addition of acid, bacterial growth is discouraged and allows urine samples to be kept at room temperature but still provide results comparable to those of refrigerated specimens.

Generally, the length of preservation capacity ranges from 24 to 72 h. Manufacturers should provide information regarding the preservation of certain analytes. Urine specimens directly transferred from collection cups into tubes containing a preservative should provide a stable environment until testing can be conducted by retarding bacterial overgrowth or breakdown of specific analytes. Non-additive tubes known as "plain" tubes do not containing any preservatives and urinalysis testing should be performed immediately following collection of the specimens.

6.4.4   Preservatives for Culture and Sensitivity (C&S) Testing

The most common and convenient preservative used for culture and sensitivity is boric acid, a product that is available in either tablet or powder. Since basic non-buffered boric acid may be harmful to certain bacterial species, buffered boric acid preservatives is preferable and should result in a better recovery rate for bacteria. The buffered form is the one most available to the laboratory when purchased from a medical laboratory supply firm. Preservatives used in urine for bacterial culture and sensitivity studies are expected to maintain a specimen in condition equal to

Table 6.2 Securing custodial samples

Special collection kits must be used that contain tamper proof seals to prevent exchange of the sample during transportation
Signed donor consent (consent is required, but in a court of law, this may not be necessary)
Photo identification establishing the identity of the donor of the specimen
Inspection and observation of the collection by a monitor to insure sample is valid for a urine specimen
Urine temperature measurement to determine if sample was freshly voided and no other fluids added
Specimen is labeled in the presence of the person being tested, before sealing the sample in an outer container, both of which will also require a tamper-proof seal
Sample is maintained under lock and key until transport to a testing facility occurs

refrigeration. Properly preserved urine specimens may be held at room temperature until time of testing. Each laboratory should carefully study the best method to insure expected results are obtained by performing duplicate methods of refrigeration and the use of acids on a regular basis for continued quality assurance. This type of process would be a good subject area for documentation in which to contribute to quality assurance committees as few laboratorians would think of the potential gained from this study.

6.4.5 Drug Screenings

Drug screenings are normally a requirement for employment in some facilities, for insurance physicals and are sometimes required by legal authorities. This process is one that requires diligence and care in providing a specimen that is not contaminated or altered in any way, and has a clear *chain-of-custody* to insure the validity of the sample. Even when a random morning sample is collected, a significant amount of documentation must accompany the sample. A detailed protocol must be followed to safeguard the identity and validity of the sample in order for the sample to be used as evidence in a court case. This documentation may be used in a court of law with persons responsible for certain steps in the handling of the sample to be possibly called as witnesses. The following list contains elements of the protocol for collection of a custodial sample (Table 6.2) to determine the presence of drugs, but is not limited to drug cases.

6.5 Specimen Collection and Transport Guidelines

- As with any type of laboratory specimen, there are certain conditions designated for handling of the specimens that need to be met in order to follow proper collection and transportation procedures for urine specimens. This will ensure stability of the specimen and lead to more accurate test results.
- All urine collection and/or transport containers should be clean and free of particles or interfering substances. They should also be either designed by color to prevent deterioration by light of certain analytes, or shielded from light during transport and storage.

- Glass containers should not be used as breakage results in contamination of the work area, producing glass shards capable of causing injury to lab personnel and custodial workers.
- The collection and/or transport container should have a secure lid and be leak-resistant to prevent loss of the specimen and to prevent contamination of the transporter and the sample.
- All types of collection containers and tubes should be properly identified and should contain any cautionary information regarding preservatives. Identification data and other information is required to accompany the specimens in clinical facilities.
- Materials used to construct the container should not deteriorate or leach dissolved materials including interfering substances into the specimen.
- Specimen containers should be disposable and under no circumstances reused for subsequent specimens. It is virtually impossible to determine if a container that has been used is free of contaminants.
- The CSLI guidelines for urine recommend the use of a collection container that is used for voiding into by the patient hold at least 50 mL. It should have a wide base that is not easily tipped over. In addition to at least a 4 cm base to prevent spillage, the wide mouth of the container provides the patient with a sufficient area for voiding into the container. A 24-h container should hold up to 3 L. This is necessary to provide for the upper limits of a normal daily volume of urine output. It is inconvenient for the patient when it is necessary to require the use of more than one container for large volumes of the specimen.
- The Clinical and Laboratory Standards Institute (CSLI) guidelines recommend sterile collection containers for microbiology specimens to prevent any surface contamination of the containers from combining with the specimen. The containers should have secure closures to prevent specimen loss and to protect the specimen from environmental contaminants such as bacteria, molds and dust.
- Transport tubes and other devices used in the procedure should be compatible with the automated systems and other instruments used by the individual labs.
- Collection containers and/or transport tubes should be compatible with a transport system that might require the use of a pneumatic tube system. A leak-proof container that is padded when necessary to avoid damage to the container is critical when specimen transport is used to convey the sample to the laboratory from another location within the health care facility.
- CSLI recommends the use of an amber colored container for specimens being assayed for light sensitive analytes such as urobilinogen and porphyrins. The colored material of the specimen container prevents the degradation of certain analytes.

6.6   Specimen Preservation Guidelines

Validity of samples is paramount in obtaining accurate test results. If samples are contaminated, bacterial growth will invariably and drastically alter test results. Some specimens are required to be maintained at a somewhat warm environment, such as bacterial cultures at normal human body temperature. Some samples are

Table 6.3 CLSI requirements for specimen collection and handling

CSLI guidelines for microbiological urine testing recommend the use of chemical preservatives if the specimen cannot be processed within 2 h of collection. If this time frame cannot be met, the specimens should be refrigerated at 2–8 °C. For urinalysis, CSLI recommends that the individual laboratories evaluate their choice of preservatives prior to using them in the facility's laboratory.
A proper ratio of the sample and the preservative must be consistently maintained to make sure the results that will be obtained from the preserved sample are accurate.
An evacuated tube system is designed to achieve proper fill volume to ensure the proper specimen-to-additive ratio and proper preservative function. Evacuated systems also reduce the potential exposure of the healthcare worker to the specimen.
Chemical preservatives should be non-mercuric and environmentally friendly. The Environmental Protection Agency (EPA) and the American Hospital Association (AHA) cites mercuric oxide used in urinalysis preservatives as a source of mercury found in waste products from medical laboratories. Some states have mandated a zero tolerance policy for the production of mercury-contaminated waste and the improper disposal of such materials.

damaged by freezing or becoming too warm, so specimen requirements must be adhered to strictly in order to protect the patient from misguided treatment or lack of timely treatment if a specimen must be recollected. The following Table 6.3 follows the guidance from Clinical Laboratory Standards Institute to insure a specimen is properly collected and handled.

> **Points to Remember**
> Preanalytical procedures, or those that must precede the testing of the sample, is as or more important that the testing procedures themselves. Following an established protocol that is systematic and similar regardless of the type of specimen being collected, is paramount in order to avoid the erroneous reporting of results.

6.7   Summary

The collection of body fluids, including the most commonly collected fluids of urine and blood, are a vital part of the quality assurance program for the clinical laboratory. Body fluids can yield valuable results to aid in the diagnosis and treatment of patients. Good quality assurance practices would mandate conscientious adherence to the procedures for collection, storage and transportation of all body fluids.

Several aspects of collection must be addressed in order to comply with good practices in the laboratory. First, the type of specimen required for the examination must be identified and properly prepared for. Then, if there is a timing requirement, a schedule that is not only convenient for the patient as well as the staff, but that is feasible with the patient's other treatment that he or she may be undergoing. The volume must be adequate and in some cases is critical for adequately performing the examination requested. The proper container that provides for safety of those handling the sample and that is constructed in a manner that would not cause deterioration of the sample. There are a variety of manufactured containers for all of the various body fluid samples that must be collected, transferred or stored. When preservatives are a requirement, proper handling of the preservative including instructing the patient on the proper handling of the container must occur. A specific protocol must be followed when collection of a specimen for drug analysis is performed.

Case Study 6.1
A 55-year-old woman who is somewhat obese and lives a sedentary lifestyle is undergoing a physical exam. The physician performs a dipstick urine examination and all the results are normal except for a small amount of glucose.

1. What other test(s) would he perform?
2. If the blood glucose values are elevated, what condition would he most likely consider?
3. What would be the best and most conservative approach for treatment of this patient?

Case Study 6.2
A urine sample in a screw cap container without a label is sent to the laboratory from the emergency. The patient's name is written on the cup with a felt-tipped marker. It is brought by a medical assistant, who requests that a drug screen be performed on the sample immediately, as the patient has been in an accident where he may be charged with vehicular homicide. She states that this is the only sample that was collected, and offers a hand-written request to test for a battery of drugs of abuse.

1. Should the laboratory technologist accept this sample? Why or why not?
2. Would the sample results stand up in a court of law? Explain your answer.

Review Questions

1. Why is it necessary to calculate the protein from a 24-h urine specimen rather than merely documenting a semi-quantitative level found in a random urine sample?
2. What is critical to remember when using a preservative for a urine sample when a bacterial culture will be performed?
3. List special requirements necessary when collecting a specimen for drug analysis, and give the reasons for these requirements when collecting, storing and transporting of the samples.

Answers Found in Appendix C

Diseases of the Urinary System

7

Objectives

Understand the relationship of abnormal urinalysis examinations and how they are used in the diagnosis of disease.

Differentiate between diseases directly associated with the urinary system and those that are metabolic and that affect other organs and systems of the body but yield abnormal results during performance of the urinalysis.

Recognize the normal appearance and test results in both normal and abnormal urine samples.

Describe metabolic diseases and how they affect the results of urine sample analysis.

7.1 Function and Diseases of the Kidney

The majority of kidney and urinary tract diseases result from infections by a large and diverse group of microorganisms. The interior of the renal organs, the kidneys, and the other anatomic structures of the urinary tract are basically sterile except for a small group of *Gram positive anaerobic* organisms that sometimes inhabit the genitourinary system and appear to cause no medical problems and function as normal flora. But it is generally accepted that the presence of microorganisms in the urinary system are a result of a bacterial infection, and in most cases, a simple urinalysis will yield clinical signs of an infectious process. In the female, an abundance of bacterial flora normally exist and reproduce in close proximity with the external opening of the urethra, and often a bacterial infection results when these bacteria find their way into the urethra. A thorough understanding of the anatomy and physiological functioning of the kidneys is essential to the understanding of disease processes manifested by abnormal findings in the results obtained in the performance of a complete urinalysis.

© Springer International Publishing AG, part of Springer Nature 2018
J. W. Ridley, *Fundamentals of the Study of Urine and Body Fluids*,
https://doi.org/10.1007/978-3-319-78417-5_7

Fig. 7.1 Structures comprising the urinary system

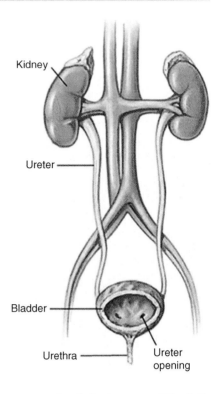

Not all diseases affecting the urinary system are of an infectious type (Fig. 7.1). Anatomical and physiological problems also affect the kidneys and other organs of the system, and may be diagnosed by tests that include the analysis of urine and other body fluids. It is critical to identify the causes of abnormalities in the urine and other body fluids that may be related to organs and systems of the body other than the urogenital system. Diseases of both the *urogenital system* and metabolic diseases of the body that result in abnormal urinalysis findings will be covered in this chapter. The term "urogenital" is used in many cases since the related systems of reproduction and urine excretion are both often included in a combination system, where a disease process of one system may be manifested in both.

7.2   Renal Anatomy and Related Functions

In review from earlier chapters, the kidney is the largest organ of the urinary system, and most individuals have two kidneys, but occasionally an individual will possess three of the organs. Of course, on the other hand some individuals due to injury or disease might have lost a kidney. However, many persons are able to function normally with only one kidney, since a single kidney will contain more than one million nephrons. The urinary system is composed of the kidneys, the ureters that empty into the bladder and the urethra and possesses sensory devices

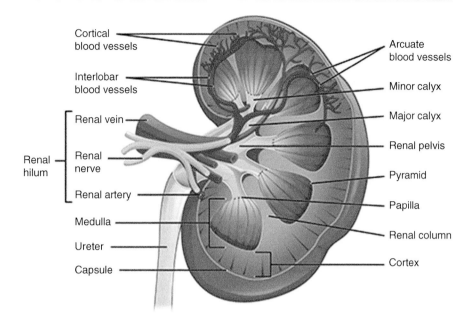

Cortical blood vessels
Arcuate blood vessels
Interlobar blood vessels
Minor calyx
Renal vein
Major calyx
Renal pelvis
Renal hilum
Renal nerve
Pyramid
Renal artery
Papilla
Medulla
Renal column
Ureter
Cortex
Capsule

Fig. 7.2   Internal view of the structure of the kidney

to warn the individual when his or her bladder is full. Sphincter muscles control the act of urination by tightening to prevent urine from leaving the bladder and relaxing to allow the urine to flow from the bladder into the urethra and to exit the body. A study of the functions of the urinary system, or more accurately the urogenital system, is important in gaining an understanding of various disease processes that may be a result of dysfunction of the entire system or of other systems and organs that result in abnormal urinalysis findings. The kidney (Fig. 7.2) contributes to a number of physiological functions vital to the health and maintenance of life.

Each kidney contains 1–1.5 million nephrons, the functional units of the kidneys where urine is formed and retention, excretion and secretion take place (Fig. 7.3). Nephrons are composed of the Bowman's or glomerular capsule where the tufts of capillaries called the glomeruli are found, followed by the proximal tubule, the Loop of Henle, then the distal tubule which enters the collecting duct for excretion. The chief purpose of the kidneys is to clear wastes from the blood selectively based on the needs of the body, while maintaining essential water, nutrients, and electrolyte balances.

The kidney is responsible for a number of important functions in order to maintain life by filtration, reabsorption and secretion. These functions include the removal of wastes from the body that occur due to metabolic processes or destruction of certain products within the body. These waste products are chiefly nitrogenous, as they contain a nitrogen atom in each waste molecule. An equally important

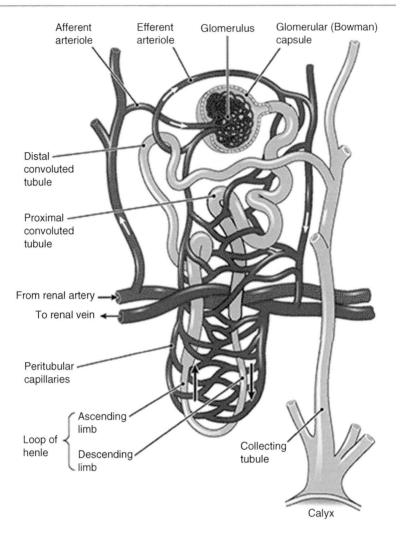

Fig. 7.3 Components of the nephron of the kidney

task the kidneys perform is to adjust the *pH* of the blood by maintaining the body's blood at a slightly alkaline state by retaining or excreting critical elements that affect the pH of the body (Box 7.1). The respiratory system and the urinary system work in tandem to regulate the pH of the body, which is maintained at a fairly consistent level of 7.35–7.45, a slightly alkaline level for the pH of the blood. The following diagram indicates how the kidneys are able to release or retain H^+ and HCO_3^- ions to regulate the pH of the body.

> **Box 7.1: Formula for Regulating pH of the Body**
> $H_2O + CO_2 \rightarrow H^+ + HCO_3^-$ or $HCO_3^- + H^+ \rightarrow H_2O + CO_2$ as a reversible reaction

When the pH of the blood becomes too acidic, H^+ ions are excreted by the kidneys and HCO_3^- ions are retained. When the pH of the blood becomes too alkaline, HCO_3^- ions are excreted and H^+ ions are retained until a normal pH is restored.

7.2.1   Renal Functions

Renal functions include four basic components in the physiological processes necessary for maintaining health and the continued existence of the human organism. A complex arrangement coordinates the urogenital system and its production of urine with the cardiovascular system, particularly with respect to the flow of blood.

- Renal Blood Flow
  Renal blood flow consumes roughly 25% of the cardiac output and is perhaps second to the liver in receiving the largest volume of arterial blood pumped by the heart. Another vital organ, the liver, receives 25–30% of the body's cardiac output. Therefore, these two vital organs together under normal circumstances would account for approximately half of the body's cardiac output, and arguably are the two most important organs in the human body other than the brain, lungs, and the heart. Cessation or diminishing of the blood flow to the kidneys and the liver, both of which are vital organs, will lead to shock. This is an extremely serious medical condition that if not remedied quickly would lead to death. Post mortem examinations of one who died of shock will show extreme pallor (paleness) of the kidney tissues as a result of decreased blood flow.
  Blood supplied to kidneys by the renal arteries enters the nephrons through the afferent arteriole. Blood flows through the glomeruli and leaves by the efferent arteriole. Arterioles are able to help create hydrostatic pressure differentials important for glomerular filtration and the maintenance of consistency in glomerular capillary pressure and renal blood flow within the glomeruli.
- Glomerular Filtration
  Blood from the afferent arteriole enters glomeruli located within the Bowman's capsule. Plasma filtrate must pass through three cellular layers of the individual Bowman's capsule. And pores found in the cellular layers serve to increase permeability of the capillaries but do not allow passage of large molecules or materials such as protein. But even in healthy individuals, a very small amount of protein and low numbers of blood cells may normally be excreted. Hydrostatic

pressure enhances the filtration of the blood though the capillaries due to the smaller size of the efferent arteriole and the glomerular capillaries. Flow of blood within the kidney is controlled through functioning by a complex hormone system of rennin-angiotensin-aldosterone system. As a result of the glomerular mechanisms, approximately 120 mL of water per minute containing low-molecular-weight substances are filtered through the millions of glomeruli found in the kidneys. A common urine function test to measure this function, called the glomerular flow rate (GFR) determined by the creatinine clearance test (mentioned earlier) and will again be discussed later in this publication.

- Tubular Reabsorption
  It would be impossible for the body to lose 120 mL of water without an intake of gallons of water per hour and containing necessary elements the body needs each minute. Therefore, reabsorption of most of the water and nutrients occurs on an almost constant basis during both day and night. Active transport includes reabsorption of glucose, amino acids, and salts in the *proximal convoluted tubule* and chloride in the ascending Loop of Henle and sodium in distal convoluted tubule (See Fig. 7.3). Substances to be reabsorbed must combine with a carrier protein contained in the membranes of the renal tubular cells. Passive transport does not require energy and also occurs as movement of molecules across a membrane caused by differences in concentration or electrical potential on opposite sides of membrane.

- Tubular Secretion
  Tubular secretion refers to a process where specific molecules are transported actively from the blood and into a filtrate from which urine is removed. In the kidneys, tubular secretion involves both waste product elimination and maintenance of the correct pH range of the body. Both of these functions that are essential for maintaining life and health. The process of maintaining the correct pH is necessary to facilitate many of the physiological processes contributing to normal functions throughout the entire body. Specifically, the actions of enzymes require a certain pH range and the promotion of the growth of normal bacterial flora within the body. Regulation of acid-base balance in the body is accomplished through the secretion or retention of hydrogen ions. This prevents filtered bicarbonate from being excreted via the urine and facilitates the return of bicarbonate ions to the plasma. This process of reabsorption of filtered bicarbonate occurs primarily in the proximal convoluted tubules. And to emphasize earlier discussions, excess hydrogen ions (H^+) leads to acidity of the body, while excess bicarbonate ions (HCO_3^-) leads to increased alkalinity of the body.

- *Osmolality* as a Measure of Urine Solute Concentration
  There are three related measurements performed in urinalysis that are based on the numbers and concentration of particles in urine, one of which is the specific gravity, a simple test performed in the routine analysis of urine. The second is that of either osmolarity and osmolality of the urine (technical descriptions provided in earlier chapter). The specific gravity determination depends on the number of particles present in a solution as well as the density of these particles. These particles are primarily urea, while sodium and chloride are also high in concentration.

The higher the number of particles dissolved in a sample, the higher the specific gravity will be. Although urea, a waste product in the urine, contributes a great deal to the specific gravity of the specimen, it is of little importance in relation to salts and glucose! The specific gravity is basically described as the mass per unit of volume compared with the same volume of pure water, which has a specific gravity of 1.000. Therefore the urine sample always has dissolved particles and will always have a specific gravity value greater than 1.000.

The specific gravity is used in the routine urinalysis to assess the level of hydration of the patient and is also affected by metabolic disorders such as *proteinuria* (protein in the urine) and *glycosuria* (glucose in the urine) among other solutes. The specific gravity is a test of convenience. But for critical measurements dealing with the ability of the kidneys to concentrate waste and other products, the determination of either the osmolarity or osmolality of a sample is used. Both osmolarity and osmolality refer to the concentration of an osmotic solution and are similar but may not be interchangeable for certain medical conditions.

The differentiation of osmolarity versus osmolality is important to gain a complete understanding of the relationship of the three measurements of concentrating ability. Both of these procedures are measured in osmoles, and refer to any non-dissociable substance. Although osmolarity is sometimes used in medical conditions, the volume of a solution will change with the addition of solutes, and when accompanied by changes in the temperature or pressure, so osmolality is the most commonly used methodology. Osmolality is the number of osmoles of solute in a *kilogram of solvent*, while osmolarity is the number of osmoles of solute in a *liter of solution*. To put it more simply, osmolarity is the concentration of a solution, while osmolality deals with the concentration of particles in a solution.

Although osmolality deals with the concentration of the particles that are dissolved in a liter of fluid such as the urine, the determination may also be used for serum and plasma samples. Serum and plasma samples are tested to determine the presence of several conditions that include shock, diabetes, and dehydration, among others. For the detection of these conditions, the osmolality of the serum is checked, and is known as plasma osmolality, where the concentration of substances such as chloride, sodium, potassium, glucose and urea are calculated. Since osmolarity is in a sense difficult to determine, osmolality does not change with volume, temperature and pressure changes, as it is based on a kilogram of solvent rather than a liter of volume. For these reasons, osmolality is the procedure most often performed on both serum (plasma) and urine.

When testing for the concentration of solutes in a urine sample, tests are performed by an instrument called the osmometer. This analytical device is extremely accurate when determining small changes in the concentration of dissolved solutes in liquids such as urine, plasma and serum. Certain physical properties called colligative properties include vapor pressure, boiling point elevation and freezing point depressions and are used to measure changes that occur due to concentration changes of dissolved substances. The osmometer utilizes the freezing point depression to measure the differences in the freezing point of urine, plasma or serum by comparing it with pure water. A previous analogy of an iceberg was provided and bears repeating as an aid to understand the concentration of solutes within a liquid and the differences between the concentrations of solutes occurs with the iceberg. An iceberg is composed of water that contains fewer solutes than the salt water of the ocean surrounding the iceberg. An iceberg as a less-concentrated solution freezes at 32 °F, while ocean water with dissolved salts requires a lower temperature (28.4 °F) before freezing. But after seawater freezes, the ice contains very little salt because only the water part freezes.

The clinical significance of osmolarity or osmolality includes the initial evaluation of the renal system's concentrating ability. The values are useful in monitoring the course of renal disease, monitoring fluid and electrolyte therapy, establishing the differential diagnosis of a high level of sodium known as *hypernatremia* and *hyponatremia* (low levels of sodium) and polyuria (higher than normal production of urine), while evaluating the secretion and renal response to ADH (anti-diuretic hormone or *vasopressin*).

Normal serum osmolality values are between 500 and 850 mOsm/kg of water. ADH is stimulated when the osmolarity of the plasma rises, so water is retained to lower the osmolarity. Not all solutes are equally effective as osmotic stimuli for ADH secretion, but sodium chloride (NaCl) is very effective, while urea has little effect. A rise in blood glucose concentration *in the presence of adequate insulin* has little or no effect at all by changing ADH secretion. In the absence of adequate insulin, glucose has a small stimulating effect on ADH secretion. Physiologically, a change in NaCl concentration as the result of water loss is probably the most important stimulus for the secretion of ADH.

One of the diseases called Liddle Syndrome is an example of extreme osmolality. This rare inherited disorder is characterized by extremely high blood pressure, or hypertension. The mutation of a gene that affects *aldosterone* results in this disease. One can imagine the impact on health since aldosterone is the hormone that regulates sodium retention by the kidneys. This causes reabsorption of large amounts of sodium with too little being excreted. The osmotic pressure or the increased osmolality of the blood, would produce hypertension.

Another disease caused by a malfunction of ADH is that of Type I diabetes insipidus (DI). Diabetes is perhaps a misnomer as it is not characterized by a lack of or malfunction of insulin, but by a disorder where ADH does not aid in retaining fluids. The term "insipidus" indicates a lack of taste and may be attributed to the practice of tasting urine by ancient medical practitioners. The urine may not have had a sweet taste to it as does in diabetes mellitus that is not under control by diet or medication. This disorder is in part diagnosed by the excretion of mammoth amounts of dilute urine of low specific gravity, and it is not unusual to void several gallons during a 24-h cycle. This loss of water causes an unrelenting thirst where inadequate secretion of antidiuretic hormone prevents the loss of fluids. Type II diabetes insipidus may be caused by a mutated form of the gene for aquaporin, where a cell membrane protein controlling flow of water out of the kidneys with reabsorption is defective. Excessive thirst and urination is often the first sign of this disease as well as glucose levels and hypernatremia, since dehydration occurs frequently.

A number of probable causes for the development of diabetes insipidus has been postulated. Trauma to the brain and neurosurgery have been blamed at least for some of those suffering from this disorder. Side effects of some drug therapies, including a specific antibiotic called demeclocycline or on antidepressants where lithium buildup has led to vomiting, dizziness and on occasion weight gain. Lithium may be toxic at elevated levels while not producing the beneficial results desired. Death of kidney tissue called an infarction related to a number of causes where the kidneys have lost their ability to prevent loss of water from the body. ADH is produced by the hypothalamus and is stored in the posterior pituitary gland along with oxytocin. An inherited genetic trait occurs where ADH is not produced by the hypothalamus in effective levels, insufficient to stimulate the ability of the kidneys to limit loss of water from the body.

Points to Remember
The testing of urine samples for diseases of the urinary system may reveal diseases not only of the kidneys and associated structures but of metabolic diseases that cause the "spilling" of certain constituents into the urine. The lack of proper circulation to the kidneys may also result in conditions that are not abnormalities of the kidneys themselves.

7.3   Diseases of the Urinary System

Components found in the evaluation of urine, physical, chemical and microscopic, are used to determine a multitude of disorders that are of a metabolic basis or that are malfunctions of the body that directly affect the renal system. The refinement of the earlier-invented microscope by Antoni van Leeuwenhoek in the seventeenth century (Fig. 7.4) enabled Thomas Addis to develop methods for quantitation of the microscopic sediment (called the Addis count), a procedure that is seldom used currently. Richard Bright was chiefly given credit for introducing the urinalysis as part of a doctor's routine patient examination in 1827, in which only a few components were tested. But by the 1930s, the number and complexity of the tests possible in a routine urine analysis had reached a point of impracticality, and the use of the urinalysis was practically eliminated from routine physical examinations. But in the 1960s development of modern and rapid testing techniques such as a dipstick that allowed performance of a number of screening tests became readily available, therefore the routine urinalysis again became favorable as being necessary and practical, and is now an important part of the patient examination.

Although disease states throughout the body can affect renal function and produce abnormalities in the urinalysis, abnormal results are frequently associated with disorders directly affecting the kidney. A basic discussion of the major renal diseases, including possible causes, clinical symptoms, associated pathology, and

Fig. 7.4 Early version of
a microscope

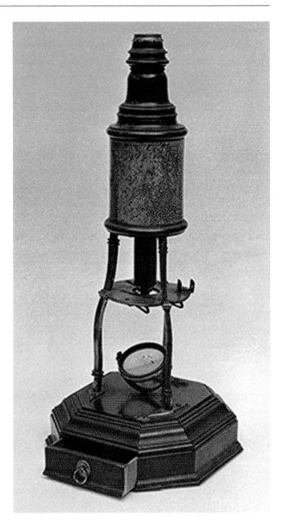

laboratory findings—is presented at this point to enable laboratory personnel to better understand the significance of test results in these conditions. The following diseases progress from the simple and more easily treated conditions to more serious and chronic disease states.

7.3.1 Cystitis and Urethritis

A number of terms are associated with cystitis and urethritis, and the onset can be sudden and acute, or it can merely cause mild discomfort. The symptoms for the two conditions are similar and may be indistinguishable from each other, and cystitis and urethritis often occur concomitantly. It is possible for that the body can rid itself of these bacteria through urination and may actually clear itself of the condition in a relatively short period of time in mild cases. Cystitis is caused most commonly by bacteria that enter the urethra and then move up to the bladder. These bacteria can lead to infection, most commonly in the bladder. Acute cystitis is usually caused by a bacterial infection of the bladder or lower urinary tract, and is a common malady for a number of individuals who suffer from recurrent bouts of cystitis. Cystitis is an infection of the bladder and urethritis is an infection of the urethra where the urine leaves the bowel.

Cystitis is rare in men due to a variable but generally a rather lengthy urethra requiring the bacteria to travel a greater distance to the bladder. Therefore women tend to get infections more often than men because their urethra is shorter and closer to the anus and during intercourse, but urination immediately following intercourse may prevent the condition from occurring. Older adults also have a high risk for developing cystitis. This is due in part to conditions such as benign prostatic hyperplasia or BPH and prostatitis in male patients and strictures (narrowing or blockages) of the urethra that may occur due to scar tissue damage from earlier infections, including sexually transmitted diseases, medical conditions that are commonly referred to as STDs.

The term "acute" means that sudden or severe symptoms may occur suddenly or in a relatively short time frame. The infection can spread secondarily to the kidneys where the bacteria adhere to the wall of either the urethra or the bladder and grow quite rapidly, enabling some bacterial organisms to remain in the bladder, causing additional problems. Most cases of cystitis are predominantly caused by *Escherichia coli* (*E. coli*), a bacterium normally found in the intestines (Fig. 7.5). Cystitis is a relatively simple condition to treat initially, but when untreated, may progress to the kidneys, causing either acute or chronic disease in which the kidneys may be permanently damaged.

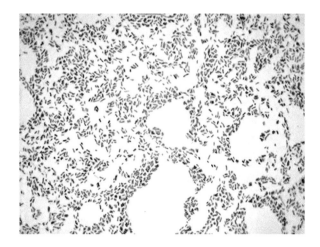

Fig. 7.5 Microscopic
view of stained *E. coli*

It should be understood that most urinary tract infections (UTIs) involve only the bladder and urethra, which is known as the lower urinary system and are known as cystitis. The symptoms of cystitis are similar to those of pyelonephritis, and is the precursor to the development of pyelonephritis. Cystitis usually begins with discomfort when voiding (urinating) and are often accompanied by a sense of urgency along with painful and frequent urination. Symptoms may include any or all of the following. Pain in the back or the flank (side), fever and chills almost always occur, along with vague feelings of nausea accompanied occasionally by vomiting, malaise (weakness and fatigue) and confusion that occur mainly in the elderly patient. Noticeable changes in the urine often prompts a patient to consult a physician, such as hematuria (blood in the urine), or cloudy and foul-smelling urine, discomfort when urinating or urgent feelings of needing to void (often without success), and increases in the frequency of urination.

7.3.2 Pyelonephritis

Acute *pyelonephritis* is most frequently seen in women, often resulting from untreated cases of cystitis or lower urinary tract infection, and does not cause permanent damage to the renal tubules. Recurrent infections caused by structural abnormalities or obstructions of the urinary tract that allow bacteria to remain in the kidney may progress to damage and chronic pyelonephritis. Urinalysis findings in both acute and chronic pyelonephritis are similar and include white blood cells that are often found as clumps of white blood cell casts, bacteria, positive nitrite reactions, and possible proteinuria and hematuria (Fig. 7.6). With the exception of the presence of white blood cell casts that are indicative of tubular involvement, similar results will be found with infections of the lower urinary tract such as cystitis.

The condition known as pyelonephritis is defined as a serious bacterial infection of the kidney that can be either acute or chronic. Other than cystitis, pyelonephritis is one of the most common renal diseases but with more serious consequences. Acute pyelonephritis is a sudden inflammation caused by bacterial infections and chiefly affects the interstitial area and the renal pelvis and less commonly the renal tubules. When acute pyelonephritis progresses to chronic pyelonephritis, a persistent and long-standing kidney inflammation can scar the tissues of the kidneys and may lead to a fatal condition called chronic renal failure, which can only be remedied by. This disease is most common in patients who are predisposed to recurrent acute pyelonephritis, such as those with urinary obstructions or vesicoureteral reflux (back flow from the bladder to the ureters).

Acute pyelonephritis is one of the most common renal diseases, and the condition results in an inflammation caused by bacteria. These bacteria are frequently from a grouping called Gram negative bacilli (including *E. coli* or *Klebsiella* sp., rod-shaped organisms), but can be the result of bacterial colonization of potentially hundreds of bacterial species. The condition primarily affects the interstitial areas and the renal pelvis, and less frequently the renal tubules become involved. Fortunately, acute pyelonephritis is almost always curable with antibiotics when

Fig. 7.6 Urine sample
exhibiting hematuria

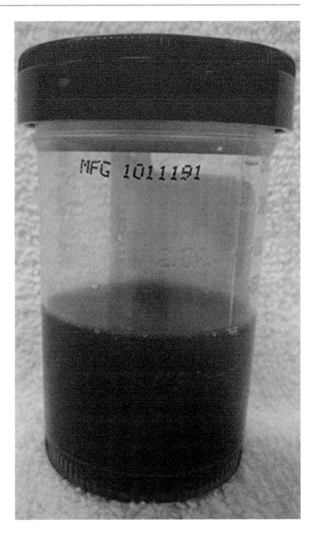

administered early in the course of the disease before damage to occurs in the filtering units of the kidneys.

Chronic pyelonephritis is potentially extremely serious and can spread to the blood, affecting other organs of the body. If allowed to become a long-standing or persistent inflammation, kidneys and associated structures of the urogenital system can become scarred and will likely lead to chronic renal failure. This disease is most common in patients who are predisposed to recurrent acute pyelonephritis due to a number of factors, one of which occurs with urinary obstructions of several types. It should be understood that most urinary tract infections (UTIs) involve only the bladder and urethra, which is known as the lower urinary system.

The symptoms of pyelonephritis are similar to those of cystitis, which may be the precursor to the development of pyelonephritis, and usually begins with discomfort when voiding (urinating) and are accompanied by a sense of urgency along with painful and frequent urination. Symptoms may include any or all of the following: pain in the back or the flank (side). Fever and chills almost always occur, along with vague feelings of nausea accompanied occasionally by vomiting, malaise (weakness and fatigue) and confusion that occurs mainly in the elderly patient. Noticeable changes in the urine are often the reasons a patient consults a physician, such as hematuria (blood in the urine), or cloudy and foul-smelling urine, discomfort when urinating or urgent feelings of needing to void (often without success), and increases in the frequency of urination.

A number of factors are related to the occurrence of pyelonephritis. Along with cystitis that progresses through the ureters and to the kidneys, bacterial contamination from the anus is most common. Less frequently, a number of bacteria from the skin or the environment may cause pyelonephritis. But conditions that result in a reduced urine flow most likely contribute to the development of pyelonephritis along with exposure to a source of bacteria. A normal urine flow from the ureters and through the urethra tends to flush out bacteria before colonization occurs. But if the urine flow is slowed or completely halted, any bacteria present in the urethra and the bladder can more easily travel up the ureters and to the kidneys.

Other common causes of urine obstruction include benign prostatic hypertrophy (BPH) in men, strictures in the urethra from previous infections such as including the previously-mentioned sexually-transmitted diseases (STDs) and abdominal or pelvic masses that result from cancer. Patients with diabetes or those with an impaired immune system may suffer from increased rates of pyelonephritis from the body's inability to rid itself of bacteria or to combat a simple infection. Bacteria thrive in an increased level of glucose, so the diabetic is commonly at risk. But another leading cause of pyelonephritis results from urinary calculi (stones) that may form in either the kidneys, the bladder or ureters. Kidney stones mechanically contribute to pyelonephritis by creating an area for bacteria to grow where the flow of urine is unable to flush the organisms from the body.

7.3.3   Acute Glomerulonephritis

Acute glomerulonephritis occurs when systemic infections by organisms that do not normally cause urinary tract infections that may result in conditions directly caused by bacterial infections such as occurs with pyelonephritis. The condition is a generalized condition but refers to a specific set of renal diseases where an immunologic mechanism triggers inflammation and proliferation of glomerular tissue that may damage the basement membrane and even the capillary endothelium (lining of the interior of the vessels). The disease was recognized in ancient literature as patients with back pain and often accompanied by reduced urine flow and gross blood in the urine.

But it required the continued evolvement of the microscope and histological studies of changes in tissues of the body before researchers were able to describe changes in the glomeruli resulting from the immunologic attack on the tissue. Glomerulonephritis may represent as much as 15% of glomerular diseases reported.

Localized increases in morbidity rates relative to glomerulonephritis attributed to post streptococcal infections will be described in the following sections. The disease has declined steadily over several decades but is still a medical problem in isolated and underdeveloped areas of the world, where effective antibiotics and other medical support efforts are scarce. This global decline in the numbers of cases is attributed to a substantial number of factors and is mainly due to the delivery of more advanced health care and improved environmental conditions.

In general, glomerulonephritis refers to a "sterile" inflammatory process that affects the glomeruli and is associated with the finding of blood, protein, and casts in the urine. The disease is called a "sterile" inflammatory process since there is no active and ongoing bacterial infection of the kidneys. There will often be no bacteria manifested in the urine sample, and cultures of the urine will most often yield a negative result. Acute glomerulonephritis, as the name implies, is a disease characterized by the rapid onset of symptoms consistent with damage to the glomerular membrane.

The secondary manifestations of the disease may include edema, hypertension, and sometimes and electrolyte imbalance based on the inability of the kidneys to excrete and reabsorb certain materials. When properly managed until the inflammation has subsided, a permanent cure may be realized. The initial urinalysis findings include marked hematuria, increased protein, and oliguria (low urine output). Microscopic findings may also yield evidence of any or all of the following: red blood cell casts, dysmorphic or poorly formed red blood cells, white blood cells, and casts that may include hyaline casts, granular casts, and white blood cell casts. As toxicity to the glomerular membrane is alleviated, the urinalysis results will return to normal, with the possible exception of microscopic hematuria that lasts until the membrane damage has been repaired. Blood tests that in particular include *blood urea nitrogen* (BUN) and creatinine that may be elevated during the acute stages but will return to normal along with the urinalysis results. Demonstration of elevated levels of streptococcal enzymes identifies the disease as streptococcal in origin and often in the past moreso than currently resulted from untreated conditions of "strep" throat or streptococcal pharyngitis.

Acute glomerulonephritis is usually manifested by a sudden onset of hematuria, proteinuria increased levels of protein in the urine), and red blood cell casts. The typical patient presents with symptoms similar to those associated with pyelonephritis but are often accompanied by high blood pressure (hypertension), edema (swelling), and decreased urine flow. The disease progresses when immune complexes where the deposition of complement and immunoglobulins (protein fraction of the blood associated with the formation of antibodies) occurs in response to the streptococcal infection. This is due to an affinity of the organism for the glomeruli and the coronary valves. Glomerular lesions in acute glomerulonephritis result from glomerular deposition in a localized site and formation of humoral immune complexes of material called complement as well as antibodies.

On gross appearance, patients with advanced glomerulonephritis might reveal kidneys that are grossly enlarged with histopathologic changes that are typically observed microscopically from stained tissue samples. There will often be swelling of the glomerular tufts of capillaries and. immunofluorescence studies reveal the components of the immune system. Subsequent infections by the streptococcal organism allow transport of the organisms through the blood to the kidneys as well as additional immunoglobulins (IgG). It is possible to determine if a recent streptococcal infection has occurred, a condition that may potentially result in further glomerular damage, by performing antibody titers (serological dilutions) for additional antigens such as *antistreptolysin O* (ASO), streptokinase and DNAase-B. Following damage to the glomeruli, these units of the kidney no longer effectively filter out certain components while reabsorbing those that should be retained. Kidney transplant or hemodialysis are usually the only choice indicated at this point.

7.3.4   Chronic Glomerulonephritis

The term chronic glomerulonephritis' has been used to describe a variety of disorders that produce continual or permanent damage to the glomeruli. The etiology of this condition is unclear and subject to debate. The onset might begin with mild symptoms such as recurring hematuria in young adults or hypertension and gradually progresses to end stage renal disease. It is a long course disease with periods characterized by asymptomatic signs and symptoms.

Depending upon damage wreaked upon the glomeruli during a substantial time period, progression to a condition called end-stage renal disease may occur. Patients endure worsening symptoms with malaise, edema (swelling0), and oliguria (low urine excretion). Significant anemia may occur due to due to kidney damage where erythropoietin (EPO) is produced that stimulates production of red blood cells. The typical urine sample of those with chronic glomerulonephritis will show microscopic red blood cells (hematuria), proteinuria where protein is lost from blood plasma, glycosuria from failure to reabsorb glucose, and several varieties of casts. Increase in measures of the glomerular filtration activity result in elevated BUN and creatinine levels. Electrolyte imbalances of sodium and potassium along with a reduced filtration rate (creatinine clearance) are significant.

> **Points to Remember**
> Serious diseases of the urinary system may originate with a simple condition that would have been easily treated, but that progressed into a chronic condition. Symptoms and signs of these conditions, particularly early in the disease process, may be mild, scarcely noticeable, and easily ignored.

7.3.5   Rheumatic Fever, An Autoimmune Glomerulonephritis

"Rheumatic fever," a general term used for a specific type of chronic glomerulonephritis, is an inflammatory disease that occurs following a Group A streptococcal infection called strep throat or scarlet fever. The causative organism, *Streptococcus pyogenes*, Group A, is Beta-hemolytic to blood agar when the organisms are grown on this type of culture media. Beta hemolysis means that the growing organisms will completely *lyse* or destroy intact red blood cells imbedded in the culture media. The disease is believed to be caused by antibody cross-reactivity that can involve chiefly the heart, but may also affect the brain, skin, and joints. The illness typically develops 2–3 weeks after a streptococcal infection. Acute rheumatic fever commonly appears in young children and ranges to the mid-teens, with only about a fifth of first-time attacks occurring in adults. Since the joints are often affected, the disease was ascribed the name of *rheumatic fever* due to some similarities in signs and symptoms to rheumatism (degenerative disease of the joints of the body).

For emphasis, again the condition is most frequently seen in children and young adults following respiratory tract infections caused by a certain strain of *Streptococcus pyogenes* called group A Beta- hemolytic streptococcus. During the course of the infection, these nephrogenic strains of streptococci are believed to form immune complexes with circulating antibodies and become deposited on the glomerular membrane, resulting in damage to the integrity of the membrane. Similar symptoms may also be seen following endocarditis (inflammation of the inner lining of the heart), abscesses, bacterial pneumonia, and other severe infections in which bacterial antigens are circulating about the body in the blood. In most cases, treatment for the underlying infection and the successful management of the secondary complications may result in a cure.

7.3.6   Berger's Disease

The most common cause of asymptomatic hematuria progressing to chronic glomerulonephritis is an IgA nephropathy known as Berger's Disease, in which immune complexes containing IgA may be deposited on the glomerular basement membrane. Patients usually present with an episode of macroscopic hematuria associated with strenuous exercise or an infection. Recovery from the macroscopic hematuria is spontaneous; however, asymptomatic microhematuria remains and serum IgA levels may be elevated. Examination of the urine in symptomatic chronic glomerulonephritis reveals the presence of blood, protein, and many varieties of casts, including broad casts, and a specific gravity of 1.010, indicating a loss of renal concentrating ability and a decreased glomerular filtration rate. Elevated serum levels of blood urea nitrogen, creatinine, and phosphorous and decreased serum calcium levels are seen in the progression to *end—stage renal disease*.

7.3.7   Goodpasture's Syndrome

Goodpasture's syndrome is a rare disease that was first described by an American pathologist, Dr. Ernest Goodpasture. The disease can involve rapidly progressive kidney failure, while at the same time is accompanied by lung disease. But some forms of the syndrome (cluster of symptoms) involve just the lungs or kidneys and not both. The symptoms often occur quite gradually at a slow pace. It is also known by the term "anti-glomerular basement antibody disease". It is used to distinguish this rare condition from other diseases with similar symptoms. The disease is an autoimmune disease that causes a type II hypersensitivity reaction that over time will cause damage to both the kidneys and the lungs. Glomerulonephritis and lung hemorrhaging are characteristic of the disease. Early symptoms are not often sufficient to warrant the depth of medical investigation required to diagnose this condition, so diagnosis is often made at a late point in the progression of the disease. A kidney biopsy (surgical excision of tissue) that reveals IgG deposition on the basement membranes of the target organs is the most effective means of diagnosis.

7.3.8   Acute Interstitial Nephritis

This is a syndrome with rapid onset of clinical manifestations of renal dysfunction, and is sometimes referred to as tubulointerstitial disease since the renal tubules and the renal interstitium are closely located. A variety of causes may contribute to the syndrome, which may include bacterial infection or reactions to medications, such as analgesics and certain antibiotics. Inflammation of the renal interstitium occurs with an absence of glomerular or vascular abnormalities, which distinguishes the condition from other inflammatory disorders of the genitourinary system.

Acute pyelonephritis may arise prior to interstitial nephritis. Septicemia (bacterial infection of the blood), drug toxicity from a number of medically-prescribed materials, graft rejection following organ transplantation, and certain immune disorders are some of the causative factors in development of the disease. Symptoms may be reversed when any underlying cause is remedied, but residual damage may remain following treatment for the initial origin of the condition. Laboratory findings include hematuria, often readily visible in the urine for drug induced cases, intact WBC's and WBC casts, and no microscopically visible bacteria, with often low to perhaps moderate excretion of protein in the urine (proteinuria). The presence of white blood cells called eosinophils normally reacting in allergic reactions may be found in the urine sediment may be useful to confirm the diagnosis but alone are not diagnostic, but should be accompanied by other clinical findings for diagnosis.

Interstitial nephritis, also called tubulo-interstitial nephritis, is a form of nephritis that impacts the interstitium of the kidneys that covers the tubules, where absorption and secretion take place. This disease can be either acute, meaning it occurs suddenly, or chronic, meaning it is ongoing and ultimately ends in kidney failure. Both acute and chronic tubulo-interstitial nephritis occur when caused by a bacterial infection (pyelonephritis) of the kidneys. The most common cause is by an allergic reaction to a drug but is not solely caused by toxicity of a medication. The onset of the disease following exposure to a drug toxic to the kidneys can range from a few days to half a year in some cases.

Sometimes the individual may present with no symptoms of disease, and when symptoms are present, they may be widely varied and can be confused with other diseases of the renal system. When symptoms arise they may occur rapidly (time frame) and gradually gather in severity. Patients who suffer from tubulo-interstitial nephritis will experience a fever in more than one-fourth of the individuals, enlargement of the kidneys in most cases as in glomerulonephritis when caused by an allergic reaction. Lower back pain, *malaise*, weight loss, problems with urination and lower back pain may occur. In some renal disorders other than infection, imbalance of reabsorption and secretion due to glomerular damage may result in an electrolyte balance.

7.3.9   Nephrotic Syndrome

The condition called nephrotic syndrome is a group of symptoms including extremely elevated levels of proteinuria (protein in the urine) as well as the loss of massive amounts of protein due to an increased permeability of the glomeruli. Increased permeability of the glomerular membrane may be caused by changes in the electrical charges in the basal lamina and podocytes of the basement membrane, permitting the passage of high molecular weight proteins and lipids into the glomerular filtrate. This loss of protein leads to low blood protein levels, due to the loss of large amounts of protein through the kidneys, high cholesterol levels, high triglyceride levels, and edema (swelling). The latter condition of edema is related to the disruptions of protein and albumin levels in the blood plasma, where both protein and albumin, a form of protein, are decreased Albumin is the protein most responsible for the excretion and reabsorption in the kidneys.

The condition is characterized by the appearance of massive proteinuria (>3.5 g/day), and circulatory disorders that affect the pressure and flow of blood to the kidney are among the most frequent causes of the signs and symptoms of nephrotic syndrome. The condition may occur as a result of the complications in cases of glomerulonephritis, toxic injury from drugs and heavy metals, as well as diseases such as vasculitis, systemic lupus erythematosus, severe infections, diabetes, *amyloidosis*, and allergic reactions. This condition may also occur as a result of infection, including strep throat, *hepatitis*, or mononucleosis, cancer, genetic disorders, immune disorders, or diseases that affect multiple body systems.

Absorption of the lipid-containing proteins by the renal tubular cells followed by sloughing or peeling off of the cells produces the characteristic oval fat bodies seen in the sediment examination that may include fatty casts. The urine may appear almost colorless, and a frothy appearance may be observed assumedly because of the large numbers of fat bodies. Tubular damage may also accompany the damage to the glomeruli. Nephrotic syndrome can affect all age groups. In children, it is most common from age 2 to 6. This disorder occurs slightly more often in males than females. Symptoms of the disease include edema or significant swelling is the most common symptom. It may occur as follows (Table 7.1).

Table 7.1 Symptoms and
signs of nephrotic syndrome

In the face and around the eyes
In the arms and legs, especially in the feet and ankles
In the belly area
Rapid gain in weight from fluid retention
Foamy appearance of the urine from fatty bodies
Anorexia or poor appetite
High blood pressure

7.3.10 Renal Failure

Acute renal failure may also be called acute kidney injury (AKI) and is described as a rapid loss of kidney function (filtering, secreting, and excreting) and may occur suddenly. Causes of the condition may be attributed to acute tubular necrosis or direct tubular damage from nephrotoxic agents such as prescribed medications or the use of illicit drugs. Renal vasoconstriction (decreased renal blood flow) may also damage the kidneys as well as direct tubular damage from a number of toxins, including food items of which the eating of toxic species of mushrooms are one such source. Trauma leading to the development of hypotension and low blood perfusion caused by thermal and caustic burns, traumatic or surgical shock, or intravascular hemolysis from a transfusion reaction or hemolytic disease are sometimes causes of acute renal failure.

Acute renal failure is somewhat common in the hospitalized patient and is characterized by anuria (cessation of urine production) or oliguria (below normal output of urine). Laboratory studies may reveal elevated blood urea nitrogen (BUN) and creatinine. In severe cases, complications of high potassium levels will result in cardiac arrhythmias, metabolic acidosis and *uremia*. Medical care should include restoration of fluid balance and treatment of the underlying condition that precipitated the development of acute renal failure. Depending on its severity, AKI may lead to a number of complications, including metabolic acidosis, increased potassium levels, and increased levels of waste products in the urine. The condition may be subdivided into three categories, based on the causative factors in the development of acute renal failure.

- Prerenal causes of include those that result in diminished blood flow (hypovolemia) to the kidney(s). Low blood pressure, low blood volume from anemia or injury and heart failure may potentially lead to kidney failure. Other less common causes include circulatory changes such as *arteriole stenosis* (narrowing), and blood clots in the renal vein that drains the kidney of blood.
- Intrinsic causes of damage to the kidney are those that cause glomerular or tubule damage, and may include glomerulonephritis, acute tubular necrosis and acute interstitial nephritis.
- Postrenal aspects of renal failure are chiefly those that prevent urine from emptying into the bladder and exiting the body through the urethra. Prostatic hyperplasia (enlargement of the prostate gland in men), kidney and bladder stones, clogged urinary catheter and strictures in the urethra are basic and common reasons for kidney failure from postrenal origins.

Chronic renal failure is not unusual as it may develop as a result of any of the forms of glomerulonephritis discussed previously. Chronic kidney disease is the slow loss of kidney function over time. Since the main contribution to the health of the human is the ability of the kidneys to remove wastes and excess water from the body, laboratory values for waste products excreted from the body from the kidneys will be affected. As in acute kidney failure, laboratory findings include decreased glomerular filtration rate (GFR), diminished renal concentrating ability, and elevated values found for blood urea nitrogen and creatinine, both as waste products of the body's metabolic processes.

The causes and incidences as well as risk factors for the development of chronic kidney disease progressively become worse over time. There may be few or no symptoms in the early stages, and loss of function often requires months to years to develop. It may delay the onset of clinical signs since significant damage may occur before symptoms appear and sometimes do not occur until kidney function is less than one-tenth of normal functioning. The final stage of chronic kidney disease is called end-stage renal disease, where the kidneys no longer function adequately and the patient is required to seek dialysis or a transplanted kidney. Chronic kidney disease and end-stage renal disease affect roughly 0.2% of the United States.

The most prevalent causes for development of these serious conditions are that of diabetes and high blood pressure. However, a significant number of other diseases are capable of seriously damaging the kidneys. Problems with the arteries including traumatic injury to the vessels that lead to or into the kidneys are vital in providing oxygen and nutrition to the specialized structures of the kidneys. Birth defects of the kidneys (such as that of polycystic kidney disease in which cysts develop in the kidneys and organs may eventually destroy kidney tissue and therefore the functions of the organs (cerebral aneurisms are also prevalent in sufferers of this disease). Some pain medications and other drugs along with certain toxic chemicals may eventually destroy the kidneys and their ability to perform their functions necessary to maintain life and health.

Autoimmune disorders such as *systemic lupus erythematosus* (SLE) and *scleroderma*, a progressive and systemic hardening of the skin, are often implicated in kidney failure. Kidney stones, certain infections of the kidneys and reflux nephropathy, a condition in which the kidneys are injured by urine that "backs up" from the bladder and into the kidneys are also considerable contributors to eventual kidney failure.

Besides an accumulation of waste products in the body, particularly in the blood, chronic kidney disease affects almost all body systems and functions, including red blood cell production, blood pressure control, and vitamin D (calcitriol decreases excretion of calcium by the kidneys) and bone health. The early symptoms of chronic kidney disease often occur with other illnesses, as well. These symptoms may be the only signs of kidney disease until the condition is more advanced. Even early in the disease course, patients suffering from kidney disease leading to end-stage conditions may have feelings of general but undefined illness, fatigue and malaise, headaches, anorexia with unintentional weight loss, nausea and dry, itchy skin (pruritus).

Other physical conditions, signs and symptoms may develop, especially when kidney function have become advanced. These include musculoskeletal pain, central nervous system signs and symptoms that include confusion, changes in skin pigmentation that may include lightening or darkening of the skin, drowsiness and confusion. Numbness mostly in the extremities may be accompanied by cramps and muscle twitching, and perhaps bruising upon experiencing light trauma. Excessive thirst and changes in breath odor, impotence and menstrual cessation along with swelling of the hands and feet may occur. Insomnia, sleep apnea, restless leg syndrome with increased hiccupping related to changes in the electrolyte balance of the blood is somewhat common.

7.4   Cushing's Syndrome

Cushing's syndrome is a hormonal disorder leading to increased *cortisol* levels that causes various morphological manifestations such as upper torso obesity, thin arms and legs and a rounded face, usually causing childhood obesity (Fig. 7.7). This disease is noted in the studies of urinalysis and body fluids as the hypothalamus, a small area of the brain that sends a chemical messenger called corticotrophin-releasing hormone to the pituitary gland. The condition is caused by prolonged exposure of the body's tissues to high levels of the hormone cortisol. The disease is somewhat rare but is usually noted in the second to fifth decades of life. Along with obesity and elevated glucose and blood pressure, patients with these clinical findings are predisposed to the development of Cushing's syndrome. In turn, the

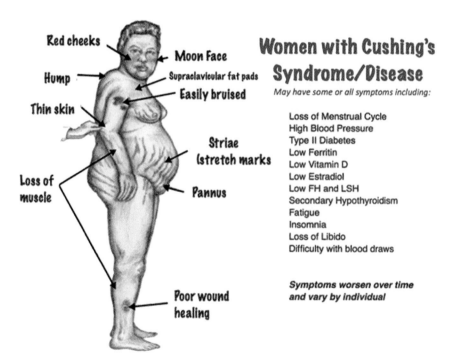

Fig. 7.7 Patient with signs of Cushing's syndrome

pituitary secretes adrenocorticotropin hormone (ACTH) which causes the adrenal glands located just above the kidneys to release cortisol into the blood.

7.5   Special Urinalysis Screening Tests

Besides the basic urinalysis screening tests and the accompanying procedures to confirm various disorders of the urinary system, other diseases that are not in themselves a disorder of the urinary system, result in findings of compounds in the urine based on metabolic disorders of the body. Many of these diseases are metabolic, meaning that there is some error in the normal metabolism of certain products in the body that may be a result of the absence of an enzyme or in the malfunction of certain tissues and organs of the body.

Inherited metabolic diseases usually result in the accumulation of abnormal metabolic substances in the urine. This increased concentration of a variety of compounds may be due to a variety of causes, and are grouped into two categories, namely the overflow type and the renal type. The most frequently encountered abnormalities are associated with metabolic disturbances that produce urinary overflow of substances that are a result of protein and carbohydrate metabolism in the body. This is understandable when the complexity of reactions in the body involving a large number of enzymes that are utilized in the metabolic pathways of proteins and carbohydrates. In addition, many of these enzymes are essential in the completion of metabolic process that are critical to life. Disruption of enzyme function can be caused by failure to inherit the gene to produce a particular enzyme, referred to as an "inborn error of metabolism," or by organ malfunction from disease or toxic reactions. The majority of the disorders discussed in this chapter are associated with errors in the metabolism of amino acids.

7.6   Amino Acid Disorders

A group of disorders called "amino acid disorders" are critical for medical intervention by screening of newborns, but in some cases is important for older children and adults, to detect inborn errors in metabolism of amino acids. Of the more than 100 known amino acids, 20 of them are utilized as "building blocks" of which human proteins are constructed. Ten of the twenty amino acids are termed "essential" amino acids and must be acquired through a balanced diet. The remaining ten amino acids are synthesized by the body from raw materials obtained through diet. Deficiencies may exist due to genetic abnormalities, or may be acquired due to certain medical conditions. When congenital enzyme deficiencies exist from birth that affect amino acid metabolism or congenital abnormalities in the amino acid transport system of the kidneys, a condition results that is called "aminoaciduria."

Accumulation of abnormal metabolic substances that may be found in the urine may be due to a variety of causes and are grouped into two categories that are classified as the overflow type and the renal type. The most frequently encountered of these abnormalities are those associated with metabolic disturbances that produce a urinary overflow of substances involved in protein and carbohydrate metabolism. Since amino acids are the building blocks of proteins of which many organs and tissues of the body are comprised, they have many important functions in the body. Diseases may be based on heredity or may be acquired, and involve amino acid processing which is in some way is defective in metabolic pathways, or in the body's ability to incorporate vital amino acids into the various types of cells where they are needed. These disorders frequently produce symptoms early in life. Some states in the United States require routine screening of neonates (newborn) for several common disorders involving amino acids. The most common amino acids screened for in the United States are for *phenylketonuria*, which all states require at birth, as well as *Maple Syrup Urine Disease*, an inherited autosomal disorder. There is a substantial number of other inherited disorders, but those screened for at birth will vary from one state to another.

7.7   Inherited and Acquired Metabolic Diseases

When an enzyme responsible for the metabolism is absent, effectively blocking the metabolism of that amino acid, the disorder is called a primary *aminoaciduria*. When the amino acid is produced but there are errors in either absorption or the transport of an amino acid to the appropriate site, the disorder is termed a secondary aminoaciduria. Both types of aminoaciduria are either inherited (congenital) or are acquired because of other medical conditions. Aminoaciduria may be grouped into two types called overflow and renal, based on the mechanism by which the amino acids accumulate in the body. In the overflow type, both the plasma level of one or more amino acids will be increased (aminoacidemia) and the urine level (renal) of the metabolic product will be increased.

A common primary aminoaciduria is that of phenylketonuria, which is usually referred to as the PKU, and is the most common overflow type of aminoaciduria. A number of other primary aminoacidurias, where an enzyme is absent, are significant. Several of these are the result of the absence of an enzyme involved in the urea cycle, produced during the metabolism of nitrogenous (nitrogen containing) foods. These cause increased blood ammonia levels and the increase of one or more amino acids. Ammonia, a nitrogen containing molecule, is derived from the decomposition of nitrogen-containing substances that include proteins and amino acids. A rise in ammonia leads to neurological symptoms of stupor and confusion, and may progress to a comatose state.

The second type of aminoaciduria is that of the renal type, where the kidneys are involved rather than an enzyme deficiency. Renal aminoaciduria is attributed to the renal tubular transport are metabolic disorders which lead to impairment in the ability of certain solutes, including salts or amino acids, to be transported through the renal tubules, resulting in disruptions of renal reabsorption. In the renal type of aminoaciduria, one or more amino acids are excreted in excess in the urine. But in the renal type, plasma levels are not increased as they included as an overflow type.

Some renal types of aminoaciduria are congenital (inherited), but most are acquired (not inherent) and secondary to other medical conditions. An example of a commonly inherited renal type aminoaciduria is that of cystinuria, a condition based on defects in the reabsorption of certain amino acids by the kidney. There is also an attendant excretion of lysine, arginine and ornithine in the urine. These products are often associated with urinary calculi (stones) in the urinary system.

7.7.1   Fanconi's Syndrome

Fanconi's syndrome has been described in various ways over a number of years by other researchers, but Guido Fanconi, a Swiss pediatrician, contributed chiefly to the knowledge of the disease during the past century. Many of the renal tubular disorders, such as that of Hartnup disease and similar tubular dysfunction, were described by Fanconi and included the transport of many different substances and not just one specific metabolite, as is the case in some of the related tubular disorders. There are differing cases in Fanconi syndrome, some of which are congenital while others are acquired. The syndrome is related to a medical condition that affects the proximal renal tubules.

The syndrome, a cache of symptoms, includes several conditions characterized by aminoaciduria. The inability of the proximal renal tubules to reabsorb amino acids along with glucose, uric acid, phosphates (may lead to rickets-like disorders) and bicarbonate (essential in acid-base balance), all of which may be excreted from the body by the urine. Polyuria is common in this condition, perhaps due to the body's efforts to rid the body of the materials that are not reabsorbed. Osteomalacia (softening of bones) and failure to attain normal stature are common manifestations of this disorder.

The disorder is X-linked, where the female is usually the carrier and the male suffers from the disorder, as is the case in a number of other medical conditions, such as hemophilia. The disease may also be acquired by a number of means. Underlying medical conditions the include tubular necrosis, interstitial nephritis, amyloidosis, myeloma, rejection of transplanted tissues or organs, and Sjogren's syndrome, an autoimmune disease that is often accompanied by rheumatoid arthritis and several other conditions may lead to the development of Fanconi's syndrome. Exposure to certain toxins such as heavy metals and recreational sniffing of glue may lead to an acquired case of Fanconi's syndrome. Therefore, the condition is manifested in a number of generalized ways rather than the presence of one specific defect and can be either hereditary or acquired.

7.7.2   Phenyketonuria

Phenylketonuria (PKU) is a disorder that causes a buildup of the amino acid *phenylalanine*, which is an essential amino acid that cannot be synthesized in the body but is present in food. Under normal circumstances, the excess phenylalanine is converted into another amino acid called tyrosine and is eliminated from the body. In the absence of the enzyme that converts the amino acid to tyrosine, phenylalanine builds up in the blood and is toxic to the brain, and is capable of causing severe mental retardation. If PKU is increased in a family and DNA is available from an individual family member affected by the condition, *amniocentesis* or chorionic villus sampling by use of a catheter that is inserted into the cervix and the outer portion of the membranes that surround the fetus. DNA analysis can be performed to determine whether a fetus has the disorder. PKU occurs in most ethnic groups so is routinely tested for all newborns in each of the United States but the incidence of the disorder varies with race and ethnic origin and includes five forms of the disease.

The most commonly encountered type is that of type I, a disorder found in roughly 1 in 10,000 births in the United States, and accounts for at least half of the diagnosed PKU cases. Because of its high prevalence, all states currently screen newborns for phenyketonuria. An inherited deficiency of an enzyme, phenylalanine hydroxylase, is responsible for the development of this condition, and is essential for the conversion of phenylalanine to tyrosine. In the absence of this enzyme, phenylalanine accumulates in the plasma where it is oxidized by phenylalanine transaminase to phenylpyruvic acid before being removed by the kidneys. The terminology for the disorder called phenyketonuria is derived from the phenylpyruvic acid, a metabolic derivative of phenylalanine which is also known as a ketoacid. The most medically important result of an untreated case of phenyketonuria will include mental retardation as well as skin disorders, neurological signs, and psychotic manifestation or behavior that mirrors autistic behavior. These conditions can be mostly avoided through the adherence to a diet that is almost totally free of phenylalanine. Those who go undetected and progress to an advanced level of the disease may be characterized by a recognizable "mousy" odor of both the body and the urine, and might be a clue to the medical examiner of a pathologic metabolic condition.

Most affected newborns are detected during routine screening tests. Newborns with PKU rarely have symptoms immediately after birth, but some infants may appear sleepy or eat poorly soon after being born. If not treated, affected infants progressively develop mental retardation over the first few years of life, which eventually becomes severe. Other symptoms include seizures, nausea and vomiting, an eczema-like rash, lighter skin and hair than their family members, aggressive or self-injurious behavior, hyperactivity, and sometimes psychiatric symptoms. Untreated children often give off a "mousy" body and urine odor as a result of a by-product of phenylalanine (phenylacetic acid) in their urine and sweat.

To prevent mental retardation, phenylalanine intake must be restricted. But it should be noted that some phenylalanine is required for healthy living so the diet must be carefully monitored to maintain a certain range in the blood levels of affected individuals. Because the natural sources of protein contain considerable amounts of phenylalanine, children with phenyketonuria cannot have meat, milk, or other common foods that contain protein. Instead, they must eat a variety of phenylalanine-free processed foods which are specially manufactured. Low-protein natural foods, such as fruits, vegetables, and restricted amounts of certain grain cereals, are essential to the diet, which must be maintained for life.

Fig. 7.8 Typical collection card for infant blood to be tested for the presence of phenylalanine

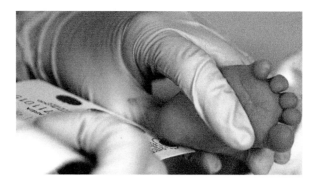

A test procedure, the bacterial inhibition test developed by Guthrie, is a routine practice for most clinical laboratories and is the best-known blood test for PKU. In this procedure, blood from a heel stick is absorbed into filter paper circles, and the circle on the filter paper is completely saturated with a single application of blood. These blood saturated disks are then placed on a culture media that has been streaked with a bacterial organism called *Bacillus subtilis*. If an increased level of phenylalanine is present in the blood, it will counteract the impact of Beta-2-thienylalanine, which effectively inhibits the growth of *Bacillus subtilis* present in the specially-prepared culture media, and growth is observed immediately adjacent to a blood-impregnated paper disk (Fig. 7.8).

7.7.3   Tyrosyluria

Tyrosine is one of the 20 amino acids that is common to a number of proteins and serves as a precursor to the production of *epinephrine, melanin*, and thyroxine. Tyrosyluria describes a condition that is an inherited metabolic defect, or it may result from an acquired and severe liver disease. The accumulation of excess tyrosine in the blood plasma that produces the urinary overflow of tyrosine is not well categorized or described as to the causes. In both inherited and acquired states, tyrosine and *leucine* crystals may be concurrently observed in urine sediment. Enhanced urinary excretion of certain metabolites of tyrosine, such as p-hydroxy-phenylpyruvic acid is commonly found in cases of present in tyrosinosis, scurvy (ascorbic acid deficiency), *pernicious anemia* as well as several other diseases. Some cases of tyrosyluria in infants may disappear spontaneously as the child ages and does not seem to result from any of the vitamin deficiencies normally attributed to the disease.

7.7.4   Alkaptonuria

Alkaptonuria is a rare inherited condition in which large amounts of homogentisic acid is excreted in the urine due to the incomplete metabolism of tyrosine and phenylalanine. The term "alkaptonuria" originated with the observation that urine from patients with this condition becomes significantly darker as the sample becomes more alkaline when standing at room temperature while exposed to air. The metabolic defect is caused by the failure to inherit a required gene necessary for producing the enzyme homogentisic acid oxidase. The condition is rare as it affects only about one to four individuals per one million, but in some geographic regions (Slovakia and the Dominican Republic) the disease is much more common. A related condition occurs after the age of 30 in some individuals, characterized by an accumulation of dark pigment in connective tissues including the cartilage and skin, called ochronosis.

7.7.5 Melanuria

A secondary metabolic pathway for tyrosine is responsible for producing melanin, protein, thyroxine, epinephrine and tyrosine sulfate. Melanin is a pigment responsible for the dark color of hair, skin, and eyes, and the deficient production of melanin results in albinism. As with alkaptonuria, increased levels of urinary melanin will also result in darkening of the urine. The excretion of urine of a dark color may also be a result of the presence of other pigments or from the action of a number of coal tar components such as phenol, creosote, resorcin, as well as others.

7.7.6 Maple Syrup Urine

This is a rare disease but is easily discovered in the department of the medical laboratory that processes urine samples. The disease is often discovered by the unique odor experienced by those working with the patient or with the specimens from the very young patient. Children with Maple Syrup disease, as well as those with other amino acid disorders, are unable to metabolize certain amino acids. In a number of states, newborns are required to be screened for this disease. Maple syrup urine disease is caused by an inborn error of metabolism, inherited as an autosomal (chromosomes other than those of X and Y) recessive trait. The amino acids involved in this metabolic pathway are leucine, *isoleucine, and valine*. Keto acids rapidly accumulate in the urine, and the disease is often detected by medical laboratory personnel or by nursery employees due to a strong maple syrup-like odor. The by-products that accumulate as a result of the build-up of amino acids may cause significant neurologic changes such as retardation and sometimes seizures. Other body fluids besides the urine, including sweat, will sometimes have a strong maple syrup odor.

There are a number of different forms of maple syrup urine disease and among the various forms, symptoms vary in severity. Neurological abnormalities are characteristic of the most severe form of the disorder, where seizures, coma, and death may occur within a few days to a few weeks. In milder forms, children may first appear normal but later develop vomiting, staggering, confusion, coma, and exhibit the odor of maple syrup during physical stress and when ill. Some children with mild forms of the disease may be successfully treated with injections of the vitamin B_1. A special diet may be used that is low in the amino acids that are affected by a missing enzyme particular to the form of the disease from which the person suffers.

7.8 Organic Acidemia

Generalized symptoms of the organic acidemias often include an early onset of severe illness. These conditions are commonly used to classify a group of metabolic disorders based on the disruption of the normal steps in the metabolism of amino acids. Some of the amino acids are called branched-chain amino acids that include isoleucine, leucine and valine, often lead to an accumulation of acids not normally present in the body. Some odd-chained fatty acids are also affected in disorders that cause organic academia. Complications that lead to acute medical conditions are often brought on by vomiting that leads to metabolic acidosis, hypoglycemia (low glucose levels in the blood), ketonuria (increased ketone bodies from metabolism of body fat), and increased serum ammonia from protein breakdown. There are three disorders that occur with some frequency in the disease called organic aciduria. The most frequently encountered disorders of this type are isovaleric, propionic, and methylmalonic acidemia.

7.8.1 Tryptophan Disorders

Tryptophan is an essential amino acid that was previously sold to the general public as supplements in health foods and preparations. A number of persons became quite ill due to high levels of the material, which is necessary for normal growth and development. However, it was believed that tryptophan would give a general feeling of well-being, since it is a precursor to both serotonin, a mood elevator, and niacin. The major concern of the urinalysis laboratory in the metabolism of tryptophan is the increased urinary excretion of metabolites indican and 5-hydroxyindoleacetic acid (5-HIAA). One of the most infamous diseases of tryptophan metabolism is pellagra, in which there is a deficiency of tryptophan. This deficiency of tryptophan causes a deficiency of niacin and was once common but is seldom encountered in patients today as it has been largely eradicated due to the inclusion of niacin in vitamins. High levels of niacin (nicotinic acid), as does the other amino acids, may lead to nausea and vomiting, occasionally along with sedation (state of calm or sleep).

Pellagra is most often manifested by cutaneous, musosal, gastrointestinal and neurological signs and symptoms. The mucus membranes of the mouth and other orifices of the body may atrophy with ulcers and cysts developing. Anemia is a common occurrence and diarrhea is almost always characteristic of the condition. When central nervous system involvement occurs, organic psychosis may lead to disorientation, memory lapses, and confusion, followed by delirium and diminished consciousness. Pellagra was seen in the Mississippi Delta in the early twentieth century

Fig. 7.9 Cutaneous
manifestation of pellagra

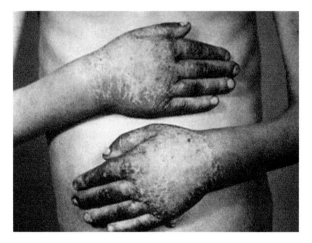

due to a tryptophan-poor diet that largely consisted of salt pork, cane syrup and corn meal, all of which have little or no tryptophan.

Today, those mostly affected by pellagra are alcoholics, who consume mostly carbohydrates and water from their alcoholic beverages. For the most part, alcoholic beverages are almost completely absent of any appreciable levels of tryptophan and it is felt that a deficiency of tryptophan may lead to more serious mental health conditions. Dementia was sometimes so severe that patients with symptoms of pellagra were confined to governmental mental institutions. A deficiency of tryptophan in the diet has led some public health authorities to attribute certain serious mental health diseases, including schizophrenia, to this lack of adequate tryptophan (Fig. 7.9).

7.8.2 Indicanuria

Another name for indicanuria is "blue diaper syndrome," a rare autosomal recessive disorder, where the infant's urine-stained diaper will turn indigo blue when oxidized by exposure to air, upon which it progresses from a colorless state to an indigo blue color. The condition is caused by a defect in the absorption of tryptophan. Under normal conditions, most of the tryptophan that enters the intestines is either reabsorbed in the production of protein. Some of the tryptophan is converted to *indole* through metabolism by the numerous intestinal bacteria, before being excreted in the stool. Some intestinal disorders occur where larger amounts of tryptophan are converted to indole. Many of the conditions where this occurs includes malabsorption, infection by abnormal enteric bacteria, and obstruction of the intestine. A rare condition, an inherited disorder called Hartnup disease results in increased amounts of tryptophan being converted to indole. Symptoms most often include digestive disorders with fever and visual disturbances. The excess indole along with other materials including water is then reabsorbed through the intestinal walls and into the capillaries before being circulated to the liver. There it is converted to indican before it is excreted in the urine.

7.9   5-Hydroxyindoleacetic Acid

A second metabolic pathway of tryptophan is for the production of serotonin uti-lized in the stimulation of smooth muscles. Serotonin is produced from tryptophan by the *argentaffin cells* in the intestine and is carried through the body primarily by the platelets. Normally, most of the serotonin is used by the body leaving only small amounts of its degradation product, 5-hydroxyindoleacetic acid (5-HIAA) available for excretion in the urine. But when malignant tumors involving the argentaffin cells develop, excess amounts of serotonin are produced, resulting in the elevation of urinary 5-HIAA levels. 5-HIAA is tested by 24-h urine samples combined with an acidic additive as a preservative to maintain the specimen at a pH below 3 (extremely acid) to prevent bacterial contamination and decomposition of the components of the urine. Certain foods and drugs are known to interfere with the measurement. 5-HIAA levels can vary depending on other complications, including tumors, renal malfunction and resection of the small bowel.

Since 5-HIAA is a metabolite of serotonin, testing is most frequently performed for the diagnosis of carcinoid tumors of the small intestine, where large amounts of serotonin are released. Serotonin is a neurotransmitter, and low levels of 5-HIAA in the cerebrospinal fluid have been associated with aggressive behavior and suicide by violent means, activities common in those suffering from low serotonin levels. In frequent occurrences, other conditions have been associated with abnormal levels of serotonin (hyperserotonemia) that include autism.

5-Hydroxyindoleacetic Acid (5-HIAA) levels are also used for determining the presence of some types of depression due to a neurochemical imbalance due to ele-vated levels of serotonin. Related tests to determine any presence of a neurochemical imbalance will often include *homovanillic acid* and vanillylmandelic acid (VMA), low levels of which may occur concurrently with high levels of 5-HIAA in certain mental conditions. High levels of VMA are often associated with a condition called pheochromatocytoma, a tumor of the sympathetic nervous system that causes heart palpitations, sweating, hypertension, anxiety, and other clinical signs and symptoms.

Serotonin competes with catecholamines, and particularly with dopamine, a neu-rotransmitter, for uptake into the brain. This leads to malfunctions of mental func-tioning, from an imbalance of serotonin. Decreased levels of dopamine coupled with increased levels of serotonin may also result from a diet low in tyrosine, the amino acid that is metabolized into dopamine, and a diet rich in tryptophan, which is converted into serotonin. Dietary restrictions and increased intake of tryptophan may serve to correct the imbalances between neurochemicals, and in some cases improve the symptoms of the condition called depression.

7.10   Porphyrinuria

Porphyrinuria refers to the excretion of large quantities of porphyrins in the urine. Porphyrins are the intermediate compounds in the production of heme, an iron-containing molecule that is non-protein, found on the hemoglobin molecule located on the surfaces of red blood cells of mammals. The basic synthesis for heme production utilizes nitrogen and carbon atoms from glycine and acetate. A number of stages during which heme is synthesized may be disrupted, leading to an excess of porphyrin compounds that contain nitrogen (N) rather than iron found in the heme molecule. Lead poisoning is the most common cause of porphyrinuria. Several types exist, and the diagnosis of the various types will require the processing of either or both erythrocytes and fecal samples, depending on the type in question.

There are seven disorders, and arguably eight, that fall under the general term of porphyria. All of the types involve a deficiency in an enzyme that is involved in the synthesis of the substance called heme, a product found in large amounts in several organs and tissues of the body including the bone marrow, liver and red blood cells. The enzyme deficiency allows normal body chemicals called porphyrins to accumulate in toxic amounts in the body. The metabolic disorders of porphyria are clinically manifested in a variety of ways and are characterized by a decreased activity of a specific enzyme or enzymes in the synthesis of heme. Characteristic patterns of the overproduction of specific heme precursors such as the porphyrins result in an accumulation of the substances in certain tissues. Porphyrias may be active clinically, with manifestations of the disease, while in some cases the condition is latent or in remission. But high levels of heme precursors that may be found in blood, urine, and stool samples regardless of the stage in which the patient falls. Most types of porphyria are based on an inherited genetic pattern, but one type, *porphyria cutanea tarda*, may be familial (inherited) or acquired.

7.11   Homocystinuria

The condition is a rare inherited metabolic disorder caused by an enzyme deficiency and is characterized by a harmful accumulation of homocystine in the body and leads to increased levels for the amino acid methionine. Children with homocystinuria are unable to metabolize the amino acid homocystine, which, along with certain toxic by-products, builds up to cause a variety of symptoms. Symptoms may be mild or severe, depending on the particular enzyme defect. Infants with this disorder may appear normal at birth. The first symptoms will often include dislocation of the lens of the eye (subluxation) that results in a significant decrease in visual acuity, and is usually evident in those three years of age. Most children have skeletal manifestations which may include osteoporosis. The child will often be unusually tall and thin with an exaggerated spinal curvature, and will possess long limbs, and long, spiderlike fingers. Mental retardation, accompanied by psychiatric and behavioral disorders are prevalent.

Homocystinuria increases the danger of cardiac and arterial disease, and makes the blood more likely to easily clot, with resultant strokes and often high blood pressure. Some state governments have laws that require screening for homocystinuria at birth, where enzyme measurements are performed. Confirmation tests following a positive screening result are performed by determining enzymatic functions in liver or skin cells. Treatment choices are limited, but some children with homocystinuria will improve with a diet rich in folic acid which tends to lower the homocystiene levels along with the administration of vitamin B_6 (pyridoxine) or vitamin B_{12} (cobalamin).

7.12 Cystinuria

The condition called cystinuria is an inherited medical condition that is an autosomal recessive metabolic disorder. Those suffering from cystinuria are afflicted by urinary calculi, commonly called "kidney stones," although they may form in the kidneys, ureters and bladder. The amino acid cystine accounts for less than 3% of kidney stones, first identified in 1810 as being responsible for producing kidney stones, is a sulfur-containing compound produced by acids reacting with proteins. Kidney stones affect slightly more than 10% of males and slightly less than 10% of females in Europe and North America. Cystinuria is the first disorder of amino acid transport where the gene responsible for the disorder has been identified.

Although the rate of occurrence of stones that contain cystine is relatively small, the frequency of recurrence of the formation of stones and the substantial size of the stones create much discomfort among the sufferers of the condition. Persons with this hereditary condition are often diagnosed by the presence of cystine crystals that may be found in the urine. An accompanying condition may occur as a disorder called cystine storage disease, resulting in deposition of cystine in the tissues of the body. This condition is a more serious medical malady than mere cystinuria, and leads to failure to grow in children, with resultant medical conditions such as rickets (bone malformation), hypothyroidism, renal tubular acidosis, and eventually may lead to kidney failure.

7.13 Melituria (Galactosuria)

The term "melituria" is an archaic term that refers to the increased level in the urine of any of the sugars that may be found in the body. These sugars include glucose, pentose, fructose, lactose, maltose, sucrose or galactose. Specific diseases related to the metabolism of sugars in the body such as that of galactosuria, must be discovered soon after birth in order to gain a positive survival rate of the infant. Galactosemia is not related to and is quite different than that of the commonly diagnosed condition of lactose intolerance, which is not as serious as galactosuria. Galactosemia is an autosomal recessive trait resulting from the absence of an enzyme necessary to convert galactose to glucose, a sugar that is required for many of the metabolic processes of the human body.

The rate of galactosemia varies between population groups, with a high rate in an Irish group (Irish Traveler). Inbreeding in isolated areas is often attributed to an increased rate of galactosuria. Galactosemia, the increased presence of galactose in the blood, is excreted through the kidneys and is detected by testing of the urine of the newborn for non-carbohydrate reducing substances. A common test of newborns is that called the *Clinitest*, manufactured by the Bayer Corporation, that is used to detect reducing substances including galactose, fructose, lactose, and a group of sugars called pentoses (Fig. 7.10). Pentose sugars contain five carbon atoms while glucose, also known as dextrose, has six carbon atoms in its molecular configuration.

Fig. 7.10 Clinitest kit used for determination of reducing substances other than glucose

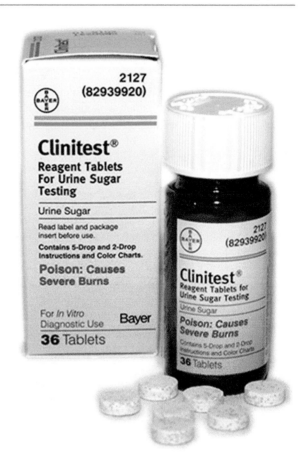

Points to Remember
Metabolic diseases that result in the finding of amino acids and other constituents are usually discovered early in life. These types of conditions are chronic, and when treatment is available, they often require a lifestyle modification.

7.14 Summary

A wide range of disorders may be attributed to conditions affecting the urinary system. Some of these are due to an infectious process and may be easily treated and quickly cured. When untreated, certain other conditions develop that lead to long-term disease of the kidneys that require scheduled treatment and medical maintenance of the health of the affected individual. Some disorders are not infectious in nature but are manifested by procedures measuring the kidneys' ability to rid the body of toxins and waste materials. A knowledge of the basic functions of the urinary system in which excretion, selective reabsorption, and secretion occurs, is essential when studying the disease processes of this system as well as those affecting other parts of the human body.

Basic screening procedures for the determination of systemic disease as well as those that primarily affect the body's ability to effectively maintain the fluid balance of the body must be diligently and properly performed. The first step toward producing meaningful results is based on a properly collected and processed urine sample. Clinical data from these results will provide a wealth of clinical information that may lead to further and more definitive testing of both the urine and other body fluids, organs and entire body systems.

Inherited metabolic diseases are significant in number, and while some are quite rare, it is important to be aware of clinical findings that may lead to a definitive diagnosis. Overflow diseases in which errors of metabolism might be hereditary, and most are, will result in the need to understand the relationship of body fluids and their impact on the health of individuals. It should be remembered that while urine is the body fluid other than blood that is most often screened for and examined for a variety of diseases, the other body fluids are equally important in the diagnosis of a number of diseases.

Case Studies

For the following case studies, it may be necessary to consult charts and clinical information from several locations in this textbook before coming to a definitive conclusion as to a diagnosis. It will also require additional information to answer some of the questions associated with the case studies.

Answers to this and other case studies may be found in Appendix D

Case Study 7.1

A 10-year-old girl received a physical exam prior to going to summer camp in a mountainous region. A midstream urine sample was performed as part of the physical. She had recently suffered from a low grade fever, lower abdominal pain and most recently, mild discomfort when voiding. The results revealed the following findings:

Urinalysis results report, case study 7.1

Physical appearance		
Color	Yellow	
Character	Slightly cloudy	
Chemical screening		
Leukocyte esterase	Positive	
Nitrite	Negative	
Urobilinogen	Negative	
Protein (test strip)	Trace	Confirmed by SSA precipitation
pH	6.5	
Blood	Negative	
Specific gravity	1.015	
Ketone	Negative	
Bilirubin	Negative	

Glucose	Negative	
Sediment evaluation		
Squamous epithelials	Few	
Renal epithelials	0	
Erythrocytes	0	
Leukocytes	20–25	
Casts	0	
Crystals	0	
Bacteria	Trace	
Other (specify)		

1. What are the abnormal values?
2. What is a reason for a negative nitrite result when bacteria were seen microscopically?
3. What is the probable diagnosis for this patient?

Case Study 7.2
A 35-year-old graduate student reported to the emergency room of a local hospital complaining of low back pain exam prior to going to summer camp in a mountainous region. A midstream urine sample was performed as part of the physical. The results revealed the following findings:

Urinalysis results report, case study 7.2

Physical appearance		
Color	Yellow	
Character	Slightly cloudy	
Chemical screening		
Leukocyte esterase	Positive	
Nitrite	Negative	
Urobilinogen	Negative	
Protein (test strip)	Trace	Confirmed by SSA precipitation
pH	6.5	
Blood	Positive	
Specific gravity	1.015	
Ketone	Negative	
Bilirubin	Negative	
Glucose	Negative	
Sediment evaluation		
Squamous epithelials	Few	
Renal epithelials	0	
Erythrocytes	10–15	Intact cells on dipstick
Leukocytes	20–25	
Casts	0	
Crystals	0	
Bacteria	Trace	
Other (specify)		

Microbiology report:

The Gram stain revealed the presence of numerous Gram positive cocci

Upon collection of a catheterized specimen, the bacterial culture confirmed a *Staphylococcus saprophyticus*

1. What are the abnormal values found in this report?
2. What is a reason for a negative nitrite result when bacteria were seen microscopically?
3. What would likely be seen upon Gram staining the urine sediment?
4. Can *S. saprophyticus* be the causative agent for a urinary tract infection?
5. What is the most probable medical diagnosis for this patient's condition?

Case Study 7.3

A 15-year-old male was brought to the emergency room of a local hospital, and his family reported increasing lethargy and complaints of headaches by the young man. A urine sample and a blood sample for a complete blood count were obtained. The blood cell count showed normal results. The results of the urinalysis revealed the following findings:

Urinalysis results report, case study 7.3

Physical appearance		
Color	Yellow	
Character	Clear	
Chemical screening		
Leukocyte esterase	Negative	
Nitrite	Negative	
Urobilinogen	Negative	
Protein (test strip)	Negative	Confirmed by SSA precipitation
pH	5.5	
Blood	Negative	
Specific gravity	1.045	Confirmed by refractometer on diluted sample
Ketone	Pos—Mod	
Bilirubin	Negative	
Glucose	Positive >2	
Sediment evaluation		
Squamous epithelials	Occasional	
Renal epithelials	0	
Erythrocytes	0	
Leukocytes	1–2	
Casts	0	
Crystals	0	
Bacteria	0	
Other (specify)	Budding yeast	

1. What are the abnormal values found in this report?
   High specific gravity, positive ketones, high level of glucose
2. What is the reason for yeast cells being found?
   Commonly found in urine of persons with glycosuria
3. Why is the specific gravity elevated?
   High levels of glucose will increase the specific gravity as a dissolved constituent
4. What is the probable diagnosis for the young man's condition?
   Diabetes mellitus

Case Study 7.4

A teenaged male suffers from recurrent bouts of pharyngitis accompanied by headaches, fever, and significant discomfort. On one occasion, he has visited an outpatient clinic where a rapid test for streptococcal infection shows a positive reaction. He is placed on a short course of antibiotics and is told to rest more frequently. He again experiences a sore throat a few weeks after completing the antibiotic therapy, but says little to his parents of these symptoms, as he is busy with school and is involved in a variety of athletic activities. A few weeks after his last sore throat, he awakes with a headache and puffiness of the face. He is taken for a physical examination, and a urine sample is collected, with the following results.

Urinalysis results report, case study 7.4

Physical appearance		
Color	Reddish-brown	
Character	Cloudy	
Chemical screening		
Leukocyte esterase	Negative	
Nitrite	Negative	
Urobilinogen	Normal	
Protein (test strip)	Positive 3+	Confirmed by SSA precipitation test
pH	6.0	
Blood	Positive 2+	
Specific gravity	1.015	
Ketone	Negative	
Bilirubin	Negative	
Glucose	Negative	
Sediment evaluation		
Squam epithelials	Occasional	
Renal epithelials	0	
Erythrocytes	25–30	Some dysmorphic structures
Leukocytes	0–2	
Casts	1–2 RBC/LPF	
Crystals	0	
Bacteria	0	
Other (specify)	0	

1. What are the abnormal values found in this report?
2. What is the clinical significance of the patient's medical history?
3. What is the probable diagnosis for the condition from which the patient is suffering?

Case Study 7.5

An 8-year-old girl has been treated for a number of urinary tract and other infections over the past year. She has most recently exhibited a change in her appearance, from that of a wiry frame to a swollen appearance, including edema of the face. Upon visiting her pediatrician due to a paleness of the face and general malaise, her urine and blood are tested for any abnormalities that may lead to a diagnosis. The results of the urinalysis are as follows:

Urinalysis results report, case study 7.5

Physical appearance		
Color	Pale yellow	
Character	Slightly turbid	Appears frothy
Chemical screening		
Leukocyte esterase	Negative	
Nitrite	Negative	
Urobilinogen	Normal	
Protein (test strip)	Positive 4+	Confirmed by SSA precipitation test
pH	6.5	
Blood	Negative	
Specific gravity	1.020	
Ketone	Negative	
Bilirubin	Negative	
Glucose	Negative	
Sediment evaluation		
Squam epithelials	Few	Many oval fat bodies in clumps
Renal epithelials	0	
Erythrocytes	2–3	
Leukocytes	1–3	
Casts	1–3 fatty/LPF	
Crystals	0	
Bacteria	0	
Other (specify)	0	

1. What are the abnormal values found in this report?
2. What could contribute to the white froth of the sample?
3. What could contribute to the general and the facial edema?
4. Explain the presence of oval fatty bodies.
5. What would be the most likely diagnosis for this patient?

Case Study 7.6

A 51-year-old female has no medical history of any urinary tract disease with the exception of a couple of cases of simple cystitis, which were quickly resolved with the administration of antibiotics. Early one morning, when no one else was home, she developed agonizing pain in her back and left side. Shortly there afterward, she began vomiting and was extremely weak and was perspiring heavily. She made her way to the door of her home, and summoned a neighbor, who took her to the local emergency room. The results of a urinalysis were as follows:

Urinalysis results report, case study 7.6

Physical appearance		
Color	Yellow	
Character	Hazy	
Chemical screening		
Leukocyte esterase	Negative	
Nitrite	Negative	
Urobilinogen	Normal	
Protein (test strip)	Negative	
pH	6.0	
Blood	Positive (Large)	
Specific gravity	1.010	
Ketone	Negative	
Bilirubin	Negative	
Glucose	Negative	
Sediment evaluation		
Squam epithelials	Few	
Renal epithelials	0	
Erythrocytes	50–60	
Leukocytes	3–6	
Casts	0	
Crystals	0	
Bacteria	0	
Other (specify)	0	

1. What are the abnormal values found in this report?
2. What could contribute to the blood in the sample?
3. What could contribute to the general nausea?
4. What would be the most likely diagnosis for this patient?

Case Study 7.7

A 60 year-old man is brought to the emergency room by police cruiser. The patient is somewhat confused and is thought to be a long-term alcoholic, as he is well known in the circle of homeless victims. He is pale and around his mouth the mucus membranes are crusty and reddened. He exhibits evidence of dementia, and is unaware of reality at times.

1. What other characteristics of this disease might be observed?
2. What dietary material is deficient in those suffering from this condition?
3. What will be the likely diagnosis of this man's condition?

Review Questions

1. The most common disorders of the urinary system are based on:
   a. Bacterial infection
   b. Viral infection
   c. Genetic manifestations
   d. Anemia
2. The basic organs included in the urinary system include all of the following except:
   a. Bladder
   b. Ureters
   c. Uterus
   d. Urethra
3. The kidney is responsible for a number of important functions. They normally include all of the following except:
   a. Reabsorption
   b. Filtration
   c. Reabsorption
   d. Formation of crystals
4. The chief functional unit of the kidney is:
   a. Nephrons
   b. Proximal tubule
   c. Loop of Henle
   d. Adrenal glands
5. The blood flow to the kidneys includes approximately what percentage of the total volume of the blood that nourishes the body?
   a. 50%
   b. 33%
   c. 25%
   d. All of the arterial blood supply
6. The flow of blood within the kidney is controlled by the functions of a complex hormone system that includes all except:
   a. Antidiuretic hormone
   b. Rennin
   c. Angiotensin
   d. Aldosterone
7. The glomerular flow rate of water containing low-molecular-weight substances that flow through the glomeruli of the kidneys per minute is:
   a. 12 mL/min
   b. 1.2 mL/min
   c. 120 mL/min
   d. None of the previous responses

8. The correct pH (acidity or alkalinity) of the blood of the human body is maintained by:
   a. Retention or excretion of hormones
   b. Retention or excretion of hydrogen ions
   c. Retention or excretion of bicarbonate ions
   d. b & c
9. Which of the following would greatly affect the specific gravity of the urine?
   a. Dehydration
   b. High levels of protein
   c. Glycosuria
   d. All of the previous responses
10. Which of the following statements is true regarding the value of using the measurement of osmolality rather than osmolarity for the measurement of non-dissociable substance?
    a. Osmolality is affected by changes in temperature, atmospheric pressure
    b. Osmolarity is not affected by changes in temperature, atmospheric pressure
    c. Osmolality is not affected by changes in temperature, atmospheric pressure
    d. Either method of measurement is equally acceptable
11. What is the physical or colligative property used to measure the concentration of solutes in the urine, serum or plasma?
    a. Boiling point depression
    b. Freezing point depression
    c. Weighing of solutions, and comparing the values with that of pure water
    d. Tensile strength of the bonds between atoms of the molecule
12. The stimulation of ADH is *most* effectively triggered by:
    a. Changes in NaCl concentration
    b. Changes in potassium concentration
    c. Insulin level
    d. Proteinuria
13. Which of the following is/are components of Liddle's syndrome?
    a. Extreme hypertension
    b. Extreme hypotension
    c. High levels of sodium excretion
    d. High levels of potassium excretion
14. A disease caused by a malfunction of ADH is that of:
    a. Diabetes mellitus
    b. Diabetes insipidus
    c. Polyuria
    d. None of these
15. The simplest and most easily treated urinary tract infection (UTI) is called:
    a. Cystitis
    b. Pyelonephritis
    c. Glomerulonephritis
    d. Prostatitis

16. Acute pyelonephritis will produce a positive nitrite reaction due to:
    a. Presence of certain bacteria
    b. Presence of white blood cells
    c. Presence of red blood cells
    d. Presence of increased glucose levels
17. The kidney condition referred to as the sterile inflammatory process is:
    a. Polycystic kidney disease
    b. Pyelonephritis
    c. Urethritis
    d. Glomerulonephritis
18. Rheumatic fever is precipitated by:
    a. Recurring cystitis
    b. Post streptococcal infections
    c. Injudicious use of antibiotics
    d. Repeated viral infections
19. Blood tests that may be elevated during the acute stages but will return to normal along with the urinalysis results are:
    a. Bacterial cultures
    b. Blood urea nitrogen, creatinine
    c. Kidney enzymes
    d. Pathological examinations of tissue
20. The disease characterized by progressive kidney failure but is accompanied by lung disease is called:
    a. Urethritis
    b. Goodpasture's syndrome
    c. Rheumatic fever
    d. End-stage renal disease
21. A condition that is characterized by massive proteinuria and associated edema is that of:
    a. Nephrotic syndrome
    b. Liddle's syndrome
    c. Diabetes mellitus
    d. Rheumatic fever
22. Acute renal failure is often characterized by:
    a. Normal urine output
    b. Decreased potassium levels
    c. Anuria or oliguria
    d. Polyuria
23. A group of disorders called "amino acid disorders" usually refer to:
    a. Enzyme deficiencies that prevent normal synthesizing of amino acids
    b. Accumulation of abnormal metabolites
    c. May be of the "renal" or "overflow" type
    d. All of the above

24. Various states within the US require tests at birth to detect hereditary metabolic disorders. The one required by all states is that for:
    a. Maple Syrup disease
    b. Alkaptonuria
    c. Phenyketonuria
    d. Diabetes mellitus
25. Fanconi's syndrome is best described as an X-linked disease that is:
    a. An acquired disease
    b. A congenital disease
    c. A cluster of symptoms and signs
    d. All of the above
26. Metabolic acidosis may progress to an acute medical condition due to:
    a. Hypoglycemia
    b. Ketonuria
    c. Increased serum ammonia levels
    d. All of the above
27. A precursor to the neurotransmitter serotonin is:
    a. Niacin
    b. Tryptophan
    c. Porphyrins
    d. Dopamine
28. Porphyrins are the intermediate compounds in the production of:
    a. Carbohydrates
    b. Enzymes
    c. Amino acids
    d. Heme

Answers Found in Appendix C

Elements Involved in the Physical Evaluation of Urine

Objectives

Develop an understanding of the appearance of a normal urine specimen.

Classify urine samples as to the clarity of the specimens.

Describe the tests used for routine measurements of metabolites found in the urine, both normal and abnormal.

Recognize certain odors imparted to urine and the significance of each.

Correlate the relationship of urine samples by color as to concentration.

Understand the reasons for correcting specific gravity values based on the presence of elevated levels of protein, glucose and opaque materials used in radiographic studies.

Describe the meaning of the specific gravity and the procedure called osmolality.

List the differences between the values for three methods of performing specific gravity determinations.

8.1   Physical Examination of Urine

The earliest known analysis of the urine as it related to health or disease was that of observing the physical properties of this body fluid. Except in certain analytical procedures, the volume of the specimen as a physical property is not normally determined, except for certain quantitative tests that require knowledge of the amount of an analyte (substance being tested for) that is being "spilled" for a 24-h period. The first examination that provides clues as to whether a urine specimen is normal is called the macroscopic examination. This means that the senses of sight and smell are used to assess the basic characteristics of the urine sample. Some of these techniques are also employed when evaluating other body fluid specimens, as appropriate. Macroscopic characteristics include several basic and simple techniques for preliminarily evaluating a urine sample, as follows. Other tests including that of the specific gravity or concentration of a urine specimen is also

© Springer International Publishing AG, part of Springer Nature 2018   143
J. W. Ridley, *Fundamentals of the Study of Urine and Body Fluids*,
https://doi.org/10.1007/978-3-319-78417-5_8

considered a part of the physical examination of urine. In some cases, the presence of mucus in the sample may cause a viscosity or stickiness of the sample, particularly when the sample is poured into a centrifuge tube or the dipstick is inserted, and should be noted. The odor of the sample is another readily discernible characteristic of a urine sample.

8.2   Visual Appearance

The first impression of a urine sample is often that of its overall appearance. A urine sample with no abnormalities will most often be completely clear when it is freshly collected and not preserved or refrigerated, the latter of which may cause the formation of tiny crystals from solutes within the sample as it cools. The immediate appearance of the sample will yield clues as to the physical components that may be present, and will be particularly apparent to the experienced laboratory technician or technologist, as well as to other medical specialists (Table 8.1). Turbidity and colors found in urine samples often provide clues to both chemical and microscopic properties.

8.2.1   Normal Appearance

Appearance is a general and subjective term that may refer to the color and clarity of a urine specimen for the purpose of screening a sample for abnormalities. In a routine urinalysis, appearance is determined in the same manner used by the ancient physicians who were limited by the necessity of merely observing the appearance of the sample. This observation would have been more challenging to the medics of that time, since clear glass containers might not have been available under all circumstances, although the presence of glass has been known from thousands of years ago. The appearance was observed by visually examining a mixed specimen while holding it in front of a light source, such as a candle, lamp or sun in the early history of man. Common terminology used to report appearance includes clear, hazy, slightly cloudy, cloudy, turbid, and milky.

The normal appearance of freshly voided urine is usually clear but a white cloudiness may be caused by precipitation of amorphous phosphates and carbonates, especially when the sample has been allowed to stand or is kept in a cool environment. Normal urine is most often acidic and may also appear cloudy because of precipitated amorphous urates, *calcium oxalate*, or uric acid crystals. The cloudiness in acidic urine will often resemble brick dust due to the formation of the pink pigment uroerythrin, a normal component of urine, on the surface of any crystals that have formed. The presence of white blood cells, red blood cells, squamous epithelial cells and mucus, particularly in specimens from women, will also result in a hazy but normal urine.

Table 8.1 Physical properties, appearance of urine based on medical conditions

Physical property	Normal	Abnormal	Potential conditions
Color	Yellow, straw, slightly amber		Normal color is due to the presence of urochrome
		Absence of color except for minimal yellow color	Dilute urine
		Dark yellow or orange-tinted	Concentrated urine
		Amber	Concentrated urine due to dehydration or presence of bilirubin from liver disease or destroyed red blood cells
		Brown	Elevated bilirubin, old red blood cells that are not lysed
		Green-brown	Biliverdin, a greenish pigment from bile is produced by oxidized bilirubin
		Orange-red to orange-brown	Formed from urobilinogen (colorless) after exposure to room air
		Brilliant orange	Aminopyrine is a painkiller and fever reducer that is now only rarely used because of its dangerous side effects for urinary tract pain, burning, irritation, urgency
		Red	Fresh blood or hemoglobin from red blood cells or myoglobin from muscle desstruction
		Clear red	Hemoglobin from destruction of red blood cells
		Cloudy red	Presence of large numbers of intact red blood cells
		Clear red brown	Myoglobin from traumatized muscles
		Red (dark) or red-purple	Porphyrins are precursors of hemoglobin that are involved in the synthesis of hemoglobin
		Dark-brown to black	Often involves old bleeding of the urinary tract, excesses of melanin, homogentisic acid and certain poisonings
		Unusual green, green-blue and deep orange	Ingestion of certain vegetables, certain medications
Character (transparency)	Clear		Normal concentration of sample
		Hazy, turbid or cloudy	Presence of mucus, crystals, bacteria, white and red blood cells, casts and fat bodies
		Foamy	Small amount may be normal while large amounts may indicate protein; yellow foam indicates presence of bilirubin

(continued)

Table 8.1 (continued)

Physical property	Normal	Abnormal	Potential conditions
Odor	Slightly pungent		Normal, slightly acid urine
		Ammonia-like smell	Bacterial breakdown of waste product urea
		Foul-smelling	Urinary tract infection
		Fruity and aromatic	Diabetes producing ketone bodies from fat metabolism

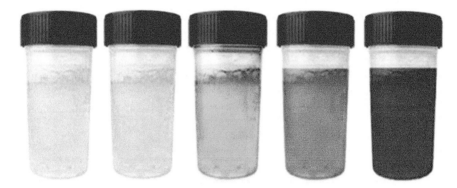

Fig. 8.1 Color variation in normal urine sample appearance

8.2.2 Color

The presence of pigmentation in urine specimens and even in other body fluids is often the first clue to the presence of certain constituents, although the presence of some abnormal materials in the urine may not alter the color of the fluid. The color of urine will vary from an almost colorless condition to one of black. The color will vary considerably at various times of the day for the same individual, although it is primarily some shade of yellow, straw or amber for most individuals, dependent on the state of hydration (Fig. 8.1). These variations may be due to normal metabolic functions, physical activity, ingested materials, or pathologic conditions. A noticeable change in urine color is often the reason a patient seeks medical advice, and it then becomes the responsibility of the laboratory to determine whether this change in color is a normal state or whether it is related to a pathologic condition. The person who examines the urine for color should be able to discern a number of colors. While some persons who are color-blind may be unable to see certain hues that are present. It may also be difficult for a color-blind person to analyze colorimetric changes on a color chart for the chemistry screening tests involved in the performance of a complete urinalysis.

8.2.2.1 Normal Urine Color

Terminology and the policies used to describe the color of normal urine may differ slightly among laboratories. Yellow is the most common description of a urine specimen but other common descriptions include pale yellow, straw light yellow, yellow, dark yellow, and amber. Care should be taken to examine the specimen under a good light source, by looking down from the top of the specimen container against a white background. The yellow color of urine is due to the presence of a pigment which was called by the term "urochrome" by Thudichut as long ago as 1864. Urochrome is a product of endogenous metabolism and is derived from urobilin, a brown pigmented product produced during the oxidation of urobilin, which in turn is derived from *bilirubin*. But under normal conditions urochrome is produced at a constant rate and the rate of fluid intake will greatly affect the concentration of the color it imparts to the urine.

The actual amount of urochrome produced is dependent on the body's metabolic state, with increased amounts being produced in thyroid conditions and fasting states. Urochrome also increases in urine that stands at room temperature. Because urochrome is excreted at a constant rate, the intensity of the yellow color in a fresh urine specimen can give a rough estimate of urine concentration. A dilute urine sample will be pale yellow, with a low specific gravity, and a concentrated specimen will be dark yellow, with a somewhat higher specific gravity. Remember that, due to variations in the body's state of hydration, these differences in the yellow color of urine are normal. Urine that would be measured as a normal output for a 24-h period would most often be normal in color, and larger volumes than normal would often be almost colorless while those of smaller daily volumes would be darker in color, as a general rule. Testing of a concentrated specimen would yield much higher levels of certain components being tested for than those urine samples that are more dilute.

8.2.2.2 Abnormal Urine Color

Straw or amber urine may not always signify a normal concentrated urine but can be caused by the presence of the abnormal pigment bilirubin. A very small amount of bilirubin may be present under normal circumstances, and will not be measured in a routine urine report. However, if it is present based on color during the chemical examination portion of the urinalysis, its presence is suspected if a yellow foam appears when the specimen is shaken (Fig. 8.2). A urine specimen that contains bilirubin may also contain hepatitis virus that would reinforce the need to follow standard (formerly universal) precautions. The conversion of large amounts of excreted urobilinogen to urobilin will also produce a yellowish to orange coloration of urine, but in the case of urobilin, yellow foam does not appear when the specimen is shaken.

Red is the usual color imparted to urine by blood, but the color may range from pink to black, depending on the amount of blood, the pH of the urine, breakdown of the blood and the length of contact. Red blood cells remaining in an acidic urine for

Fig. 8.2 Urine containing bilirubin, evidenced by yellow foam after shaking

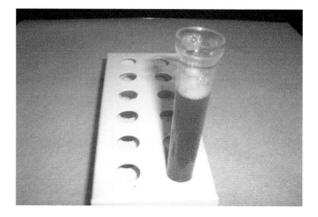

several hours will produce a brown to black urine due to the denaturation of hemoglobin to methemoglobin. A fresh brown to black urine containing blood may also be indicative of' glomerular bleeding. And in addition to RBC's, two other substances, hemoglobin and *myoglobin*, will produce a red urine and may yield a positive result when tested for blood. Myoglobin is released when there is muscle damage, and is a valuable adjunct in diagnosing a coronary attack. Hemoglobin is released when red blood cells are destroyed, and the hemoglobin from the surfaces of the red blood cells is released into the blood stream from which it is at least partially removed from the blood though the urinary system.

Many abnormal urine colors are of a nonpathogenic nature and are caused by the ingestion of highly pigmented foods, medications, and vitamins. Eating fresh beets will produce a red colored urine in certain genetically susceptible persons, and asparagus may give urine a green hue as well as sometimes imparting a characteristic odor. Even the chewing of Clorets breath deodorants can result in greenish-tinged urine. An orange color may result from high levels of carotene from the eating of large amounts of carrots, a plant product also capable of staining the skin of the hands and feet an orange color. Highly colored urine samples are often attributed to the ingestion of certain medications, vegetables, fruits, vitamins, dyes, and chemicals but offer little of diagnostic value. Azo dyes (those with double-bonded nitrogen atoms) impart an orange color to the urine specimen (Fig. 8.3). These dyes are bacteriostatic, meaning they inhibit the reproduction of bacteria but do not actually kill the organism. The color by azo dyes may be confused with the presence of abnormal levels of bilirubin, and either of these often will cause difficulty in reading test strip results, the most common manner of determining the presence of elevated levels of certain analytes.

8.2.3   Odor

Although it is seldom of clinical significance and is not a part of the routine urinalysis, urine odor is a noticeable physical property. Freshly voided urine will have

Fig. 8.3 Urine sample containing bacteriostatic dye

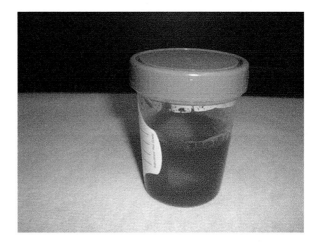

only a faint odor of aromatic compounds. As the specimen stands, the odor of ammonia becomes predominant. The breakdown of urea is responsible for the characteristic ammonia odor. Causes of unusual odors include bacterial infections, which cause a strong, unpleasant odor, and diabetic ketosis, which produces a sweet or fruity odor. A serious metabolic defect results in urine with a strong odor of maple syrup and is appropriately called maple syrup urine disease. Ingestion of particularly asparagus as previously noted can cause an unusual or pungent urine odor. The ingestion of multiple vitamins will often be noted, imparting a "pharmacy-like" odor. This is due to the fact that most vitamins that are ingested in a tablet or capsule form are readily excreted from the body, unlike those derived from a balanced diet.

8.2.4 Turbidity

The character of a specimen is the term used for the clarity of a urine sample. A number of materials will cause turbidity of a urine specimen. Some of these are abnormal but many are not and are found routinely in a percentage of samples examined. The physical examination should include turbidity and color in the initial screening of the sample, prior to performing other tests. For some procedures, it may be advantageous to remove the constituents that are causing turbidity prior to performing chemistry tests and other procedures that may affect the results. Besides amorphous crystals, the four most common substances that cause turbidity in urine are white blood cells, red blood cells, epithelial cells, and bacteria. Other causes of turbidity include the presence of lipids, semen, mucus, lymph fluid, crystals, yeast, fecal material, and extraneous contamination with materials such as vaginal creams, talcum powder, and even radiographic contrast media. Many of these substances are nonpathogenic and are not reported on the laboratory test results. However, because white blood cells, red blood cells, and bacteria are indicative of pathogenicity, a fresh, turbid specimen can be cause for concern.

Infection Control Flash
Urine is not considered as a means of transmitting infectious materials to those who work with the specimen, even when bacteria, yeasts, and other organisms may be contained in the sample. With rare exceptions, such as with certain parasites that occupy water during the stages of their life cycle, no serious infections have been transmitted through the urine, including HIV.

8.2.5   Specific Gravity

Specific gravity is the density of a substance compared with the density of a similar volume of distilled water at a similar temperature. There are essentially three methods of determining the specific gravity of a sample. One is by use of the *refractometer* (Fig. 8.4), where the sample is compared with light. The value is observed when light passes through the sample placed over a prism, which enables the determination of the concentration of solutes in the sample. The second is performed with the use of a urinometer. This device is a small cylindrical flask with a flotation bulb with a scale on a top stem that corresponds with the specific gravity of the specimen. This method compares urine with pure water. The third is the most commonly used method and involves the use of a chemistry dipstick which measures the dissolved ions in the sample. It is sometimes necessary to confirm the screening results where the chemistry dipstick method has been used, by one of the other methods as previously outlined.

The specific gravity assesses the kidneys' ability to reabsorb dissolved components of the urine. A normal specific gravity, dependent upon the hydration status of the individual, is from 1.000 to 1.040. The use of the refractometer may entail several steps to ensure an accurate value is obtained. When using the refractometer, a refractive index is used. This is a comparison of the velocity of light in air with the velocity of light in a solution. The velocity is dependent on the concentration of dissolved particles present in the solution and determines the angle at which light passes through a solution. Calibrating the refractometer is a necessary component

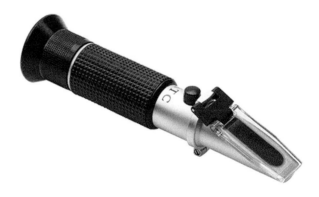

Fig. 8.4 Urine refractometer

of quality assurance programs and should be accomplished on a regular schedule. Calibration of the refractometer requires placing distilled or *deionized water* on the surface of the glass chamber as is done for an actual urine sample. The scale is then adjusted by use of a small tool provided with the refractometer to a 1.000 level on the visible scale. This should be done each day before initiating testing of samples and following every ten samples or a predetermined number specified in the procedure manual to ensure that the calibration is accurate.

When the temperature of a urine sample is warm, or if it is cold, it may also be necessary to correct the urinometer reading, since a urinometer is calibrated to read exactly 1.000 using distilled water at a specific temperature. The calibration temperature for the urinometer is printed on the instrument and is usually about 20 °C. When the specimen is cold, 0.001 must be subtracted from the reading for every 3° that the specimen temperature is below the urinometer calibration temperature, ie. 20 °C in most instances. And conversely, 0.001 must be added to the reading for every 3° that the specimen measures above the calibration temperature.

Corrections are also necessary when the urine contains abnormally high levels of either protein or glucose values. A gram of protein per *deciliter* (g/dL) of urine will raise the urine specific gravity by roughly 0.003 and will need to be adjusted accordingly. A gram of glucose per deciliter will require the deletion of 0.004 to the uncorrected reading for each gram of glucose. Keep in mind that glucose is usually measured in milligrams (mg) so a fraction of the 0.004 for each gram will need to be adjusted as applicable, perhaps as a fraction of a gram. So, to correct a specific gravity discrepancy that is due to the presence of glucose, the correction might be more or less than the 0.004 ratio. For instance, one gram contains 1000 mg. Therefore, if the glucose estimate on a screening procedure indicates a 500 mg value, the specific gravity value to be reported would be only one-half of the 0.004 adjustment, or 0.002.

8.3   Chemical Analysis of Urine Specimens

Following the visual examination of the urine sample, the presence of certain chemicals are tested for, most often by the use of a test strip containing chemically reactive pads that yield a color based on the intensity of the reaction. The chemical dipstick was developed to avoid the time-consuming tests used prior to the 1950s for detecting the presence of specific constituents. This method of using chemically treated pads on a plastic or paper strip has evolved from those that detected the presence of only a few components to one that is more accurate and that gives fewer false positive or false negative results. The modern chemistry dipstick provides a simple and convenient method for performing 10 medically significant chemical components commonly found in the urine. This methodology provides an analysis for significant chemical analytes including pH, protein, glucose, ketones, blood, bilirubin, urobilinogen, nitrite, leukocytes, and a screening test for the specific gravity. Some reagent strips are designed to measure only certain components, and not all of the 10 analyses listed.

Table 8.2 Urine test strips used for screening of samples for chemical constituents

Manufacturer	Location	Name of test strips
Arkray Inc.	Kyoto, Japan	Aution Sticks
Iris Diagnostics	Chatsworth, CA, USA	vChem Srips
Roche Diagnostics	Indianapolis, IN, USA	Chemstrips
Siemens Healthcare Diag., Inc.	Deerfield, IL, USA	Multistix

Some constituents tested for through the use of the test strips may also require confirmation by other methods as false negative and false positive results are possible, giving misleading clinical information to the physician or other health care practitioner. These confirmatory tests include urobilinogen, bilirubin, protein and albumin, as well as glucose in some cases, where reducing substances other than glucose may be of clinical interest. Reagent strips are available for routine testing from a number of medical supply providers (Table 8.2). This has helped to improve the testing the presence of chemical substances. The routine testing for chemical examinations of the urine has changed dramatically since the early days of urine testing, due to the development of accurate reagent strip method for screening tests for the chemical analysis of urine.

8.4   Reagent Strip Technique for Urinary Chemistry

Testing methodology consists of dipping the strip completely, but briefly, into a well-mixed urine specimen, removing excess urine by touching the edge of the strip to the container as the strip is withdrawn. The various analytes that are tested for will require different reaction times. Strip readers are available that "read" the results, using programmed times for each of the components contained on the test strip. A manual procedure requires that the evaluator wait the specified amount of time for the reaction to occur before comparing the color of each segment of the strip with a color chart found on the container holding the strips. For the best semi-quantitative results, the manufacturer's stated time should be followed but in the event that precise timing cannot be adhered to, it is recommended that reactions be read at 60 s but never later than 120 s. Those with the shortest reaction (found on the chart accompanying the strips) should be read first, with the leukocyte esterase reaction (a test for the presence of white blood cells) read last. A good light source is, of course, essential for accurate interpretation of color reactions. Color blind individuals should always use a semi-automated strip reader that prints the results, rather than trying to interpret the various color changes of the strip.

Specimens that have been refrigerated must be allowed to return to room temperature prior to reagent strip testing, as the enzymatic reactions on the strips that are used to detect some of the chemical components are temperature dependent. Certain components of the urine are present at small levels even in the urine of normal individuals who are free of disease. This requires that the strips be adjusted for sensitivity of these analytes to prevent the reporting of positive results for those components that are present in trace amounts for all patients. Adjustment of the sensitivity of the results is necessary to prevent medical treatment of normal patients or the diagnosis of a pathological condition where none exists. Many screening tests require careful attention to measure the appropriate levels to gain significant data from large population groups. Appendix B provides a chart for the routine chemistry tests for urine which contains clinical data pertinent to the individual reactions along with precautionary notes for each of the test strip values.

8.5   Quality Control and Storage of Reagent Strips

In addition to the use of correct testing technique, reagent strips must be protected from deterioration caused by moisture, *volatile* chemicals, heat, and light. All of the various brands of reagent strips are packaged in opaque containers with a desiccant designed to absorb moisture that would cause deterioration of the chemically-impregnated strips. When not in use, and between uses, these bottles should be tightly closed and kept stored in a cool area, away from extreme light and heat sources. Bottles should not be opened in the presence of volatile fumes, as the chemically-treated strips are capable of absorbing vapors. All bottles are stamped with an expiration date that should be observed on a routine basis to avoid the use of strips that may no longer be capable of reacting with certain constituents being tested for.

8.6   Automation in Urinalysis Procedures

Typically, the analysis of urine samples has been a tedious and time-consuming process with a great deal of subjectivity between individuals and health care facilities in the evaluation of urine samples. Other body fluids that required even more diligent testing have also been automated to an extent, although abnormal samples may require analysis by a human for some of the systems developed to automate the process. But over the past few decades, more quantitative procedures particular for urine analysis in the manual procedures has led to more automation and has improved the professional perception of automated examination of urine samples and of other body fluids. However, most laboratories still utilize a manual method of testing, with the semi-automated strip reader as an adjunct to the testing of urine samples.

The value of the urinalysis has grown progressively since the first crude and simple observations were developed individually by medical practitioners. But medical practitioners have developed a growing respect for the valuable information that may be obtained from a properly performed urinalysis that has evolved from a simple "look and smell" that has historically been used for diagnosis of a variety of diseases. Urinalysis instruments that are connected by "track" systems to move samples around the lab to the various diagnostic areas are enabling more timely and accurate results. This track system is also used for blood samples and other body fluids samples to facilitate the movement of samples to the proper testing area or department within the laboratory. The complete urinalysis examination that is performed consistently and that meets accepted standards are gaining a renewed stature as a laboratory diagnostic test that is equal to the other more glamorous tests that utilize blood for testing.

Although chemistry, hematology, and blood bank procedures are best known in the clinical laboratory, the use of the urinalysis is gaining stature. As a screening test that provides clues to serious metabolic illnesses, the results of a complete urinalysis may signal the need for further and more definitive testing. The urinalysis procedure uses an easily collected sample that is relatively cheap and quick to perform for determining a host of disease states or even the health status of large numbers of patients. While disease detection and prevention by the urinalysis has not been in the forefront as a valuable component as a screening tool, it would be advantageous for the previously mentioned reasons.

When a urinalysis is performed using manual methodology, there is much more subjectivity in the interpretation of results than for most laboratory tests. Significant variation exists in the "reading of chemistry dipsticks" as to color change and when assessing the physical properties of samples. Well-written procedures with standardized protocol for reading, confirmation of reports of results will serve to remove some of the subjectivity. But there is significant variation in how a procedure is performed from one laboratory professional to another.

The education of the laboratory professional should emphasize the potential for subjectivity in the performance of all laboratory tests, and not just for the urinalysis or the examination of other body fluids. A valuable resource for both seasoned laboratory professionals and the laboratory student is that of the package inserts for each of the procedures. Knowledge of the theory of the tests and standard reporting formats where acceptable standards are applied for color, evaluating the strength of a reaction, and avoiding the use of confusing terms will improve the validity and accuracy of the results being transmitted to the person in charge of the care of the patient.

Technological advances in all areas of industry and the advent of manufacturing processes where greater quantities of smaller instruments can be made cheaper has revolutionized the health care industry in the past few decades. Medical devices such as the automated strip reader for urine chemistry determinations have made the instruments an essential component of the clinical laboratory rather than a luxury. These instruments are found in laboratories ranging from physician office laboratories (POLs) to almost all clinical laboratory settings throughout much of the world. It was only a relatively small step before these semi-automated dipstick readers were paired with an instrument that was capable of transporting samples to several stations within the instrument and to show the microscopic results of the urine sample on a computer screen.

Today, the large chemistry analyzers that sample hundreds of blood samples for multiple analytes have contributed the technology to do the same for large volumes of urine samples. The semi-automated dipstick reader became paired with a semi-automated microscopic analyzer, and has changed the practice of the analysis of urine to a consistent and highly efficient instrument. It is essential in the development of technology within the laboratory to avoid sacrificing quality for the sake of quantity. Since flow cytometry and automated hematology and chemistry analyzers have been a reality for at least 50 years, the automation of urinalysis was a logical step. But due to the lack of attention to the value of urinalysis, the development of a truly automated urine analyzer has lagged behind those for other laboratory departments.

In the beginning of automation, some practitioners relied on an instrument such as the *Bayer Diagnostics Clinitek*, a semi-automated strip reader. After determining values from the dipstick chemistry constituents, no further testing was performed when these values yielded normal or negative results. In some cases, the chemistry component results may be normal while abnormal components that would have been discovered upon microscopic examination may not. Some facilities have a protocol where the physician or designate could request a simple chemical evaluation, or the chemistry tests along with a microscopic. Procedures offered by some medical institutions could offer more extensive testing to include a bacterial culture when either chemistry or microscopic results indicated a need for further testing beyond that of the chemistry determinations. One limitation imposed by the initial testing which includes only the chemistry dipstick components is not sensitive to some bacterial infections of the urinary tract. For instance, the *leukocyte esterase* test only suggests the presence of white blood cells or fragments of the cells which might or might not be related to a urinary tract infection (UTI). The nitrite portion of the dipstick indicates the presence of bacteria that are capable of reducing nitrates to nitrites, but not all bacteria that are capable of producing a UTI are those that can metabolize nitrates to nitrites.

The reproducibility of the results of physical constituents between competent technologists using the manual microscopy method does not correlate well. Only a small amount from the total urine sample is used in the examination and may fail to contain certain critical elements from specimen to specimen. Infections from the upper urinary system, with the glomeruli of the kidneys as a factor in the disease, will provide differing results from those of the lower urinary tract involving the bladder and the urethra. The newer automated systems use the same applications as those offered by the flow cytometer and may be combined with similar features that a hematology analyzer uses for cellular differentiation. Formed elements that may be recovered from the urine sample using one of the newer analyzers, such as blood cells, by staining the cells with a fluorescent dye that provides markers for nucleic acids and membranes that the instrument can "see." In most of these systems, a laser measures the size and pattern of the stained cells and is designed to determine the presence of light scatter characteristics when coordinated with impedance measures where differing sizes and shapes of cells impede an electrical current as they pass through a small aperture. This sophisticated information enables the instrument to detect different forms of white and red blood cells, tubular casts formed in the renal tubules, epithelial cells from the kidneys, bladder, and urethra. Other formed objects including sperm, yeasts, molds, and bacteria can also be quantitated by the use of an automated system for urine or body fluids analysis.

Automated urinalysis systems have been in existence for more than 25 years, and studies by clinical laboratories have determined a significant change in the efficiency of performing urinalyses when automated systems are used. It is not always necessary to assign a dedicated technologist to the performance of urinalyses, but the technologist must be available to troubleshoot and to make the decision to override certain results from the instrument. Automated systems do require confirmation of a number of results that may fall outside the parameters of the instrument or where results may not correlate with the various components of the complete analysis of body fluids. Past efforts to standardize the procedure for a complete urinalysis have been challenging, but automation is now making these attempts more feasible.

Efforts to utilize current technology has led to the potential of using the automation employed in urinalysis to screen patient populations for other categories of diseases rather than those commonly found on a broad basis during the performance of a urinalysis. An automated means for determining the presence of tumors of the bone marrow, leukemias and *lymphomas* when combined with existing technology which utilizes specific antibodies for a number of tests, may become possible. Ongoing research is targeting methods in which to screen large groups on a routine basis for the early detection of cancer. Due to the obvious advantages of early detection of malignancies, there will no doubt be many innovations of technology similar to that employed in automated urinalysis and body fluids studies to accomplish the processing of various types of samples for abnormal cells.

Cutoff values for the numbers of white blood cells which would indicate the need for a bacterial culture is not yet standardized. In many cases, the numbers of white cells present do not correlate with the severity of the infection and does not indicate the source of the infection. Previously, the manual enumeration of white blood cells in urine and other body fluids samples could not be reproduced even between experienced technologists and technicians. A consistent result showing an accurate estimate of the numbers of white blood cells before a bacterial culture is indicated would provide for a great deal of efficiency and accuracy in the requests for cultures. This would save money and time in the practice of effective medicine.

The presence of bacteria in a sample is an alternate means for determining the presence of bacteria in not only urine but in other body fluids and would effectively reflect a need for a bacterial culture and antibiotic sensitivity. But meaningful bacterial enumeration from body fluids has also been a challenge for many years for several reasons. For urine samples as well as other body fluids where testing is delayed will have a higher bacterial count than those tested immediately after voiding. In addition, a urine sample that is not a "clean catch," sample, or one that is collected by catheterization, will quite often have a high count of skin contaminants, particularly in samples from female patients. Therefore, bacterial counts from urine and other body fluids that are used to indicate the need for a bacterial culture would appear to be meaningless without microscopic correlation by a laboratory technologist.

A small number of automated and semi-automated instruments are currently available for use in performing a urinalysis or an evaluation of other body fluids. Some of these commonly available are automated analyzers that include the Clinitek and Atlas (Miles), Sysmex UF-100 (Sysmex America, Inc.) available through Siemens Medical Solutions Diagnostics (Fig. 8.5), the Chemstrip Urine Analyzer

Fig. 8.5 Sysmexca-1500
fully automated urine
analyzer

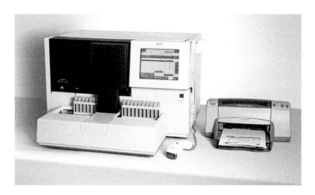

(BMC), and the Rapimat II (Behring). The iQ200 Automated Urine Microscopy Analyzer, made by Iris Diagnostics is another instrument widely available and in use in a large number of clinical sites. Since the composition of this work, later versions and new versions of similar equipment may have occurred. An instrument called the Yellow IRIS is one that has evolved over the years from the first system developed by International Remote Imaging Systems (IRIS) in 1979. This system is a sophisticated instrument that provides for some input from the operator of the instrument. This operator-attended work station can quickly provide specific gravity determinations, the chemical analysis of the sample, and a complete microscopic examination. The microscopic evaluation by this instrument eliminates several time-consuming steps required when performing a manual microscopic examination requiring centrifugation of a certain volume of urine.

While manual methods of urinalysis are very much technologist-dependent, the automated instrument generally avoids the need for hands-on handling of the samples. Many of the automated procedures can be used not only for the examination of urine but other blood-based body fluids. This eliminates steps in which the laboratory professional could contract an infectious disease from body fluids other than urine. And in addition, one technologist may be able to process up to 200 samples an hour with available technology, an impossible task when using manual methodology. When Iris Diagnostics developed the iQ200 automated urinalysis system, manual microscopy was no longer needed except for manual confirmation as the machine performs the task of "dipping" the chemically-treated dipstick before transferring the rack of urine samples between the chemistry analysis component to the part of the instrument where the microscopic procedure is performed.

In addition to screening for tumor cells, as mentioned previously, the urinalysis analyzers could have an even larger impact as they start to include other body fluids on their menus. Processing of body fluids is labor-intensive, and the Iris (iQ200) is programmed and approved by the *Federal Drug Administration* (FDA) for the analysis of a variety of other fluids including semen, bronchial washings and *cerebrospinal fluid* (CSF). Urine samples as well as other body fluids may be easily processed simultaneously in an automated fashion with no intervention by the laboratory personnel. Even viscous fluids such as synovial fluid from joints of the body can be analyzed by the iQ200 but not by the automated analyzer for hematological procedures due to the possibility of clogging the apertures through which the cells pass, but some fluids such as CSF can be processed using a hematology analyzer.

8.7   Chemical Constituents

Under normal circumstances, approximately 90–95% of the volume of urine is water. Although only a small percentage of urine consists of solutes (materials dissolved in the water), they are nonetheless necessary for ridding the body of excess materials and products of metabolic processes as a result of biochemical reactions in the cells and tissues of the body. A minute percentage of the solutes may be due to medications, such as vitamin supplements and other materials that originated outside the body. Some of the solutes are classified as ions, or single chemical elements that may carry a positive or a negative charge from the electrons surrounding them. Others are positively charged due to the presence of fewer electrons than the individual atom can potentially possess. Larger compounds are composed of a number of atoms that are bonded together to form molecules.

Both organic as well as inorganic molecules are found in the urine, sometimes as ions, which are positively or negatively charged components. Organic molecules are those that form rings or chains of carbon atoms, a characteristic that distinguishes organic molecules from inorganic molecules that do not contain carbon. The organic compounds called amino acids comprise the building blocks of the cells of the body. And other organic materials are excreted as a result of the breakdown of protein, where urea, uric acid and creatinine are formed through metabolic processes and are then excreted in the urine. Some of these organic molecules are nitrogenous (contain a nitrogen atom or atoms) and are end products of reactions that involve nitrogen metabolism. There are literally hundreds of substances that may be found in urine and other body fluids but many of them are not indicative of a pathological (disease) state.

8.7.1   pH

Importance of the pH lies primarily as an aid in determining the existence of systemic *acid-base disorders* of metabolic or respiratory origin. The pH is affected mainly by the excretion of hydrogen ions (H^+) and bicarbonate (HCO_3^-) ions, chemical constituents that help to maintain the pH of the body at an optimum level that is required by many metabolic processes.

8.7.1.1 Clinical Values for pH
The normal range for a urine sample is from 4 to 8, compared with a neutral value of 7.0. Certain dietary components may affect the pH of the urine, a valuable consideration when changes in the pH may be necessary to treat or prevent calculi of the urinary system that require a narrow pH range in order to form and to remain as

hardened crystals. An acid pH of 4–6 will also discourage bacterial growth, while an alkaline pH will provide a favorable for most bacteria to survive. Some bacterial growth will contribute to the production of an alkaline pH. Urea is normally found in the urine and when converted to ammonia, this is a condition that may drastically change the pH of the urine to a markedly alkaline state.

Points to Remember
The chief component of urine is water, but the products of metabolism that are found in urine is indicative of hundreds of metabolic processes. Some excreted materials are waste products, but others are reflective of selective reabsorption in the tubules of the kidneys, or excretory processes that are balanced by the body to maintain equilibrium of the body. Some constituents of the urine point toward a pathologic condition only when they show increased levels, while others indicate a disease state by their mere presence as abnormal elements of the urine.

8.7.2 Proteinuria

The finding of significant amounts of protein in the urine is called "proteinuria." In addition to the presence of glucose in the urine, a positive test for protein is one of the most important clinical signs of the presence of disease that may affect the urinary system. Of the routine chemical tests performed on urine, the most indicative of renal disease is the presence of protein. The presence of proteinuria is often associated with early renal disease, making the urinary protein test an important part of any physical examination. More advanced renal disease as well as a number of metabolic conditions may also contribute to elevated levels of protein found in the urine. It should be added here that a false positive result me be obtained for an extremely alkaline urine sample. Body fluids other than urine have differing levels of protein for both normal and abnormal medical conditions.

8.7.2.1 Clinical Values for Urinary Protein
Normal urine samples contain very little protein and most often less than 10 mg/dL or 100 mg/24 h is excreted, so the sensitivity of the dipstick or automated methods for measuring the protein will not yield a clinically significant result when the level found in the urine is less than 10 mg/dL. Demonstration of proteinuria in a routine analysis does not always signify renal disease. But its presence in significant amounts may indicate a need for additional testing or confirmatory testing to determine whether the protein represents a normal condition or is suggestive of a disease that results in the excretion of elevated amounts of protein.

Specimen concentration must also be considered in the finding of a trace amount of protein in a dilute specimen, as this would be of more medical significance than if found in a concentrated specimen. Major pathologic causes of proteinuria include glomerular membrane damage which may be transient or may show a chronic medical state. Other causes of proteinuria include disorders affecting tubular reabsorption of filtered protein and other materials as well as increased serum levels of proteins of low molecular weight that are excreted into the urine. Following conditions that result in glomerular membrane damage, filtration for selected components is impaired, allowing increased amounts of albumin and large globulin molecules from the blood plasma to pass through the membrane and to be excreted in the urine. Several types of protein are indicative of specific disease processes and some of the clinically important types are described.

- Disease Contributions to Excretion of Protein in Urine
    1. Glomerular membrane damage
        a. Repeated infections resulting in immune complex disorders
        b. Amyloidosis, with deposition of protein-containing materials in tissues
        c. Exposure to toxic agents
    2. Diabetic nephropathy from uncontrolled diabetes
    3. Decreased tubular reabsorption
    4. Malignancy such as multiple myeloma
    5. Conditions of pregnancy, to include pre-eclampsia
    6. Orthostatic or postural proteinuria
- *Bence Jones Protein*
    One of the common contributors to proteinuria is a result of the disease called *multiple myeloma*, where a light chain protein called *Bence Jones protein* is excreted in the urine due to a predominance of the *immunoglobulins* called *gamma globulin*. Multiple myeloma is a myeloproliferative (bone marrow), malignant disorder of the immunoglobulin-producing plasma cells. In this condition, the low molecular weight categories of protein are filtered into the urine in amounts that exceed the ability of the tubules of the kidney to reabsorb the proteins, and the excess is excreted in the urine. When Bence Jones protein is suspected, a screening test is available where the urine is heated gradually to a temperature up to 100 °C. This procedure utilizes a unique solubility characteristic of the specific protein, where the material coagulates between 40 °C and 60 °C, and then dissolves when the temperature reaches 100 °C. The process is a reversible procedure where the sample can be heated, cooled and reheated to duplicate this phenomenon, as other proteins are irreversibly coagulated. The sample can also be tested for Bence Jones protein through a procedure called *electrophoresis*, where the proteins migrate in a pattern when exposed to an electrical field.
- *Tamm-Horsfall Protein*
    A high molecular weight of protein, as opposed to the light chain proteins, is found in the urine and does not originate in the blood plasma as do other proteins found in the body fluids. This glycoprotein is secreted by the renal tubular cells, the location where tubular casts are found in certain conditions, some of which are pathological. Most urinary casts are associated with proteinuria, and *Tamm-Horsfall* protein comprises the structural matrix of the urinary casts of various types.

- *Microalbuminuria*

  The detection of *microalbumin* is a procedure developed in the past few decades and is currently used as a special dipstick chemical reaction. The measurement of small but perhaps consistent amounts of albumin that is routinely excreted by diabetic patients occurs early in the disease process. Routine chemistry evaluations using the dipstick method are not sensitive enough to detect the presence of microalbumin, so a special strip is used for this procedure. The development of *diabetic nephropathy* leading to reduced *glomerular filtration* is a common occurrence in persons with diabetes mellitus (Fig. 8.6). Onset of renal complications can first be predicted by detection of this portion of total protein called microalbumin. The progression of renal and ocular disease as well as other types of damage to the diabetic can be delayed through strict monitoring and stabilization of blood glucose levels during early stages of the disease.

- *Orthostatic (Postural) Proteinuria*

  The discovery of protein, particularly in a random sample, is not always of pathologic significance, inasmuch as several non-renal or benign causes of proteinuria exist. Benign proteinuria is usually transient and can be produced by conditions such as exposure to cold, strenuous exercise, high fever, dehydration, and in the acute phase of severe illnesses. A more persistent benign proteinuria occurs frequently in young adults and is termed *orthostatic*, or postural, proteinuria occurring following periods spent in a vertical posture and will disappear when a horizontal position is assumed. Increased pressure on the renal vein when in the vertical position is believed to account for this condition. A negative reading will be seen on the first morning specimen, and a positive result may be found on any following specimens for the remainder of the day.

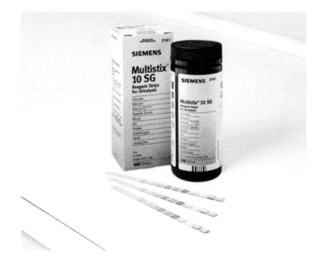

Fig. 8.6 Strips for determining presence of microalbumin

Table 8.3 Turbidimetric subjective estimate of proteinuria

Appearance of solution	Subjective turbidity	Estimate of protein excreted
Clear	None	Negative for protein
Noticeable	Trace	Minute levels of protein
1+	Print legible through mixture	Small amount of protein excreted
2+	Turbid, slight flocculation	Moderate amount of protein excreted
3+	Turbid, granules, flocculation	Large amount of protein excreted
4+	Clumps of protein	Extreme excretion of protein

- *Reagent Strip Reactions for Protein*
  Reagent strip testing for protein utilizes the principle of the "protein error of indicators" to produce a visible colorimetric reaction. Contrary to the general belief that indicators produce specific colors in response to particular pH levels, certain indicators change color in the presence or absence of protein even though the pH of the medium remains at constant levels. Readings are usually reported in terms of negative, trace, 1+, 2+, 3+, and 4+. This methodology, when employed for highly alkaline specimens may result in false positive results and must be confirmed by the following method (See following note).
- *Reaction Interference for Protein Determinations*
  Several substances and conditions are often capable of introducing interference when either the reagent strip or the precipitation method is employed. The major source of error with reagent strips occurs when highly alkaline urine specimens are being tested, resulting in an overriding of the buffer system that is incorporated into the test strip. The resulting measurement is merely that of the production of a rise in the pH and a color change occurs that is not related to the true protein concentration of the sample.
- *Confirmatory Tests—Precipitation*
  The earliest tests that were developed to determine the presence of protein were those called *precipitation* tests. This procedure utilizes heat to denature the protein and produce a visible precipitated material. Currently, most laboratories have replaced the heat and acid test with the less cumbersome cold protein precipitation procedures where *sulfosalicylic acid* (SSA) or *trichloroacetic acid* (TCA) will immediately form a precipitate, where the amounts can be semi-quantitatively determined (Table 8.3). Various concentrations and amounts of SSA can be used to precipitate protein, and methods may be subjective and vary greatly among laboratories. In general *equal amounts* of urine and SSA or TCA are placed in a test tube and the level of precipitation is graded as follows:

8.8   Glucose

The term indicating the presence of significant levels of glucose in the urine is "glycosuria." The presence of varying levels of glucose in body fluids other than urine may be equally critical in diagnosing and treating disease states other than those of the urinary tract. Glucose is the basic energy source for most living organisms, particularly mammals, a group of organisms in which humans are classified. The finding of glucose in urine occurs for significant quantities of pathological conditions, including diabetes mellitus, the most commonly encountered pathological condition, as well as others. A small amount of glucose of less than 30 mg/dL is routinely excreted by the kidneys via the urine. The renal threshold is a measure of the ability of the functional units of the kidneys to reabsorb a certain amount of glucose that is filtered into the tubules of the kidneys. The average renal threshold for most persons is approximately 180 mg/dL but varies within a few units of measurement between individuals. When the amount of glucose excreted from the kidneys exceeds this level, excess glucose is "spilled" in the urine. Some individuals have a somewhat lower threshold and even the drinking of a carbonated beverage containing a significant amount of glucose will result in the presence of glucose in the urine.

8.8.1 Clinical Implications Related to Glucose Levels

The finding of a detectable glucose in the urine by urinary glucose by use of the chemical dipstick is not a normal condition. Although the blood glucose is between 70 and 120 mg/dL, and glucose is initially excreted from the kidneys, reabsorption in the proximal tubules of the kidney diminishes the excretion of glucose in the urine, except in cases of diabetes mellitus. The normal accepted ranges will vary between individuals and the ranges may depart from this range depending on the method used for testing a population group. Other causes of glycosuria (glucose in the urine) are reduced glomerular flow from occlusions or damage to the vascular system perfusing the kidneys, and a reduced urine flow causing concentrated urine.

Because of its value in the detection and monitoring of diabetes mellitus, the glucose test is the most frequent chemical analysis performed on urine. It is estimated that due to the nonspecific symptoms associated with the onset of diabetes, over half of the cases in the world are undiagnosed. Therefore, urine glucose tests are included in all physical examinations and are often the focus of mass health screening programs. Early diagnosis of diabetes mellitus through blood and urine glucose tests provides a greatly improved prognosis. Using currently available reagent strip and tablet testing methods, patients can monitor themselves at home in order to avoid serious complications.

8.9 Hematuria (Blood)

Blood that is found in the urine may be a result of damage to the kidneys, or may be the means for excreting blood that results from a disease process in other organs of the body, although the blood cells may not be intact when they are excreted if they originate in organs and tissues other than the kidneys. Therefore, blood may be present in the urine either in the form of intact red blood cells (*hematuria*) or as the red blood cell destruction product hemoglobin hemoglobinuria). As discussed in an earlier chapter, blood present in large quantities can be detected macroscopically (by the naked eye) as well as microscopically and by use of a chemically treated dipstick.

Gross hematuria produces a cloudy red urine due to intact red blood cells and hemoglobinuria often appears as a clear red specimen, unless accompanied by other metabolic products. However, because any amount of blood greater than 5 cells per microliter of urine is considered clinically significant, and will not be detected macroscopically, it is not possible to rely on a gross visual examination to detect the presence of blood. Microscopic examination of the urinary sediment will show intact red blood cells, but free hemoglobin produced either by hemolytic disorders or lysis of red blood cells in the urinary tract will not be detected by this method. Therefore, chemical tests for hemoglobin provide the most accurate means for determining the presence of blood, and once blood has been detected, the microscopic examination can be used to differentiate between hematuria and hemoglobinuria.

8.9.1 Clinical Implications Related to Presence of Blood in Urine

The presence of red blood cells, or hematuria, in the urine may result from bleeding at some area of the urinary tract. The condition may be produced by the presence of calculi (stones) that have formed in the kidneys, by certain hemorrhagic infections caused by certain bacteria, use of an anticoagulant to prevent vascular clotting, or a hereditary or acquired coagulation disorder. The presence of a small amount of blood should be investigated as to the cause and the potential occurrence of renal disease.

8.10 Hemoglobin

Although the condition may be related to the presence of lysed (destroyed) red blood cells that are damaged by hypotonic (dilute) urine, the presence of hemoglobin may have arisen from a systemic loss of blood that has occurred elsewhere in the body. Haptoglobin is a hemoglobin carrier that is found in the plasma of the blood and when sufficient hemoglobin has been bound by haptoglobin so the carriers are saturated, hemoglobin may be found in the urine. As hemoglobin is absorbed in the renal tubules, ferritin (iron storage compound) and hemosiderin (iron-containing pigment) may be found in the urine. This constituent of urine can be detected by staining the compounds or the cells in which they are deposited with Prussian blue, but will give a negative result for blood by dipstick.

8.10.1 Clinical Implications Related to Presence of Hemoglobin in Body Fluids

Hemoglobinuria may be found in any pathological condition where red blood cells have been destroyed and hemoglobin is released in large quantities into the blood plasma, and excreted into the urine through the kidneys. Certain immunological conditions such as paroxysmal cold hemoglobinuria (PCH) and other conditions categorized as *coagulopathies* (clotting disorders) along with the transfusion of incompatible types of blood may produce this condition. Although this is a rare medical condition, it is usually discovered in young children. In this type of condition, bilirubin from the destroyed and damaged red blood cells may be excreted normally, providing high levels of urobilinogen which is reabsorbed in the intestines and excreted in the urine.

8.11 Myoglobin

Myoglobin is an iron-binding protein that is found in muscle cells and stores oxygen required for muscular activity that reacts positively with the chemical test for blood and also produces a clear red to brown coloration of the urine, similar to that imparted by red blood cells. Myoglobin is found in all muscles, including the heart and musculoskeletal system. When a muscle is exercised, it uses up available oxygen. Myoglobin has oxygen attached to the muscle, which provides extra oxygen for the muscle to maintain a high level of activity for longer periods of time. When muscle is damaged by any means, the myoglobin in muscle cells is released into the bloodstream. The kidneys help to remove myoglobin out of the body.

8.11.1 Clinical Implications Related to Presence of Myoglobin in Urine

Myoglobin is present in small amounts in the urine of all patients even under normal conditions, and the usual results for normal patients are less than 1 mg/L. Only in rare cases will increased levels of myoglobin be found in the urine. When large amounts of myoglobin are present in the blood, the protein can damage the kidney and break down into toxic compounds, causing kidney failure.

Patients with urine myoglobin greater than 15 mg/L are at increased risk of contracting acute renal failure. Increased levels of myoglobin should be expected in patients with conditions associated with muscular destruction, such as trauma, prolonged coma, convulsions, muscle-wasting diseases, and extensive exertion. *Rhabdomyolysis* is the term for acute destruction of muscle fibers and myoglobin that is usually rapidly cleared from the blood and is excreted in the urine. Large amounts of excreted myoglobin are culpable in damaging the kidneys. Diagnosis of myoglobinuria is usually based on the patient's history, and serum tests for enzymes elevated by muscle destruction. The appearance of the patient's serum can sometimes aid in the differentiation between hemoglobinuria and myoglobinuria, due to the pink or red hue of the plasma that is seen with hemoglobinuria, and the colorless plasma that is found in the presence of myoglobin. However, more specific tests are available that are effective in detecting the presence of abnormal amounts of myoglobin. In addition, other muscle enzyme tests will correlate with an increased level of myoglobin.

8.12   Bilirubin

Bilirubin is normally found in the blood in small amounts and is therefore excreted through the urine in small amounts. Red blood cells that have fulfilled their life spans, which may be shortened by certain anemias and other conditions, are destroyed and ingested by large white blood cells called macrophages. These cells are found in the liver, spleen and even in the bone marrow where the blood cells originate. Bilirubin found in other areas of the body is transported to the liver by the vascular system and is excreted in bile. In the gut, bilirubin is reduced to urobilinogen by bacterial action, and most of the urobilinogen is excreted in the feces.

8.12.1 Clinical Implications Related to Presence of Bilirubin in Urine

Small amounts of bilirubin found in the blood is tested for to determine the normal amount of blood destruction or the presence of liver disease. Hyperbilirubinuria signals that the liver is diseased or damaged, or that a hemolytic process is occurring. Atypical colors that may stain the urine a bright red to orange color may present a false finding with the chemistry dipsticks used for testing urine. These reagent strips are difficult to analyze some results and all too frequently false positive and false negative results may be present. Exposure to sunlight and even to fluorescent lights will reduce the level of bilirubin in the specimen. This technique is used for neonates who suffer from bilirubinemia, where light therapy is used to decrease the level of bilirubin in the blood of the infant.

Confirmation of a positive color change on the reagent strip requires a test called the Ictotest Tablet method and is available from the Bayer Corporation. The color produced in this reaction should be a purple or bluish color, although other colors such as pink will occur in the presence of certain non-bilirubin compounds and should be reported as a negative result.

8.13   Urobilinogen

As in the measurement of bilirubin, urobilinogen is a colorless bile pigment that results from the degradation of hemoglobin from red blood cells by bacterial action. It is produced in the intestine from the reduction of bilirubin by the normal flora that consists mostly of bacteria that dwell in the intestinal system. Approximately half of the urobilinogen is reabsorbed from the intestine into the blood before recirculation to the liver and is then secreted into the intestine through the bile duct into the duodenum. The urobilinogen remaining in the intestine is excreted in the feces, where it is oxidized to urobilin, the pigment responsible for the characteristic brown color of the feces. Urobilinogen appears in the urine because, as it circulates in the blood enroute to the liver, it may pass through the kidney before being filtered by the glomeruli. Therefore, a small amount of urobilinogen—less than 1 mg/dL or 1 Ehrlich unit- is normally found in the urine.

8.13.1 Clinical Implications Related to Abnormal Levels of Urobilinogen

Urobilinogen is seen in the urine for those conditions where red blood cells are destroyed. The compound is also typically found in a number of liver disorders, where bilirubin is increased due to a dysfunction of bile excretion into the gall bladder.

8.14 Porphobilinogen

Porphobilinogen is an intermediate product in the production of heme. It is a normally occurring and colorless bile pigment and is a precursor to porphyrins that are utilized in the production of hemoglobin. Porphyrins contain nitrogen (N^+) and no iron (Fe^{++}) while hemoglobin incorporates iron into the hemoglobin molecule. Ferroprotoporphyrin 9 is a porphyrin found in the heme portion of hemoglobin molecules. Porphyrins are normally excreted from the body in the urine and stool as *uroporphyrins* and *coproporphyrins*, respectively, which results from the degradation of hemoglobin from red blood cells via bacteria in the gut.

8.14.1 Clinical Implications Related to Increase in Porphyrins

A variety of clinical conditions result in increased excretion of porphyrins. Urine containing high levels of porphobilinogen may appear normal when freshly voided, but upon heating with dilute HCl to 100 °C may change to a port wine color. Certain enzyme deficiencies, along with other diseases may be responsible for elevated levels of porphobilinogen that are excreted in the urine. Hereditary conditions are often reported as causative factors and those that are precipitated by the use of various drugs and alcohol along with poisoning by heavy metals. Several forms of the disease are characterized by anemias and skin conditions.

8.15 Nitrites in Urine

This reagent strip test for the presence of nitrites provides a useful and rapid screening test for considering the presence of a urinary tract infection (UTI). It is not intended as a substitute for a urine culture and should be correlated with the presence of leukocyte esterase values. The value of the procedure would only determine the possible existence of a urinary tract infect for certain groups of bacteria capable of reducing nitrates to nitrites, since not all bacteria are capable of this process in their metabolism. The test is valuable in enabling the elimination of the need for culturing a urine sample for bacteria and is not clinically useful in the diagnosing of and monitoring of the course of a bacterial infection.

8.15.1 Clinical Implications Related to Nitrites in Urine

The majority of UTIs originate in the urethra and extend into the bladder due to contamination from external sources, such as bacteria found around the anal region. Urethral and bladder bacterial infections that go untreated may progress upward through the ureters to the kidneys and the functional structures such as the *nephrons* of the kidneys. The nitrite test is valuable for detecting initial bladder infections before patients begin to show overt symptoms or in the case where only vague symptoms are present. This procedure would then narrow the possibilities that the physician would consider in deciding the necessity for a urine culture.

8.16 Leukocyte Esterase

A frequent finding in the routine urinalysis is that of the presence of leukocytes (white blood cells), is an indication of a possible infection of the urinary tract. These cells are elevated in number for conditions including nearly all diseases of the urinary system. However, in certain cases, white cells may be present in conditions other than those of an infective nature. Strong oxidizing agent reactions may produce interference and provide erroneous results.

8.16.1 Clinical Implications Related to Leukocyte Esterase Presence in Urine

A positive result for leukocyte esterase is not specifically indicative of an infection of the urinary tract. Non-intact white blood cells will also yield a positive result, when none are visible upon microscopic evaluation. Leukocyte esterase results are specific in a limited way, as lymphocytes, a type of white blood cell, erythrocytes (red blood cells), bacteria and renal tissue cells do not contain esterases and therefore will provide negative results. Some antibiotics, including *tetracycline*, will give false negative results in high concentrations, and false positive results may be obtained in specimens that are contaminated by vaginal fluids.

8.17 Ketones

Normally, ketones are negative by chemical strip methods when levels are less than 2 mg/dL. There are three components included in ketones for which urine is tested. A test is positive only in the presence of acetoacetic acid but does not react with acetone or Beta-hydroxybutyric acid. Under conditions of ketonuria, components include predominantly Beta-hydroxybutyric acid (more than three-fourths) with perhaps 10% as acetoacetic acid, and only a small percentage as acetone.

8.17.1 Clinical Implications Related to Ketones in Urine

Abnormal metabolism of carbohydrates and lipids (fats) will often yield a positive result. In cases of *ketoacidosis* found particularly in diabetics and starvation which results in the metabolism of fatty tissues for energy will give positive results. Because of the lack of insulin or when an insulin form present is ineffective in metabolizing glucose, the body may resort to a form of glycogenesis involving fat catabolism. Ketones results by dipstick are positive only if the urinary levels are greater than 10 mg/dL. Traces of ketones may be obtained during physiological stress and strenuous exercise, and sometimes in pregnant persons.

8.18 Specific Gravity

The pad on the dipstick to screen for specific gravity is a time saving procedure. However, it is not recommended to replace osmometry or refractometry for critical fluid monitoring. The chemical strips measure only dissolved ions, and therefore may not correlate well with values obtained by refractometry or by use of the urinometer. This methodology is useful as general screening for dehydration and to emphasize the presence of protein, glucose and some other constituents of the urine that may cause an increase in the specific gravity. One advantage in the use of this chemically reactive method lies in the fact that the value obtained is not affected by the presence of *radiopaque dyes* that cause erroneous determinations when using the refractometer or a urinometer.

8.18.1 Clinical Significance of Specific Gravity Levels in Urine

Urine specific gravity measurements are valuable for determining the concentrating ability of the kidneys. When the specific gravity reading exceeds 1.020, it may be assumed that the kidneys are operating effectively in secreting and reabsorbing of appropriate components of the urine. More definitive tests for the proper functioning of the kidneys would include other clinical tests such as that of *creatinine clearance* and osmolality. The presence of high levels of various chemical constituents such as glucose and protein may dramatically affect the specific gravity of a specimen.

8.19   Interfering Substances

As in most laboratory procedures, certain substances may present interferences when evaluating urine test strips, although clinical procedures other than tests performed on urine and body fluids are also problematic. The use of urine reagent strip testing is a reliable method for screening specimens for glucose, protein, ketones, and bilirubin. Alternate methods are available for some of these tests and confirmatory tests should always be performed in certain circumstances. It is occasionally necessary to employ a secondary method to confirm a result, and in some cases, based on physical examination, other constituents may not be included on the reagent dipstick.

Ascorbic acid, also known as vitamin C, has been known to affect results of some tests that are routinely performed on urine. Ascorbic acid is not an abnormal finding but is present when the patient has ingested vitamin C or multiple vitamins that include large amounts of vitamin C or large amounts of citrus fruits. Vitamin C is not routinely tested for, but one brand of test strip is Rapidnost, available from Behring Diagnostics, Inc. contains a test for ascorbic acid, and when positive, may be used to indicate potential erroneous results obtained by dipstick analysis. Major manufacturers of test strips have included additional reagents or have changed their methodologies to prevent the effects of high levels of ascorbic acid on the testing of urine specimens for levels that would be normally encountered in most patients. The most important constituent tested by reagent strip that is affected by ascorbic acid is that of blood. In this case, the test strip results for blood may be negative, but intact RBCs are found in the sediment of a centrifuged urine sample.

Another consideration that is important arises when testing for protein in a specimen with a highly alkaline pH. The result by test strip may be positive, but clinically the patient should be negative for protein by dipstick. This situation is easily remedied by performing a protein precipitation test using sulfosalicylic acid or trichloroacetic acid as a confirmation of the results obtained from a chemically-treated dipstick.

The use of bacteriostatic dyes and certain substance may impart significant color to the urine sample. Reasons for unusual colors of the specimen often result from diet, medical condition of the patient or from taking medications, and may challenge the laboratory professional's abilities when attempting to visually evaluate the results of the chemical test strip. Dark amber colored urine may indicate the presence of bilirubin and the Ictotest can be used to confirm the presence of bilirubin.

Delayed processing of urine samples which are exposed to sunlight or fluorescent lights may result in inaccuracies in results of urinalysis, particularly in the artificially low levels of bilirubin and urobilinogen that may be obtained. Bacterial contamination of the body fluid sample may also impact on the laboratory professional's ability to obtain accurate results by chemical test strip. Additional information that may require alternate methods to avoid false negatives or false positive results from interfering substances will be included in the procedures that are discussed in a later chapter.

8.20 Summary

The physical examination of urine and later other body fluids dates back for thousands of years. The physical appearance of urine often correlates with the results obtained from chemical tests performed on urine in particular, and to a lesser extent, the other body fluids. The physical findings chiefly include the use of the senses of sight and smell to evaluate the normal or abnormal appearance of the body fluid.

Chemistry tests were initially cumbersome and were performed by the physicians themselves on an individual basis. During the mid-twentieth century, rapid screening tests were developed for major constituents of urine that were necessary to evaluate the health of the patients. This was accomplished through the evolution of the manual tests to simple reactions with chemically-treated pads that reacted colorimetrically in the presence of certain constituents of the urine.

As the predictive value of urinalysis results became more understood, simple strip "readers" that quickly evaluated the color changes from the dipsticks were developed. The physical examination was followed by this process that involved the chemical evaluation of the specimens, which was followed by a microscopic study of the centrifuged sediment to complete the complete urinalysis. Many of these tests were somewhat subjective, and results and reporting units varied between laboratories and even between technical laboratory personnel. It was an obvious step for the process to become standardized, where the same volume of urine was concentrated and the same protocol for reporting results was established.

Upon the standardization of the procedure, further evolution occurred through the development of analyzers with multiple functions. Color and clarity was read spectrophotometrically, and then the specimen was tested by an automated "dipping" system, and then the test strip was "read." The next step consisted of displaying the presence of microscopic elements and the quantifying of them. Today, busy laboratories are able to produce hundreds of complete urinalyses in an efficient and time-effective manner. Only extremely abnormal findings are required to be confirmed by a laboratory professional.

Case Study 8.1
A 5-year-old girl frequently plays in the park near her house. She sometimes complains of being tired particularly after playing in the cold weather and has had a recent cold. Her mother decided to seek medical advice as to her child's condition, but silently chastised herself for being over-cautious. The pediatrician especially

paid attention to the fact that the condition seemed exacerbated by exposure to cold weather. A complete blood count and a urinalysis were performed which showed a mild anemia manifested by a borderline hemoglobin and hematocrit determinations. The urinalysis showed the following results.

Urinalysis report, case study 8.1

Physical appearance		
Color	Pinkish hue	
Character	Clear	
Chemical screening		
Leukocyte esterase	Negative	
Nitrite	Negative	
Urobilinogen	2 Ehrlich units	
Protein (test strip)	Negative	
pH	6.0	
Blood	Positive 1+	
Specific gravity	1.015	
Ketone	Negative	
Bilirubin	Positive 2+	Confirmed by Ictotest
Glucose	Negative	
Sediment evaluation		
Squam epithelials	Occasion	
Renal epithelials	0	
Erythrocytes	2–3	
Leukocytes	1–2	
Casts	0	
Crystals	0	
Bacteria	0	
Other (specify)	0	

1. What are the abnormal values found in this report?
2. If the urine were shaken, what would the laboratory technician expect to see?
3. Explain the differences between high levels of urobilinogen and of bilirubin.
4. What is the probable diagnosis for the condition from which this woman is suffering?

Case Study 8.2

A 50-year-old male is undergoing an annual physical. Blood is collected for a biochemical profile, a complete blood count and a test for an enzymatic evaluation of the prostate. In addition, a midstream urine sample is collected. Analysis of the urine sample is delayed so the medical assistant places the sample in the refrigerator until the technician is able to perform the urinalysis. The results of the urinalysis are as follows:

Urinalysis report, case study 8.2

Physical appearance		
Color	Pale yellow	
Character	Slightly turbid	
Chemical screening		
Leukocyte esterase	Negative	
Nitrite	Negative	
Urobilinogen	Normal	
Protein (test strip)	Negative	
pH	8.0	
Blood	Negative	
Specific gravity	1.020	
Ketone	Negative	
Bilirubin	Negative	
Glucose	Negative	
Sediment evaluation		
Squam epithelials	Few	Many oval fat bodies in clumps
Renal epithelials	0	
Erythrocytes	2–3	
Leukocytes	1–3	
Casts	0	
Crystals	4+ amorphous	
Bacteria	0	
Other (specify)	0	

1. What are the abnormal values found in this report?
2. What could contribute to the turbidity of the sample?
3. Explain the presence of the amorphous crystals.
4. What would be the most likely diagnosis for this patient?

Review Questions

1. Arguably, the most important constituent found in urine that may cause the majority of interferences with accurate results, is that of:
   a. Azo dyes
   b. pH of the sample
   c. Disinfectants
   d. Ascorbic acid
2. Measurement of the specific gravity of the urine is important in:
   a. Determination of state of hydration
   b. Concentrating ability of kidneys
   c. Amount of dissolved ions in sample
   d. All of the above

3. Which of the following could affect the evaluation for protein in a urine sample?
   a. Acid pH
   b. Alkaline pH
   c. Ascorbic acid
   d. Red blood cells
4. Which of the following may be most important in assessing kidney damage?
   a. Glucose
   b. Nitrites
   c. Leukocyte esterase
   d. Protein
5. The presence of nitrites in a urine sample is indicative of:
   a. Azo dyes
   b. Presence of leukocytes
   c. Certain bacteria
   d. Interfering substances
6. The test pad on the dipstick for measuring blood would be negative in the presence of:
   a. Hemoglobin
   b. Lysed red blood cells
   c. Myoglobin
   d. Hemosiderin
7. Light chain immunoglobulins in the urine would be indicative of:
   a. Myelocytic leukemia
   b. Massive urinary tract infection
   c. Multiple myeloma
   d. Prerenal conditions
8. Glycosuria, or glucose in the urine in abnormal amounts, would be present in:
   a. Starvation
   b. Diet rich in carbohydrates
   c. Diabetes insipidus
   d. Diabetes mellitus
9. The finding of glucose in the urine would not be affected by:
   a. Testing refrigerated urine
   b. Increased bilirubin
   c. Testing concentrated urine
   d. All of the above
10. The confirmatory test for bilirubin in the urine is:
   a. Precipitation tests
   b. Clinitest
   c. Ictotest
   d. Bilirubin glucuronide

11. Which of the following is not one of the three ketone bodies?
    a. Acetone
    b. Prednisone
    c. Acetoacetic acid
    d. Beta-hydroxybutyric acid
12. Precipitation tests are used to test for:
    a. Carbohydrates
    b. Ketones
    c. TCA and SSA
    d. Proteins
13. A test for urobilinogen would indicate:
    a. Liver disease
    b. Presence of intact red blood cells
    c. Destruction of red blood cells
    d. Poor kidney function
    e. All of the above
    f. a & c
14. Tests for bilirubin in the urine would include evaluation for:
    a. Hormone function
    b. Kidney damage
    c. Liver disease
    d. White blood cell destruction

Answers Found in Appendix C

Considerations for Microscopic Examination of Urine

9

Objectives

Discuss the advantage of using standardized procedures for evaluating microscopic, formed elements of the urine

Describe the process of measuring and centrifuging a body fluid sample for microscopic analysis

List the three types of microscopes commonly used and the reasons for using the brightfield type for most microscopic evaluations

Prepare a microscope for use in evaluating the microscopic components of urinary sediment

Understand the presence of "normal" microscopic elements that are found in small numbers

Discuss the correlation of physical properties of urine with the microscopic evaluation

Discuss the correlation of chemical properties of urine with the microscopic evaluation

List the physical steps involved in the testing of a body fluid sample

Correctly perform microscopic urinalysis to include identification of significant elements in urinary sediment from a centrifuged sample

Understand clinical conditions and causes for the formation of casts

List common artifacts and how they may be confused with significant forms

Name crystals found in alkaline and in acid urine samples

Describe the use of stains for significant constituents of urine and tissues

9.1 Introduction to a Microscopic Evaluation of Urine

The microscopic analysis of urine and other body fluids is perhaps the most important and most commonly utilized process used to determine the presence of renal and urinary tract disease. Other body fluids are treated in the same manner as urine

© Springer International Publishing AG, part of Springer Nature 2018
J. W. Ridley, *Fundamentals of the Study of Urine and Body Fluids*,
https://doi.org/10.1007/978-3-319-78417-5_9

Fig. 9.1 Conically-shaped tube for obtaining urine sediment

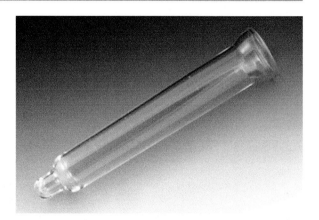

samples to an extent, as pertinent procedures depending upon the particular components of each body fluid may mirror in part those performed on urine. A predetermined amount of urine is centrifuged with a resultant "button" of *urine sediment* that is deposited in the bottom of a conically shaped and graduated tube in a standardized procedure (Fig. 9.1). Not all body fluids other than urine require centrifugation except to look for elements that may be found in small numbers. The acceptable levels of certain constituents such as white blood cells may be lower in number than those found in a normal urine sample, and could be enumerated on an uncentrifuged specimen. For example, samples such as cerebrospinal fluid (CSF), only a few white blood cells may be significant on an uncentrifuged sample.

9.2   Macroscopic and Chemical Evaluations

A thoughtful physical, or macroscopic, evaluation of a urine sample will greatly contribute to expected findings from the final step in the examination of a urine or body fluid sample. Color and clarity of the sample will provide clues as to certain physical components that may be present when examining the sediment from a portion of the sample microscopically. Renal functions that include adequate renal blood supply, glomerular filtration, tubular reabsorption, and tubular secretion all play a role in the health of the individual. These physiological functions, if abnormal, will most often be reflected in the three steps involved in the complete analysis of a urine sample. These same three steps, with modifications, may also apply in whole or in part to other body fluids. The chemistry portion of the urinalysis may also contribute helpful information that may correlate with and enhance the microscopic findings.

9.3   Microscopic Analysis of Urine and Other Body Fluids

The policies of some facilities state that the microscopic examination of urine, in particular, is not done when the macroscopic and chemistry portions of the urinalysis yield no abnormal results. The patient's medical condition may also weigh in on

Table 9.1 Microscope use and techniques

Technique used	Purpose
Bright-field microscopic examination	Routine examination of centrifuged urine sediment
Darkfield microscopic examination	Used basically in determining presence of organism called *T. pallidum* that causes syphilis
Phase-contrast microscopic examination	Microscopic elements that are colorless (low refractivity) are more easily visualized (include mucus, hyaline casts, and hematological procedures such as platelet counts)
Polarizing microscopic evaluation	Useful in visualization of crystals, fat bodies, casts with fatty constituents
Fluorescence studies	Used in techniques where microorganisms are "tagged" with a fluorescent dye, also based on immunological techniques where specific antibodies may be employed

the decision of whether to perform the microscopic analysis or not. The screening of samples and the decision to perform the microscopic analysis of the sample based on other factors as described provides for cost effectiveness and efficiency, but may result in "missing" some important finding that is not evidenced by chemical and physical evaluations.

The Clinical and Laboratory Standards Institute (CLSI) is a nonprofit organization devoted to the developing of meaningful standards that lead to the establishment of standards and guidelines for the clinical laboratory. The position of CLSI is that the decision for performing a microscopic evaluation of urine on routine urinalyses is a voluntary decision to be made by each laboratory with respect to the type of patient and the care rendered by the facility. It should be noted that a microscopic evaluation will be performed if the physician requests such tests, regardless of screening results. Specialized microscopes and techniques may be employed for specific and uncommon microscopic components of urine and body fluids (Table 9.1). It should be noted that basic bright-field microscopy is sufficient for most routine examinations of urine sediment.

9.4   Waived Procedures

A policy instituted by the Clinical Laboratory Improvement Amendments of 1988 categorizes the physical and chemical portion of a urinalysis as a "waived" procedure that can be performed by uncertified healthcare employees. A number of manufacturers provide supplies and kits used for primarily a qualitative measurement of certain analytes of the blood and body fluids (Table 9.2). Certain categories of tests are considered as being "waived" regardless of methodology employed. The microscopic analysis of urine and other body samples are classified as "moderately complex" procedures and must be performed by personnel that are skilled in the use of the various types of microscopes and possess knowledge of the purpose of each of these types, among other technical requirements. A written procedure must include

Table 9.2 Selected tests granted waived status—CLIA regulations

Test name	Manufacturer	Procedure
Dipstick or table reagent urine chemistry, non-automated	Includes various suppliers	Screening of urine for monitoring, diagnosing diseases and conditions of the urinary system
Urine pregnancy test, color comparison method	Includes various suppliers	Diagnosis of pregnancy
Fecal occult blood	Includes various suppliers	Diagnosis of or screening for colorectal cancer
Blood glucose—instruments designed for home use as approved by FDA	Includes various suppliers	Determining estimates of whole blood glucose for diagnosis and prognosis of diabetes
Hemoglobin—color scale comparison or copper-sulfate flotation	Includes various suppliers	Determine hemoglobin level indicative of anemia or hemorrhage
Ovulation status by visual color	Includes various suppliers	Determine optimum timeframe for conception following ovulation
Red blood cell estimation by hematocrit	Centrifuged blood specimen by use of microhematocrit	Screening methods for anemia or blood loss
Erythrocyte sedimentation (manual method)	Various manufacturers	Non-specific screen for inflammatory conditions related to infection and other disease states

components that ensure consistency between specimens where the analysis includes all aspects of specimen preparation, identification, steps in the analytic processes, and the accurate reporting of results. Resources must be available for troubleshooting and the identification and resolution of complex issues, and the healthcare employee must know the correlation between the various steps, as well as the significance of the physical components that may be found in the urine sediment.

9.5   Urine Specimen Preparation

Compositions of urine specimens are chiefly water that contain urea, other organic and nonorganic chemicals dissolved in water, as well as various cells, *casts*, and crystals. Steps must be taken in the transport, storage, and testing of these samples to prevent deterioration of not only the physical, formed elements but also the chemical components of the specimen. A part of specimen preparation also entails the assuring that the sample is adequate for testing, and in some cases, that the sample provided is actually that of urine.

Changes in urine specimens that are stored in collection containers are often neglected or not understood. For some procedures, a preservative is required to avoid the occurrence of changes in the specimen. But all preservation methods are not foolproof, and any of them will have advantages or disadvantages depending on the procedure and the test methods employed. The most common method of preservation for specimens to be tested by a simple urinalysis procedure is by storage in a refrigerator. Freshly voided and refrigerated specimens should be tested as soon as possible following collection.

9.6   Methods of Urine Collection

It is important to use a properly collected urine specimen, as those that are contaminated or where a delay in testing occurs, or exposure to high temperatures or sunlight will cause test results to be meaningless or even erroneous, leading to improper and unnecessary treatment. Where the sample has been refrigerated, the urine specimen should be returned to ambient (room) temperature in order to allow amorphous substances to dissociate, and to prevent interference with the pH (alkalinity or acidity of the sample). The determination of the pH of a sample changes with bacterial growth and the methodology is also standardized for performing the procedure at a particular temperature. Clean catch specimens, where a midstream specimen is collected in a clean or sterile container after using an antiseptic cleansing of the tissue surrounding the urethral opening for women, is the most convenient method of collection. But the best method that virtually eliminates skin contamination is that of the catheterized specimen, where a sterile tube is inserted into the bladder through the urethra for collection of a urine specimen.

Another less frequently employed method is by suprapubic aspiration, where a sterile needle is used to puncture the cleansed skin of the pubic region and to enter the bladder. Negative pressure from a sterile syringe plunger accomplishes the aspiration of the sample. There is an attendant negative side effect that often results in the introduction of occupational bacteria from the environment into the bladder with an attendant spread of infection to the urinary tract. In addition, a poorly performed puncture may damage the skin tissues as well as the structures of the bladder along with blood vessels, musculature and other nearby tissues.

9.7   Specimen Requirements per Procedure

Acceptable samples must meet various criteria established by the laboratory before the sample will be processed. A list is provided in this section to establish the various types of collection methods that will meet the testing requirements for each given procedure. In addition to the collection methods, a minimum amount of sample for urine specimens as well as for other body fluids testing will be established. But the volume of some body fluids will be difficult to assess as acceptable, and will vary dependent upon the type of sample and the patient providing the sample. The container for the various samples will be easier to mandate than will the volume, especially for samples other than urine. The type of specimen and the time of collection must be verified to avoid using a sample that may have components that have deteriorated and where bacterial contamination would most likely have occurred. Urine samples must generally be tested within 2 h of collection, and are refrigerated if this is not possible.

Red and white blood cells, and particularly casts, will disintegrate quickly in a dilute sample. Refrigeration will slow the rate of destruction, but cooling of the specimen also contributes to the formation of amorphous phosphate deposition in alkaline specimens and amorphous urates in acid specimens. Some preservatives such as formalin will interfere with the results for certain chemical constituents, and others will destroy pathogenic bacteria that should have led to a bacterial culture to determine if a urinary tract infection is present.

Specific sample collection methods are vital for certain determinations. While a random sample is the most commonly used type because of the convenience of the collection of the specimen and may easily be used as a screening tool, certain procedures will require a specific collection type. Abnormalities discovered during the screening tests must be confirmed by repeat collection using certain protocols for cleansing of the female's urogenital area, catheterization, or more commonly by collection of a mid-stream sample. The various collection methods are as follows:

- Random samples for screening for basic abnormalities
- First morning specimens to insure concentration of particular analytes
- Fasting specimens to prevent dietary effects
- Two hour post-prandial sample to gauge the effect of a meal on the test values
- Twenty four-hour or timed specimens to determine the quantity of a metabolite over a length of time
- Catheterized sample to avoid skin contaminants for microbiological procedures
- *Mid-stream clean catch* specimen to flush skin contaminants from the external urethral opening called the meatus
- Suprapubic aspiration is performed when a catheterization is impossible due to physical abnormalities or urogenital surgery
- Three-glass collection used to determine the location of the urogenital tract where infection related to prostatic condition is suspected

9.8   Standardization of Microscopic Procedures

Several systems are available for standardizing the manual method for the performance of a microscopic evaluation of urine sediment. It should be understood that a few of the constituents to be determined when testing urine samples are similar to those found when performing procedures on body fluids other than urine. A dipstick chemistry test is not performed on body fluids other than urine since a qualitative analysis is accomplished on urine samples, where only an estimate of a metabolite is obtained. Quantitative tests are performed on other body fluids where a somewhat exact measurement is critical when determining a diagnosis based on specific body

Box 9.1: Standardized System for Urine Microscopic Exam

Method name	Company providing system
UriSystem	Fisher Scientific, Pittsburgh, PA
KOVA	ICL Scientific, Fountain Valley, CA
AimStick 10-SG	MarketLab, Inc., Caledonia, MI

fluids other than on urine, where the test results vary with the state of hydration. A majority of the accredited laboratories that do not have an automated system for performing complete urinalyses will utilize a standardized system. Some of the systems available are (Box 9.1):

The systems are not limited to the above businesses and generally provide the following:

- Graduated centrifuge tubes (volumes may vary between systems)
- Specially designed pipettes used following centrifugation to mix and load suspended formed elements
- Standardized slides that include a reservoir of a specified depth, and overlain with a transparent "slide cover"
- *Supravital stain* that is optional and is used to stain elements of the centrifuged sediment

The slides will vary in the number of specimen wells, the depth and surface area of each well, and the material used to construct the slides (materials must be completely clear and transparent for accurate descriptions and identification). In comparison with non-standardized methods still used by some, changes in methodology may require adjustment when transitioning from the old, traditional method of a plain microscope slide and a separate cover glass. The depth of the newer standardized slides will as a rule possess a reservoir of greater depth than the older method, requiring the laboratory professional to focus at several levels so the technical personnel can properly enumerate the cellular elements, in particular. Some of the slides also have an imbedded grid for those that wish even more standardization, a method which may require a calculation (Fig. 9.2). Regardless of the system employed, the CLSI guidelines require that the following factors be consistently observed by the facility employing a specific system.

- A consistent volume of at least 10 mL (CLSI recommends 12 mL, the volume required by most systems)
- Centrifugation time should be standardized, with 5 min being the norm for most methods
- Centrifugation speed should be an RCF (*relative centrifugal force*) of approximately 400 g (gravities); most documents recommend a range of 400–450 g's.

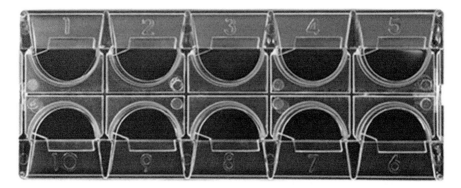

Fig. 9.2 Standardized slide for identification and enumeration of urinary sediment

Box 9.2: Calculations for Relative Centrifugal Force
$RCF = 1.118 \times 10^5 \times$ radius in centimeters $\times$ rpm^2

When necessary, the g's can be calculated from the distance (radius) between the center of the centrifuge shaft to the bottom of the well that holds the specimen tube. *RCF* is dependent on the speed of rotation in rpm and the distance of the particles from the center of rotation. *RCF* can be calculated by using the *formula* in Box 9.2 Centrifuges should be calibrated routinely. Use of the braking system will dislodge sediment prior to decanting the liquid portion of the sample and should not be used. Corrections for differences in length of the arms of the centrifuge to RCF or relative centrifugal force of 400 is accomplished by the formula in Box 9.2.

- Dilution factor based on the volume of the mixed sample before centrifugation and the final volume of liquid containing the sedimentary button
- Volume of sample is contained in the well over which a transparent covering is designed. The volume to be analyzed is calculated by figures based on the volume of sediment on the slide, the area of the cover slide and the diameter of the microscope objective used to view the sediment and the concentration of the dilution factor of the initial and the final volume of specimen
- Reporting of results should use the same criteria for reporting format as well as consistent reference ranges against which actual derived values are measured

Normally, few or no formed elements will be found in a normal urine sample except for a small number of *squamous epithelial cells* that are found in the urine of females. The main constituents of interest in the microscopic examination of urine and other body fluids include several types of blood cells. Renal epithelial cells originate in the convoluted tubules of the kidney, and increased numbers of these cells may be found in some renal diseases and in particular tubular injury. White blood cells, or leukocytes, indicate a disease process in most instances when they are increased in number. An increased number of *polymorphonuclear* neutrophils is often indicative of a bacterial infection. *Mononuclear* white cells, either monocytes or lymphocytes may be a result of infections by other organisms. Cells found in the urine and other body fluids will include erythrocytes, leukocytes, sperm, yeasts, fungi, and one-celled organisms termed as parasites.

9.9   Microscopic Examination of the Urine

Following the physical or macroscopic examination of the urine sample as well as that of other significant body fluids, the results of these clinical findings will normally correlate with the microscopic entities found in the centrifuged sediment of urine. Biological components are also called organized components, a term meaning that they may be a part of the tissues of the body, including blood cells, epithelial cells, and invading organisms such as bacteria, molds, yeast and fungi, as well as certain parasites, may be found in the sample. When spermatozoa are found in the urine of a male, inflammation of the prostate gland should be evaluated. But when spermatozoa are present in the urine of a female, they will not be reported unless it is specifically required due to legal circumstances such as alleged rape.

Only a few constituents will most often be found in the urine but in certain medical conditions, abnormal analytes and increases in elements that are normally present in only small numbers may be evident. Chemical components of a urine sample which are tested for by chemical test strips are based on waste products which are those originating from the metabolic functions of the body. These may be referred to as unorganized sediment that in addition to metabolic constituents as well as waste product, but also include crystals that form as a result of the presence of certain chemicals, usually in excess, and certain conditions that lead to the formation of crystals. Abnormal crystals may be formed due to metabolic errors that may be a result of serious hereditary conditions. Others may be iatrogenic, meaning they are acquired as a result of medical procedures such as administering of drugs.

The careful examination of a centrifuged urine and of other body fluids (usually uncentrifuged) will provide evidence leading to the diagnosis of a variety of kidney and urinary tract diseases. The study of the sediment may also indicate the presence of metabolic disorders that are hereditary and systemic conditions. Microscopic elements may originate from a variety of body sites, ranging from the blood, the kidney, the lower urinary tract and even from environmental sources. In order to control costs, many medical facilities do not perform a microscopic examination of all urine samples, when the physical and chemistry portions of the urinalysis are negative. It should be remembered that quality control and standardization of microscopic reports are important to insure accurate and meaningful results.

9.9.1   Commonly Encountered Elements of Urine Sediment

The following forms are representative of significant findings, when present in increased levels, may reveal the presence of disease. Normal numbers of these forms may be found in most specimens and are insignificant. Others are incidental to the collection of the specimen, and are sometimes confusing for the new laboratory professional or student. It should be remembered that the significance of numbers for body fluids other than for urine will be different, and in some cases none at all should be present. Some formed elements will be reported as numbers per low power field (LPF) and others will be reported as numbers per high power field (HPF). The terms *LPF* and *HPF* refer to the power of the objective used for examining the urinary sediment. LPF indicates that the 10-power objective is used, and HPF indicates use of the 40-power objective.

The presence of cellular components of urine and body fluids, both red and white blood cells, may provide a useful clue that could confirm or dismiss certain diagnoses of the urinary tract (Table 9.3). Other cells such as those originating in the kidneys, the tubules and the bladder, as well as those lining the ureters and urethra, are likely of diagnostic value.

Table 9.3   Microscopic cellular components of urine and body fluids

Component	Normal values	Identification	Clinical significance
White blood cells (Leukocytes)	0–5/HPF	Enhanced by addition of dilute acetic acid is done to enable cellular structures such as nuclear morphology and granules in the cytoplasm. Some white cells are called "glitter cells" as they tend to absorb water and the granules of the cytoplasm reveal "Brownian" movement. Cells with a single round nucleus may be lymphocytes, and those with segmented nuclei are neutrophils	Typically morphonuclear neutrophils are the most significant of leukocytes In pyuria, or infections of the urinary tract, leukocytes may move by amoeboid movement (*diapedesis*) through tissues to site of infection or inflammation Also present in glomerulonephritis, cystitis, prostatitis, and urethritis
Squamous epithelial cells	Few/LPF (enumerated as few, moderate or many)	Most numerous of the epithelial cells, these large flat cells with a single distinct nucleus, no larger than a red blood cell, line the urethra and the genitourinary system. It is not unusual to find a small number of these cells in a urine specimen, but sometimes abnormal forms are found	In substantial numbers may indicate a contaminated specimen

Table 9.3 (continued)

Component	Normal values	Identification	Clinical significance
Clue cells (squamous epithelial cells)	None	Clue cells are squamous epithelial cells from the vaginal region that are coated with a short bacterial rod called *Gardnerella vaginalis*	Cytoplasm of some squamous epithelial cells have inclusions of hyaline granules that may appear as bacteria adhering to the surface are will not be indicative of any infectious disorder as are true clue cells
Transitional epithelial cells	Usually not found in significant numbers (few/hpf) but are increased in urinary tract infections	Transitional epithelial cells are slightly smaller than squamous epithelial cells and may be round with a tail-like structure or may be pear-shaped. They have the ability to absorb large amounts of water	These cells assume varying shapes and are indicate and involvement of the renal pelvis, bladder, and upper urethra
Renal epithelial cells	Normally found only in small numbers (few/HPF) in the normal urine sample	Renal epithelial cells are also called renal tubular cells and are smaller and rounder than transitional epithelial cells. In addition, the nuclei will cover more of the cytoplasmic portion of the cell than in squamous and transitional epithelial cells	Renal epithelial cells are the most significant as they indicate tubular *necrosis* and are important in graft rejection of transplanted kidneys
Red blood cells	0–2/HPF	In unstained specimens, red blood cells (RBCs) appear as pale and biconcave discs that have no nucleus. Dilute urine will cause RBCs to appear as colorless circles (ghost cells) and hypertonic urine will cause crenation of the RBC, where the surface appears to be covered with spikes	Red blood cells in the urine should correlate with the chemistry results for blood. Other procedures may be necessary to determine the lack of RBCs in the urine when the chemical test strip is positive, or vice versa. Usually glomerular damage results in the presence of microscopic RBCs, or damage to vascular tissue as in renal calculi (stones). The abnormal shape of RBCs is called *dysmorphia* and would indicate a referral for cytology by a pathologist

9.9.2   Quantification of White and Red Blood Cells

Only a semi-quantitative count of blood cells is necessary in most instances. When performing a manual microscopic examination, components of the urine are enumerated using at least a ten low-power (LPF) or high-power objective (HPF) objective. Crystals, mucus, and bacteria are quantified per field of view

Table 9.4 Semi-quantitative descriptions for field of view

Terms and descriptions for elements per FOV		
Term		Description
Rare	1+	Present but not present in each field
Few	1+	One or more present in most fields of view (FOV)
Moderate	2+	Relatively easy to find, but number varies between FOV's
Many	3+	Large numbers present in all fields
Packed	4+	FOV is overcrowded with cells touching each other

(FOV) in somewhat descriptive terms (Table 9.4). Terms and definitions of elements and their estimated numbers are decided by each laboratory. Red and white blood cells along with casts are reported as a range of the formed elements viewed, for instance, 0–2, 3–5, or 6–10). These numbers are *averages* determined from viewing several fields as determined by each respective laboratory. It may be necessary to use a higher power of magnification for definitive identification, but constituents counted are reported as a number per low power (LPF). These parameters are established for providing consistency of reporting as an intralaboratory policy.

Two factors must be considered during a microscopic examination. The values determined per FOV is dependent upon the optical power lenses used and the volume of sediment/liquid mixture, determined by the volume for the particular standardized microscopic slide used. The greater the size of the FOV, the greater the number of components that will be viewed. So for reproducibility within the laboratory with more than one microscope used for urine sediment evaluation, the diameters and depths of the FOV's called ocular field numbers require consistency upon microscope and slides used. For correlations with automated microscopy systems, each laboratory should report urine sediment numbers as the number present per volume of urine and not as a value per low- or high-power field. It is possible to convert the number of elements observed per low- or high-power field to the value present per milliliter of urine tested.

It may be necessary to enhance elements observed in urine for characteristics difficult to see using the brightfield microscope. Several stains in common use when visualization and differential identification is necessary are often of inestimable value when preliminary identification leaves doubt (Table 9.5). An additional tactic to aid in identification of low-refractile elements is the simple process of changing the type of microscopy. Using a lower illumination level or the use of phase microscopy or special stains may be required and could mean the difference of 'missing' an element that could lead to a quick diagnosis for the physician.

Table 9.5 Techniques for visualization of microscopic urine sediment

Techniques	Features
2% acetic acid	Enhances leukocyte and epithelial cell nuclei
Fat stains (Sudan III)	Stains neutral fat such as triglycerides, confirmation of fat bodies
Prussian blue	Identifies hemosiderin (iron) as free crystals or in cells and casts
Dilute toluidine blue	Nuclear detail, differentiating WBC's, renal tubular epithelial cells
Sternheimer-Malbin	Cast inclusions, hyaline casts and mucus
Phase-contrast microscopy	Enhances translucent or low-refractile elements
Gram stain	Identification of bacteria as gram positive or negative

9.10   Cast Formation

Casts are formed structures which may be of several types, and are the only elements found in the urinary sediment that are completely unique to the kidney (Table 9.6). This is due to their being formed in the tubules of the kidney. In order to correlate normal and pathological macroscopic and microscopic characteristics of elements encountered during the examination of urine sediment, the student must be able to identify casts correctly. Casts are formed due to a number of pathological conditions, although a few hyaline (clear) casts may be found in the urine samples from normal individuals.

Kidney tubules secrete mucoproteins that are proteins which are characterized by becoming gel-like during conditions where an acidic pH is present. Coupled with an increased solute concentration in the tubules and a sluggish urine flow through the nephrons, casts are able to form. When gelled, impressions of the contents of the tubules form these structures may be compared with the formation of fossils in the sediment in the earth when organisms have trapped and their body structures have been preserved. Any materials, usually organic, that are present in the tubules at the time where urine flow is decreased, becomes trapped in the casts that will incorporate any types of cells or other materials that are found in the tubules during a particular period of time. They are cylindrical in shape and are defined by their contents or size.

Some types of crystals may be normal and possess no clinical significance. Others may be abnormal and lead to diagnosis of metabolic disorders as well as the likelihood of urinary calculi (kidney stones) to form in the kidneys and associated organisms found in the urinary tract found in (Table 9.5). Many crystals frequently found in urine are seldom of clinical significance, as most are precipitated salts. When these crystals are subjected to changes in pH, temperature, or concentration, the patterns of solubility may change, giving clues to their identity (Table 9.7).

Table 9.6 Casts in urine and body fluids

Type of cast	Frequency	Components of cast	Causative condition
Hyaline casts	0–2/LPF	As the most frequently seen cast, the hyaline casts contain a globulin called Tamm-Horsfall and are not detected by the protein portion of the urine test strip	This cast may be present in significant numbers following a traumatic event where urine flow has been slowed, as in an accident. Although thought to be normal in small numbers the cast may be increased in acute glomerulonephritis, pyelonephritis, chronic renal disease, and congestive heart failure
RBC casts	None	RBC casts are red to orange-brown, due to hemoglobin derived from RBCs. Under certain conditions, RBC cases may appear as granular casts. Free RBCs are often observed along with the RBC casts	The presence of RBC casts indicate bleeding from the nephrons and is associated with glomerulonephritis. But any condition that damages glomerular basement membrane, tubules, or renal capillaries may cause production of RBC casts
WBC casts	None	White blood cell casts are somewhat difficult to visualize. They possess rounded ends and the contents of the casts may reveal intact WBCs. A clear matrix in which the WBCs are imbedded will aid in differentiating WBC casts from clumps of WBCs	WBC casts are found primarily in severe inflammation due to infection. Pyelonephritis, interstitial nephritis, nephritic syndrome, acute allergic reactions and post-streptococcal infections that may lead to destruction of the kidney tissues by an immune reaction will cause formation of WBC casts
Epithelial cell casts	None normally present	Epithelial cells that have been dislodged from tubular linings adhere to secretions from the tubules, and form the cast that contains a somewhat random arrangement of cells. Large round nuclei are visible with a decreased amount of cytoplasmic ratio when compared with the size of the nucleus	During a medical condition where clumps of epithelial are sloughed from the tubules may result in the formation of epithelial casts. A number of medical conditions may lead to the formation of epithelial casts. These conditions include infection by the viruses called cytomegalovirus and from those causing hepatitis. Acute tubular necrosis and the ingestion of toxins such as heavy metals, *salicylates* (aspirin), and antifreeze will result in the formation of these casts

Table 9.6   (continued)

Type of cast	Frequency	Components of cast	Causative condition
Granular casts	None normally seen	Granular casts are called finely granular and coarsely granular. Originally, where blood cells, in particular WBCs disintegrated and were visible only as granules enmeshed in a protein matrix of secretions from the tubules, they were known as coarsely granular casts. In those called finely granular casts, it is believed that renal tubular cells, as they disintegrate, form finely granular casts Terminology used today is chiefly that of granular and finely granular casts	Compared with the presence of other casts, the second-most common type of cast found in the urine is that of granular casts. These casts result either from the breakdown of cellular casts and the inclusion of aggregates of plasma proteins such as albumin or immunoglobulin light chains. Depending on the size of the inclusions, they can be classified as finely or coarsely granular, but the distinction between the two has little or no diagnostic value. Their appearance is generally more cigar-shaped and more highly refractive than found in hyaline casts. These casts are most often indicative of chronic renal disease, and as with hyaline casts, can also be seen for a short time following strenuous exercise
Waxy casts	None normally seen	Waxy casts are characterized by further deterioration than those of the granular variety. The protein becomes brittle and fractures easily in the manner in which a sheet of wax breaks, hence the name. Edges and ends of casts may become serrated (sharp edges) and will have an opaque surface	Waxy casts are found in extreme cases of renal disease, where chronic renal disease has led to chronic renal failure. The presence of these casts indicates tubular obstruction where urine flow has practically ceased. Waxy casts are included in a general term called "broad" casts, to indicate a wider cast originating from a dilated tubule and is seen chiefly in chronic renal failure
Fatty casts	None normally seen	These casts are hyaline casts with fat globules incorporated in the matrix. They are usually yellowish to tan in color and in the presence of cholesterol, may exhibit a "Maltese cross" sign when viewed with polarized light	Patients with nephritic syndrome will excrete large amounts of urinary protein. These casts may form with extreme cell death of the epithelial cells for a variety of reasons as well as in the disease called *systemic lupus erythematosus* (SLE) where organic-specific immune action is directed toward the kidneys, and diabetic nephropathy may result in the formation of fatty casts. Lipiduria is always considered as being clinically significant

Table 9.7 Microscopic components of urine and body fluids normal crystals found in acid urine

Crystal	pH of urine	Shape and color	Distinguishing features
Uric acid	Low pH	Yellow to reddish-brown; shapes vary from whetstone shape, thick cubes, rhombic prism forms, small rectangles, large barrel-shaped forms, elongated lemon-shaped, six-sided plates resembling cystine crystals	Heating to at least 60 °C will cause crystals to dissolve; glacial acetic acid will also dissolve uric acid crystals
Amorphous urates	Acid	Pinkish to smoky red, very small and shapeless crystals	Heating to at least 60 °C will cause crystals to dissolve; 10% sodium hydroxide will dissolve crystals
Calcium oxalate dihydrate (common form)	Acid or alkaline urine	Colorless envelope-like form	Soluble in dilute hydrogen chloride
Calcium oxalate monohydrate (less common)	Acid or alkaline urine	Colorless, and may assume oval shape, rectangular or dumbbell shaped	Solubility at pH of 8–8.5 in solution buffered with EDTA
Monosodium urates (uncommon)	Acid	May appear as amorphous (without shape) precipitate or as slender needle shapes	

Table 9.8 Microscopic components of urine and body fluids normal crystals found in alkaline urine

Crystal	pH of urine	Shape and color	Distinguishing features
Amorphous phosphates	7.5 or greater	Colorless to pale gray amorphous (shapeless) and "pebbly" granules	Insoluble with heat, soluble in glacial acetic acid
Triple phosphates	Alkaline or neutral	Somewhat colorless and shapeless granules that contain calcium, magnesium	Soluble with glacial acetic acid
Calcium phosphate	Alkaline	Colorless and prism-shaped or may appear as rosettes and rarely as flat plates	Combined with calcium, magnesium; soluble with glacial acetic acid
Ammonium biurate	Alkaline	Dark tones of yellow or brown urates often found in older specimens from hours of standing	Soluble with acid and heat
Calcium carbonate (uncommon)	Alkaline	Colorless and occurs as tiny spheres (balls) and in pairs or "fours" that resemble crosses	Soluble in glacial acetic acid; effervesces (bubbles) during the reaction

Since some crystals are appear under normal conditions, they are not indicative of any particular pathological condition. The pH of the urine is the most contributory factor establishing the compositions and appearance of certain crystals. Crystals found in alkaline urine are normal and often occur with no significance as to and disease process (Table 9.8). But it should be remembered that certain conditions causing alkalosis of the urine may be attributed to other conditions that are not normal, such as that of a bacterial infection of the urinary tract that results in urine with an alkaline pH.

There are relatively few crystals that are formed because of errors in the metabolism of certain amino acids. Other crystals form due to the administration of certain medications, in which the metabolic constituents of the drug form as crystals (Table 9.9). Those that form as a result of treatment are known as iatrogenic in origin. These types are found following administration of the antibiotics ampicillin and those of the sulfonamide class. Antiretroviral therapy may also result in urinary crystals, and contrast media used in radiographic procedures may cause elongated, flat crystals when administered intravenously and in other types such as retrograde infusion for studies of abnormalities of the

Table 9.9 Abnormal crystals of metabolic errors and drug administration found in urine

Crystal	pH of urine	Shape and color	Distinguishing features
Cystine	Acid	Colorless with transparent and often refractile crystals that are six-sided plate like structures of varying thickness that will affect polarization of light	Qualitative test called Brand's test, provides confirmation for presence of cystine in urine. The addition of fresh sodium cyanide formed from sodium nitroprusside to a sample of urine produces a stable red to purple color in the presence of cystine
Leucine	Acid	Yellow, circular structures with concentric or radial striations	Separation through tests that separate amino acids
Tyrosine	Acid	Generally colorless but may appear to be black when focusing; shapes are often similar to fine needles radiating from the center or rosettes	Orange to wine color is produced when urine is added to nitrosonaphthol solution in presence of leucine
Bilirubin	Acid	Yellowish brown and needles without consistent shape; may appear as fragments but the color is characteristic	When uric acid crystals are present, they may be colored by bilirubin
Hemosiderin	Acid/ neutral	Golden brown granules, free floating in clumps; may be found in cells and casts	Rarely found but following hemolytic even; confirmed tithe Prussian blue stain
Sulfonamides	Acid	Yellow to brown in structure that are characteristic for the type of drug administered; may assume shape of uric acid, urates and biurate crystals	Heat and acid will hydrolyze the crystals; diazo (double-bonded nitrogen) reagent will react with crystals to form a magenta hue
Radiographic dye	Acid	Form varies with drug administered; flat, elongated rectangular plates	Elevated specific gravity of urine containing these dyes; precipitation test for protein may yield false positive results for cholesterol crystals

salivary gland (experimental at this time). It is important to determine the origin of these crystals before the determination of a metabolic disease can be established.

9.10.1 Bacteria and Yeasts

Bacteria are not normally present in urine but may be observed when an acute medical condition such as cystitis is present. Bacteria are not considered important when seen during a microscopic examination of the urine except where urine specimens are collected under sterile conditions. Bacterial contamination is often seen when a specimen is randomly collected without prepping the urethral opening of the patient, particularly in female patients. Bacteria are most often reported only when WBC's accompany them and when urinary tract infections are present. When urine specimens contain more than six squamous epithelial cells/hpf, specimens should be rejected and then recollected, as they are not suitable for bacterial culture or for microscopic analysis.

For body fluids other than urine, bacteria seen on a microscopic examination may be clinically significant as many of these fluids are collected by sterile needle aspiration and should not contain contaminants found on the skin. In addition, for certain body fluids, only a few organisms may be important in determining the need for a bacterial culture. In a specimen such as cerebrospinal fluid (CSF), the finding of a few bacterial organisms would warrant aggressive treatment due to the sensitivity of the central nervous system (CNS) to infection. Identification of the bacterial species is accomplished by culturing the specimen on a Petri dish containing a nutrient agar (a gel) that enables chemical testing of the individual colonies for specific ID. An antibiotic sensitivity may also be performed to determine the antibiotic that is capable of eliminating the infection.

Yeast cells may be seen in specimens from patients with diabetes and women with vaginal *moniliasis*, which is also known by the term, *candidiasis*. The most common yeast that infects humans is that of *Candida albicans*, an organism also known for causing "*thrush*" in infants. Thrush occurs in infants who have been on antibiotic therapy most commonly, in which case the normal bacterial flora of the mouth has been artificially altered. Women often contract a yeast infection of *C. albicans* when normal vaginal flora has been altered by antibiotics or by douching. The organism is also considered a sexually transmitted disease (STD). In addition, those patients under treatment with steroids may encounter infections by yeast, including those with underlying diseases that negatively impact the immune system.

The presence of yeast is often established by microscopically examining a specimen from the affected area of the body by direct visualization. Scrapings from the mouth or other affected areas are placed on a slide with a small amount of saline, if necessary. *C. albicans* will grow rapidly, producing buds that are readily visible. It is easy to confuse the individual yeast cells with red blood cells, but the yeast cells are generally a bit smaller, and red blood cells do not multiply by budding.

Candidiasis can occur in almost any area of the body, and when it becomes systemic, it is difficult to eradicate.

Sediment stains are used to increase the differentiation of structures leading to identification of cells and ease of visualizing them. Some elements found in urine sediment, particularly some that are artifacts of no biological origin do not absorb stains. Crystal violet and safranin O are used in conjunction with each other in a number of commercial stains available from biological supply distributors. The most common brands for general use in urinalysis procedures are those of KOVA, which also provides a complete system for urinalysis procedures, and is manufactured by Hycor Biomedical of Garden Grove, CA. Another is that of Sedi-stain, produced by Becton-Dickinson of Parsippany, NJ. Other specific stains used would include a 0.5% toluidine blue solution for the differentiation of white blood cells and renal tubular epithelial cells but is also used for examination of cells found in other body fluids. Two percent acetic acid is used to better define nuclear morphology in white blood cells but is not used where red blood cells must be enumerated, since they will be destroyed. Hansel stain is a methylene/eosin Y stain that is useful in determining the presence of eosinophils (type of white blood cell) found in the urine. This phenomenon makes acetic acid useful, however, where large numbers of RBCs would obscure the visualization and enumeration of white blood cells. (Table 9.10) condenses the staining characteristics of these and other stains used for specific purposes.

9.10.2 Artifacts

The term "artifacts" is a general term for small particles that may be confused with urinary elements that may be medically significant. Many of the artifacts found in urine are preanalytical, meaning that they usually come from contaminants resulting from specimens that are collected in dirty containers. The most common artifacts include the following:

Table 9.10 Characteristics of particular stains

Types of stain	Purpose	Characteristics
Gram stain	Enables basic differentiation of bacteria (gram positive or negative)	Used for identification of bacteria in urinary casts
Crystal violet/ safranin O	Provides contrast between nuclei of various blood and body cells	Aids in identifying white blood cells, casts and epithelial cells
Toluidine blue	Distinguishes nuclear characteristics	Differentiates renal tubular cells from white blood cells
Sudan III, oil red	Valuable in staining of fat-based elements (neutral fats, triglycerides)	Stains cells and casts containing lipids and suspended free fat droplets
Prussian blue	Stains any ferrous (iron) inclusions	Yellow-brown clumps of hemosiderin (blood iron) may be found in casts and cells such as phagocytes

Fig. 9.3 Starch or talcum powder granules often found in urine

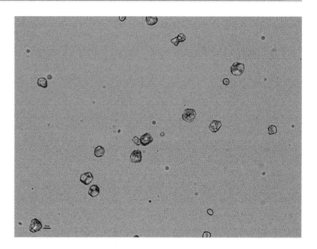

9.10.2.1   Starch or Talcum Powder Granules

These items appear as irregularly shaped spheres with indented centers. The presence of these artifacts is usually the result of the use of body powder, but may also occur through handling of supplies, specimens and equipment when wearing powdered latex gloves.

These items can be easily confused with cholesterol droplets since both appear as elements said to be birefringent and that polarize in a pattern that is similar to Maltese crosses. Starch granules are best identified by use of a brightfield microscope and are a somewhat rounded particle with a centrally-located dimple or radiating, striated slits extending from the central depression found in each granule (Fig. 9.3). Recent research seems to indicate an increased risk of cancer of female reproductive organs with prolonged use of talcum powder, but this link has not been completely agreed upon by medical authorities.

9.10.2.2   Pollen Grains

Pollen grains are uniquely shaped based on the type of plant from which they originate. These microscopic elements will present in a variety of shapes and forms and will have a singularly well-defined and thick cell wall, but are easily confused with the eggs of parasites, particularly when examined by inexperienced microscopists. Pollen grains will be found frequently in urine during the growing seasons as an environment contaminant. Since pollen grains are found on a seasonal basis for many plants, they may be of a predominant type during certain specific periods of time, leading to easier identification if necessary. They often look like crystals with parallel and concentric circles, are very large, and may appear as being out of focus even when other urine elements are in focus.

9.10.2.3   Hair and Fibers

Many kinds of fibers such as hair and fabric threads appear in the urine. However, hair and fibers have very dark, harsh-looking outlines (casts have outlines that blend

Fig. 9.4 Plant fiber such as cotton

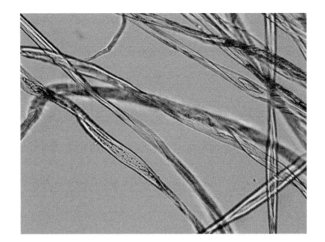

into the background). They are often moderately *refractile* and may be large. Fibers are flat (casts are cylindrical) with thicker margins (casts are thicker in the middle) (Fig. 9.4). Fibers will polarize light rays but casts are not known to do so. A beginning microscopist often confuses hair and fibers of all types with *casts*.

9.10.2.4 Debris from Diaper

Baby diapers of the disposable type are composed of a variety of materials. Some of these materials will break down into shapeless pieces of material when exposed to the urine for an extended span of time. The materials appear as elongated fibers that show birefringence with polarized light. The presence of diaper debris is an unusual finding and may require elimination as a pathological particle when encountered since it may strongly resemble waxy casts and thus confused with them.

9.10.2.5 Air Bubbles

This type of artifact will be visualized as an almost perfect circle with a dark rim around the circular structure. The bubble most often has no inclusions within the boundaries of the bubble, and they are highly refractile and are most often introduced onto the microscope slide during the process of pipetting the sample into the wells before examining them.

9.10.2.6 Fat Body (Oval Fat Bodies)

Fat bodies, which are often called oval fat bodies, are not artifacts in the strictest sense, as they may be a pathological finding. Oval fat bodies are cells that contain birefringent (split ray of light into two rays) fat droplets incorporated into their cytoplasm. When viewed under low power, the oval fat bodies may appear as large brown spots (sometimes almost black) elements due to a brownish pigmented fat that comprises the makeup of the droplets. These cells are usually seen concurrently with high levels of protein in the urine.

Fat droplets may arise from the degeneration of membranes found within the cytoplasm that separate various functioning units of the cells. This demonstration of fatty degeneration is frequently observed when certain metabolic diseases are present. Although the testing of urine samples should be done shortly after collection, if the specimen is stored for a few days, cells containing fat droplets will develop as vacuoles within the cytoplasm of the cell. Phagocytosis by specialized cells called phagocytes may occur, where oil droplets are intracellularly visible from the digestion of materials from cells and organisms along with chemical constituents that have been ingested by these cells. These cytoplasmic oil droplets are broken down by specialized structures found within the cells that are called lysosomes.

For the identification of oval fat bodies, a typical "Maltese cross" will appear when viewed by use of a microscope employing polarized light. This phenomenon of birefringence is due to a crystalline structural arrangement of the esterified cholesterol in a liquid crystal state and cholesterol-free droplets will not be birefringent. It is also easy to perform another simple technique in which the fat droplets are commonly stained with a fat stain such as Sudan, Fat Red 7B, as well as by other stains that are commercially available. However, staining with Sudan stains may produce errors in the interpretation of oval fat bodies, since some degenerated cells may stain in a pattern similar to that of oval fat bodies.

9.10.2.7   Oil Bubbles or Droplets

Frequently, these artifacts will be the result of the use of vaginal creams, mineral oils, bath oils, and even from lubricants that are used to insert urinary catheters. Oil droplets are often confused with red blood cells and yeast cells, but sometimes are fat globules that originated during normal physiological functions of the body. For this reason, oil bubbles should be differentiated from fat globules. When lipiduria or presence of lipids (fats) in the body are determined, results should be correlated with the presence of oval fat bodies, fatty casts and protein in the urine. Oil will float on urine, which is composed primarily of water, so the bubbles may be chiefly found on the underside of the cover glass on standardized slides and on the bottom of the cover glass when using a basic cover slip. This requires an additional step in performing the examination of urine sediment, following the determination of other elements found in the urinary sediment, by focusing on several layers of the specimen.

9.10.2.8   Glass and Plastic Fragments

These artifacts arise from the manufacturing process for collection and testing supplies. The elements are *pleomorphic* (many shapes and forms) and are somewhat colorless and highly refractile. Most pathogens, crystals, casts and even some artifacts will exhibit a similar appearance microscopically, while these bits of man-made materials will not be uniform when viewed as part of the urinary sediment.

> **Points to Remember**
> Proper collection of the urine sample and the handling and storage of the specimen are absolutely vital to obtaining accurate results. Standardized procedures for collecting and concentrating the samples for microscopic identification of a variety of elements will result in values that are clinically useful for diagnosis and treatment.

9.11 Summary

The microscopic examination of urine and the other major body fluids often correlates with the physical and chemical findings and may be the single most important step in the evaluation of body fluids. For obtaining accurate and useful results, a standard approach is required by using a system designed to improve the collection and processing of results. The thoughtful and proper collection techniques, the preparation of the patient for the procedure, and the storage of specimens that will not be immediately processed are important links in the laboratory's ability to provide meaningful values leading to diagnosis and treatment.

Standardization of the concentration procedure for the examination of urinary sediment includes the correct volume of sample and the proper centrifugation and chambering of the sediment. Professional organizations including the Clinical and Laboratory Standards Institute contribute to the development of standards leading to accurate testing and reporting. Formed elements of the urine and other body fluids vary with the particular body fluid being analyzed.

Except for the types of cells or items such as casts or crystals that are being quantitated and the dilution factors used, if any, the procedure when using the hemocytometer for counts per volume of body fluid is the same. When used carefully and when the steps of the procedure are followed, the resultant counts are quite accurate.

Case Study 9.1
Red and white blood cells, and particularly casts, will disintegrate quickly in a dilute sample. Refrigeration will slow the rate of destruction but cooling of the specimen also contributes to the formation of amorphous phosphate deposition in alkaline specimens and amorphous urates in acid specimens.

A 38-year-old female is a patient at the local hospital and was admitted for severe lower back pain and difficulty in voiding. Urine production had been scant for some time, but the patient was busy and had not made the effort to seek medical attention. A urine sample was collected by the nurse who had responsibility for the woman's care, and she was busy that day with several other critically ill patients. Urinalysis results revealed the following findings.

Urinalysis Results Report, Case Study 9.1

Physical appearance		
Color	Dark yellow	
Character	Cloudy	
Chemical screening		
Leukocyte esterase	Positive	
Nitrite	Negative	
Urobilinogen	Normal	
Protein (test strip)	Positive 2+	Confirmed by SSA precipitation
pH	8.0	
Blood	Positive	
Specific gravity	1.030	
Ketone	Negative	
Bilirubin	Negative	
Glucose	Negative	
Sediment evaluation		
Squam epithelials	Occasional	
Renal epithelials	0	
Erythrocytes	Rare	
Leukocytes	Negative	
Casts	0	
Crystals	4+ amorphous	
Bacteria	0	
Other (specify)	0	

1. What are the abnormal values found in this report?
2. What could contribute to the turbidity of the sample?
3. Explain the presence of the amorphous crystals.
4. What would be the most likely reason for the disparity in the chemical analysis and the microscopic findings? Please explain fully.

Review Questions

1. In the examination of urine sediment, which of the following would be the most prominent indicator of *early* renal disease?
   a. Red blood cells
   b. Aminoaciduria
   c. White blood cells
   d. Uric acid crystals

2. Which of the following statements would not be true regarding findings in urinary sediment?
   a. The presence of white blood cells indicates an infectious process in most cases
   b. Bacteria is always found microscopically in cases of cystitis
   c. The presence of bacteria indicated an active bacterial infection
   d. The presence of nitrites indicates the presence of white blood cells
3. Those suffering from the nephritic syndrome will always exhibit:
   a. Edema of tissues
   b. Albumin in the urine
   c. Lipids in the urine
   d. Elevated blood albumin
4. The most predictive of the severity of renal disease would be the presence of:
   a. White blood cells
   b. Bilirubinuria
   c. Waxy casts
   d. Hyaline casts
5. For confirming the presence of fat globules in the urine, which of the following would be included in completing the microscopic examination?
   a. Phase contrast microscopy
   b. Electron microscopy
   c. Staining with a Sudan stain
   d. Radiography of the kidneys
6. Renal epithelial cells originate from the:
   a. Bladder
   b. Urethra
   c. Ureters
   d. Collecting ducts
7. Urinary casts are formed in:
   a. The distal convoluted tubule and collecting ducts of nephrons
   b. The ureters
   c. The bladder
   d. None of the above

Answers Found in Appendix C

Procedures for Complete Urinalysis/ Confirmation Testing

10

Objectives

Upon completion of this chapter, the reader will be able to:

List the equipment and basic instrumentation of a urinalysis department that is not automated

Discuss the differences between microscopic and macroscopic components for a urine analysis

Relate the reasons for performing confirmatory tests when certain screening tests results are significant

Perform the physical and rapid chemical examinations within 20% accuracy after demonstration by instructor or preceptor

Complete the macroscopic, chemical, and microscopic examination of urine sediment, and record the results accurately

Ascertain the need for confirmatory tests for certain positive chemistry results

Perform basic confirmatory tests

10.1 Introduction

From an understanding of information presented in Chaps. 8 and 9, the procedure for a complete urine analysis and performance of confirmatory tests will complete the understanding by the student of the components of a complete evaluation of a urine sample. It should be remembered also that some information that is gained from a urinalysis utilizes similar processes for examining other body fluids. Some information in Chap. 10 will mirror to an extent that of Chaps. 8 and 9, but Chap. 10 relates to the practical use of that knowledge. Some of the information may appear repetitious, but is not identical. This is intentional in an attempt to reemphasize coverage of information found in earlier chapters. *Recall and review may be the best teacher!*

© Springer International Publishing AG, part of Springer Nature 2018
J. W. Ridley, *Fundamentals of the Study of Urine and Body Fluids*,
https://doi.org/10.1007/978-3-319-78417-5_10

Since the procedure is not a simple "how-to" explanation, references are made to clinical information presented earlier in this text. The student or practitioner should refer to narrative regarding identification of diagnostic findings and confirmation of a number of elements throughout this text. Testing personnel should remain aware of potential pitfalls involved with improper collection and handling of the specimen(s). It should also be understood that no single test is 100% error proof, and there are always variables involved with testing of which the knowledgeable laboratory professional should be aware. A brief summary from earlier study should insure proper groundwork has been laid for further learning and practical experience.

The urinary system plays a vital role in the maintenance of the body's health by excreting or reabsorbing certain constituents found in the blood for maintaining a healthy state of homeostasis. Metabolic conditions where excessive amounts of certain chemical components are found in the urine provide valuable insight into medical conditions perhaps of greater gravity than simple infections of the urinary organs and tissues. Therefore, a good understanding of the functions and physiology of the urinary system are necessary for the accurate assessment of a urine sample.

10.2   Relationship of Macroscopic to Microscopic Urine Sample Examination

Basic laboratory examinations are performed on almost all patients who have a medical appointment or an emergency visit for treatment, regardless of the symptoms and signs the patient exhibits. The complete urinalysis is one of these basic tests that is performed at one time or another on almost all patients. A urinalysis gives the physician or other category of medical practitioner such as a nurse practitioner or physician's assistant a "screening" test that may immediately indicate an ongoing or imminent disease process. An abnormal finding on a random urine specimen will often necessitate further testing and evaluation to rule out any number of diseases that cause changes in various systems of the body. This is particularly true for those designed to rid the body of excess water and waste products.

Sometimes metabolic end-point products that indicate genetic disorders or organ failure are detected during a routine urinalysis on rare occasions. But specific clues from an initial set of procedures may indicate need for further investigation. Clinical findings in the complete urinalysis may reveal a need for more specialized or specific tests not routinely performed in the general laboratory. These somewhat esoteric tests are sent to a reference laboratory equipped to perform specialized testing. Often a good screening of urine will reveal suspicious results that may lead to diagnoses not specifically related to the genitourinary system. A review of the renal system and the anatomy and physiology of the genitourinary system insures a thorough understanding of the role the kidneys play in health and disease. Just the "how to" knowledge of the steps in performing a simple laboratory test is insufficient for educating future professionals as effective clinical sleuths.

It is obvious that urine samples are relatively easier to collect as a body fluid than practically any other and the results may manifest many changes in the body by signaling problems with the functions of the body. Knowledge of the anatomy and physiology of the renal system will be helpful, yielding important information when performing basic tests using urine as the sample. While a large number of tests may be available, the most basic ones are presented here.

Specimens may be random, giving a snapshot of the current condition of the patient, but sometimes a more dilute sample may give erroneous results where the patient may be overhydrated. So it is sometimes necessary to collect an early morning sample that is concentrated. The laboratorian should be alert regarding this and other conditions capable of affecting the results that the attending physician might not be aware of. Dissemination of wrongful results that should be obvious to the observant testing personnel could delay or prevent diagnosis of a serious medical condition. Being observant would give a more accurate picture of a medical condition, including the presence of certain components that even in small amounts would be discovered in an unhealthy patient.

Other tests may require an accurate quantitative level of certain constituents of the urine that may require a timed specimen for a required number of hours, sometimes for a 24-h period. The results for the levels may require calculating totals for certain components based on the volume excreted. Certain hormones control blood formation and help to retain or excrete various ions (chemical components), and damage to the kidneys may affect the body's functions in many ways. Some specimens may require preservatives to prevent growth of bacteria or a change in the pH which might destroy components being tested for. Some of these conditions will be covered specifically in this textbook.

10.3   Rationale for Performing a Complete Urinalysis

The urinalysis is one of the most commonly used procedures for obtaining an overview of the health of a patient. Clinical findings in the urine lead to definitive diagnoses or clues to more challenging medical conditions. These test values are a tool for insuring adequacy or validity in the chosen therapeutic course of treatment. It is rare that anyone can escape a routine urinalysis when seeking medical care. Certain screening tests are performed by a variety of personnel, some of whom are not trained or educated in laboratory practice. Often a practitioner other than a lab professional is unaware of certain conditions where confirmation of results is necessary, or the possibility that results are either a false positive or false negative result with routine testing. When screening tests are performed by other than laboratory professionals, abnormal results should be referred to a licensed laboratory for further evaluation and confirmation.

A urine sample is comprised primarily of excess water, although a number of substances are found normally in small amounts are excreted through the urinary system. The level of concentration of these substances contributes to the determination as to the normality or abnormality of the test results. Chronic and acute conditions may be discovered through specialized tests performed on urine samples not covered during a routine urinalysis procedure, but results from a basic urinalysis may prompt further studies. Management of chronic conditions where kidney damage has occurred will require periodic testing of urine to insure a patient is receiving proper care. Testing of a urine sample should be performed on a fresh urine sample for optimum results.

However, if it is not possible to immediately evaluate a urine sample, appropriate preservatives or refrigeration may be used, which sometimes leads to further development of conditions that must be attributed to storage and preservation methods. As a precaution, preservatives may adversely affect test results, so the laboratorian must be aware of this potentiality. Many collection techniques for specialized tests must be tailored to the type of procedure to be performed, as some preservatives may cause the sample to be invalidated for some tests. Often, product inserts from test kits will provide information regarding interference with test results.

A great deal can be determined by an initial examination of a urine sample. The color and clarity of the sample is the first determination to be made. A scant specimen with a volume of only a few drops or mL's might be indicative of a medical problem. In addition to manual test procedures, large instruments such as the "Iris Yellow Eye" are utilized in the largest laboratories for urine examinations including both gross macroscopic and microscopic evaluations. Significant samples performed by this complex instrument require manual examination for confirmation of results. Three separate areas of evaluation for a complete urinalysis are required for a complete examination.

Macroscopic
1. Color
2. Foam
3. Volume
4. Character (turbidity, cloudiness, foam)
5. Specific gravity (by TS meter, urinometer or dipstick)

Chemical
1. Urine chemical concentrations of protein, glucose, ketones, bilirubin, blood, nitrite, urobilinogen, leukocyte esterase, and pH using methodology of Multistix or other brands of reagent strips
2. Confirmation of protein by sulfosalicylic acid
3. Ketones by Acetest tablet method
4. Bilirubin by Ictotest tablet method
5. Reducing substances by Clinitest tablet method

Microscopic
1. Preparation of concentrated sample for sediment evaluation
2. Examination for common microscopic components include
   Red and white blood cells
   Epithelial cells—squamous, renal and transitional

Casts—specify type
Microorganisms, bacterial, fungal, protozoal
Crystals—identification, either normal or abnormal forms
Artifacts and other identifiable components
Any other component not readily identified

10.4 Equipment and Supplies

Equipment and supplies must be suitable to the facility where testing occurs (Table 10.1). Some proprietary health care facilities purchase supplies and equipment in bulk and the individual facilities have little input toward types and brands of equipment and supplies required. Certain basic equipment and supplies vary little between facilities. For those facilities with large automatic urinalysis instruments, the following supplies should also be available for individual testing and confirmation in the event the automatic instrument becomes nonfunctional.

For listing the three components tested for in the urinalysis, physical characteristics, chemistry screen, and the microscopic analysis, the following sample report form is provided (Urinalysis Report Form 10.1). Results are recorded for the three areas of testing, and confirmatory tests are performed as appropriate. The previous information provided for these three levels of testing, in order to provide for accurate and valid results that are clinically significant.

The sample condition must first be evaluated prior to testing. This is the macroscopic portion of the three-part examination of urine for a complete analysis (Table 10.2). The macroscopic exam is sometimes used as a cost effectiveness measure where the physical examination of a sample does not require further testing if it meets established protocol. Others rely on the chemistry dipstick to determine if results warrant further testing. Abnormalities discovered during physical, macroscopic screening and chemistry analysis are sometime called *chemical sieving*, where samples that don't meet the parameters established by the laboratory for color, clarity, and certain positive chemistry results such as blood, protein, nitrite, leukocyte esterase and glucose are reported as normal. As the astute clinical laboratorian would readily deduce, it is possible that an occasional significant finding might be missed with this protocol in place. Certain

Table 10.1 Basic equipment and supplies

TS Meter or urinometer	Multistix reagent strips
Urine controls	Color charts—Multistix, Acetest, Ictotest, Clinitest
Transfer pipets, 5 ¾ inch size	3% sulfosalicylic acid
Acetest tablets and product insert	Ictotest tablets, absorbent pads and product insert
Clinitest tablets, tubes, product insert	Sediment system or microscope slides, cover slips

Table 10.2 Recommended physical evaluation of sample	Always use a *well-mixed* sample to insure consistency of the sample
	Use a clear plastic or glass collection container for viewing the clarity of the sample
	View the sample against a white background for observing any significant color
	Always use a consistent depth and volume of sample
	Use adequate and consistent lighting in room where testing is conducted

parasites could be present, as well and perhaps clue cells indicating vaginitis might be overlooked.

10.5   Points to Be Observed

Earlier information provided for components of the three parts of the complete urinalysis indicated the physical, chemical and microscopic analyses, are all important aspects for accuracy and it should again be stressed that the three areas should correlate. In some instances, the medical practitioner will only require a portion of the complete urinalysis. If the lab worker observes an abnormality not included in the request for testing, results should be relayed to the individual responsible for treating the patient. Brief discussions of each step in performing a complete urinalysis is outlined as an adjunct to more descriptive narratives of each of the three components provided in Chap. 8. The basic steps of a complete urinalysis, beginning with each step of the process, will be listed here. More specific information was included in previous chapters devoted to each of the three parts included in the procedure and should be included as an adjunct for completing the procedures provided here. Confirmatory tests are required to quantify the chemistry values or to insure the results are not the result of conditions that might yield false positive and false negative results and greatly reduces erroneous reports to the medical practitioner.

10.6   Physical Characteristics of Urine Samples

Physical characteristics are those initial observations for each urine sample tested. They are traits that can be detected by the basic senses of smell and sight. These are the only components tested using a portion of the five senses endowed upon humans in general. An exception occurs with use of the sense of taste, a vital portion of the physical examination of urine in ancient history. Almost everyone would agree pending further reserch that this portion of urine evaluation should be avoided currently.

10.6.1   Odor

Normal urine samples from well-hydrated patients will not possess an unpleasant odor. However, there is a slightly pungent odor to all normal specimens. Changes due to diseases, diet and infectious processes may impart a characteristic odor to the samples. *Urine odor is not normally noted on the urinalysis report form*, but may be used as additional signs that abnormalities may be present. However, not all urine samples that possess an unusual odor are abnormal, but those that do might alert the laboratorian to respond reasonably to his or her findings.

Unrefrigerated urine samples left at room temperature for some time may contain bacteria that degrade urea to ammonia. When a freshly voided urine sample emits a foul odor, it is generally attributed to bacterial infection. The urine of diabetic patients experiencing the metabolism of fats because of insulin deficits in the cells often exhibit a fruity odor, where ketones are produced in the breakdown of fat molecules used for energy when glucose is not available in the cells. Urine samples from newborns with a musty odor may signal presence of a genetic disease known as phenylketonuria, when there is a disruption in the metabolic pathway for the metabolism of phenylalanine. This condition must be reported to the physician or other health care professional for treatment, since mental retardation may ensure in short order. The presence of large amounts of ketones may also occur in starvation or those with anorexia nervosa, dieting, malnutrition, excessive exercise and vomiting perhaps accompanied with diarrhea.

Less common than phenylketonuria but no less important is that of a specific odor of the urine that resembles the sweet smell of maple syrup, and the disease if present is called Maple Syrup Urine Disease. Branched chains of the amino acids leucine, isoleucine, valine and alloisoleucine are all involved and when the condition is detected, usually in the first few weeks of life for the infant, a parent often notices the characteristic odor when changing the infant's diapers. However, some foods can produce abnormal odors that are not attributed to any disease. Ingestion of certain foods, particularly asparagus, garlic and others may impart an unusual odor after heavy intake of the foods. Odors other than those presented (Table 10.3) are of an unusual nature and should be reported, followed by further testing. Some descriptive odors of an unusual nature are: mousy; rancid; rotting fish; sweaty feet; or other odors that are quite noticeable.

Table 10.3 Common urine odors

Faintly aromatic	Normal odor
Ammonia like	Urine kept at room temperature for period of time
Fetid (acrid)	Infection of urogenital system
Sweet and fruity	Ketone development
Menthol odor	Ingestion of medications containing phenols

10.6.2 Color

The normal colors for urine samples range widely from pale yellow to amber but practically all are of some shade of yellow. Table 8.2, Chap. 8, gives more information relative to both normal and abnormal urine colors. Variations in color may be attributed to diseases, as well as to medications and diet. The hydration state (amount of water in urine) is important in evaluating the color of the sample. The pigment that produces the shades of yellow to amber is that of urochrome. The urochrome, a pigment that is derived pigment is derived from urobilin derived from the oxidation of urobilinogen, which in turn originates from bilirubin that is broken down by bacteria of the gut.

10.6.3 Appearance of Urine

The clarity or transparency of urine may yield clues to medical conditions that affect the urine and result from disease of the associated organs of the urinary system. Clear urine is generally considered to be free of solid constituents that may be suspended in the sample. When a urine sample is clear upon voiding but after standing at room temperature or upon refrigeration becomes cloudy, most often will be as a result of amorphous (without shape) crystals called sediment. The amorphous sediment is identified as to whether it is phosphates (alkaline) or urates (acid) due to the acidity or alkalinity of the sample. Substances contributing to the lack of clarity which is described as turbidity may be found as either pathologic or nonpathogenic upon further testing.

Samples may be cloudy or turbid as a result of disease processes (Table 10.4). The most commonly encountered reason for a cloudy specimen is that of the presence of increased levels of white blood cells (leukocytes). Bacterial infections usually are manifested by large numbers of white cells, and may frequently be

Table 10.4 Substances contributing to urine turbidity

Pathological condition	Non-pathological condition
RBC's and WBC's	Crystals—urates, phosphates, calcium oxalate
Bacteria in fresh, clean catch specimen	Squamous epithelial cells (even if numerous)
Yeast	Mucus, mucin
Trichomonas	Radiographic media
Renal epithelial cells	Semen with prostatic fluid[a]
Fats—Lipids	Contaminants—talcum powder or pollen
Abnormal crystals	Feces
Semen with prostatic fluid[a]	
Feces	
Calculi	
Mucoid pus	

[a]Possibility of being pathological or non-pathological

accompanied by increased numbers of red blood cells, due to bacteria that produce hemorrhagic reactions. Large numbers of red blood cells without leukocytes may be indicative of urinary calculi, also called kidney stones. In addition to red and white blood cells, epithelial cells and bacteria may cause turbidity of the samples, and large amounts of mucus may also cause a cloudy appearance. The presence of fats may cause a milky appearance in the urine.

10.6.4   Specific Gravity

The specific gravity refers to the relative concentration of solids that are dissolved in the urine. The specific gravity may be performed by use of a refractometer, where the urine sample is compared with air and its ability to refract light. The greater the level of dissolved constituents in the liquid, the greater the refractive index of the solution. The refractometer has an internal scale that is also capable of measuring the total protein of blood serum or plasma (Fig. 10.1).

Another method uses a simple device called a urinometer containing a flotation device to determine the specific gravity and compares the concentration of urine with that of pure water. In healthy individuals, the specific gravity and the osmolality of a specimen should correlate with respect to relative values obtained. In a diseased individual with kidney damage, correlation is usually non-existent. The urinometer is calibrated at 1.000, and the specific gravity of urine samples will fall somewhere on a scale from just above 1.000 up to 1.030 for normal urine samples. The density of urine, when measured by specific gravity by urinometer, is determined by dividing the density of urine by the density of an equal volume of pure water (Eq. 10.1). It should be remembered that the specific gravity as measured by a refractometer through dividing the density of the sample versus air and not water, so a slight difference may exist between the two methods.

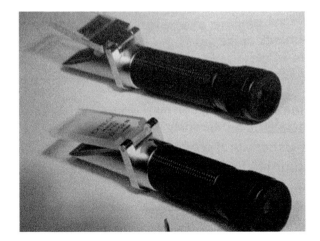

Fig. 10.1 Two similar types of refractometer, or total solids meter

Equation 10.1 Measurement of SG by Urinometer

Specific gravity (SG) = Density of urine / density of equal volume of pure water

Fig. 10.2 A refractometer scale that measures both urine protein and that of blood serum

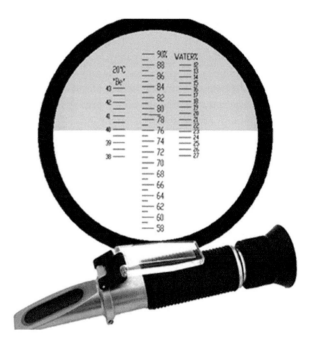

The urine dipstick method is used merely for screening large numbers of samples, and chiefly measures the amount of ions that are dissolved in the urine sample. These ions that are charged solutes include sodium, chloride, potassium and ammonium ions. Values obtained by the three methods for measuring the specific gravity of urine will vary significantly. For specific medical conditions, one method of determining the specific gravity of the urine, either by refractometer or by urinometer, should be used, as the dipstick method is an estimate only (Figs. 10.1, 10.2, and 10.3). A refractometer is designed to measure the specific gravity at 20° C.

10.7   Chemical Analysis of Urine, Strip Reaction Times

Since several major manufacturers of reactive "dipsticks" provide simplicity and ease of screening, detection of metabolic and infectious diseases is readily available. The information provided in this section generally adheres to the

Fig. 10.3 Urinometer, a special glass cylinder with flotation device

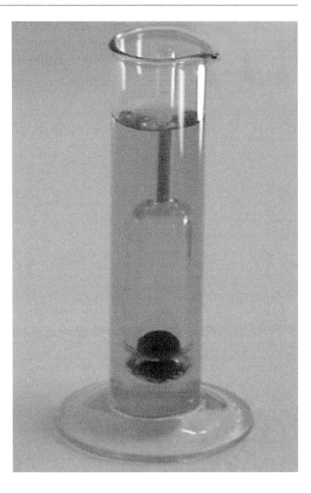

specifications for testing based on the Bayer Multistix 10 SG brand of test strips. Varying numbers of tests are available on these strips, with the most comprehensive types containing at least ten separate tests. The chemically treated pads on these strips react with somewhat specific analytes and provide a color change in the presence of the components of the urine that are being tested.

In some situations the results from these strips may be inaccurate due to the presence of other chemicals or sample conditions and must be confirmed by other tests before being reported to the physician or other practitioner. For instance, a pH of 8.0, a highly alkaline state, will produce a false positive value for protein. The sensitivity of these pads is adjusted to prevent reporting certain constituents that occur in urine samples in low levels. The confirmatory tests are performed by a variety of methods that are more specific for the particular component for which a positive or abnormal result was obtained.

Use of these strips, and knowledge of the chemical principles of the strips, must be observed and adhered to carefully for accurate results. Basic tests found in the strips are discussed individually as follows. Note that the test order is conformed to the time required for the various reactions, and ranges from the first constituent, glucose, that requires a 30 s time period, to the last, leukocyte esterase, a process that requires 2 min for a complete reaction. When complex systems are used, or a simple test strip reader, the reaction times are programmed into the instruments.

Glucose

Reaction time: 30-s before reaction is complete.

Test Strip Reactants: The enzymes, glucose oxidase and peroxidase, are imbedded in the test pad and will react specifically for glucose. Chromogens or chemicals that provide color to the reaction are visually observed in the presence of glucose. Urine samples from normal individuals do not contain measurable amounts of glucose.

Clinical Data: Glycosuria, the term used for high levels of glucose in the urine, is based on the amount of glucose "spilled" into the urine through the glomeruli, where the threshold level of glucose that can be reabsorbed by the kidneys is exceeded. High levels of plasma glucose results in an elevated specific gravity in the voided specimen. Diabetes mellitus is the most common medical condition where this condition occurs, although others such as gestational diabetes and some other metabolic conditions.

Bilirubin

Reaction Time: 30 s before reaction is complete.

Test Strip Reactants: Bilirubin is detected from coupling of bilirubin with a diazonium salt to provide a color change from a purple to brown color.

Clinical Data: Bilirubin is the product produced from the breakdown of red blood cells, and possibly in cases of liver damage and obstruction of the common bile duct. *Urine samples should be protected from sunlight and from fluorescent lights* to prevent breakdown of bilirubin. *No* detectable levels should be detected in urine of normal individuals.

Ketone

Reaction Time: 30 s for determining ketone presence.

Test Strip Reactants: Reaction sodium nitroprusside yields buff pink to a darker maroon color

Clinical Data: Ketones are found in cases of starvation and severe diabetes where fatty tissues are being incompletely metabolized as a source of energy, a condition called ketonuria. The major ketone found in the urine is acetoacetic acid and is often found in cases of ketoacidosis.

Specific Gravity

Reaction Time: 45 s for determining pH.

Test Strip Reactants: Color change occurs in reaction with methyl vinyl ether/maleic anhydride with a color developer called bromothymol blue.

Clinical Data: The specific gravity of urine samples may be falsely decreased using the dipstick method for highly alkaline specimen, requiring use of a refractometer or urinometer. The ability of the kidney to concentrate the urine in the collecting tubules is measured by this procedure. The ionic concentration of chiefly electrolytes is measured.

Blood

Reaction Time: 60-s reaction is required.

Reactants: Chromogen and a peroxidase type enzyme is the reactive mechanism that provides for a color reaction in the presence of blood.

Clinical Data: Blood is measured as both intact red blood cells and as lysed or dissolved cells on two separate pads. The presence of intact RBCs is indicated by a "dotted" pattern on the appropriate pad, while lysed cells will provide a uniform color reaction over the entire pad. Trauma or urinary calculi (kidney stones) and some infections will cause hematuria (blood in the urine), Myoglobin, a molecule providing oxygen to muscles, and is similar to hemoglobin on RBCs, will give a false positive result, as will certain vegetable constituents. Urine may be clear pink when myoglobin is present.

pH

Reaction Time: 60 s is necessary for the completion of this reaction.

Reactants: Colors of orange to yellow-green or blue occurs by reaction with bromothymol blue and methyl red.

Clinical Data: This procedure measures the alkalinity or acidity of the urine sample. Medications and diet, as well as medical conditions of the kidneys and certain medications will affect the pH of urine. Only ions or charged particles are measure, including sodium, potassium chloride and ammonium ions.

Protein

Reaction Time: A 60-s time must be allowed for this reaction to be completed.

Reactants: The pH of the pad is buffered to an acid pH with a dye that may include tetrabromophenol blue.

Clinical Data: Proteinuria is a valuable indicator of kidney disease but can be frequently attributed to infections of the urinary system. As in tests for protein in blood, proteins can affect the color of some indicators used to determine an acid-base reaction. Strips are adjusted to provide a negative result when only minimal amounts of protein are excreted in the urine, which is consistent with normal individuals.

Urobilinogen

Reaction Time: The urobilinogen test requires a 60-s wait for the reaction to be completed.

Reactants: Diazo reaction using 4-methoxybenzene-diazonium-tetrafluoroborate.

Clinical Data: Urobilinogen is produced in the intestine from bacterial action on bilirubin that is excreted through the bile duct and into the gut. The reaction is graded using measurements called Ehrlich units. Urobilinogen and bilirubin are affected by light. Urobilinogen forms a pink color and can detect levels as low as 0.1 Ehrlich unit. Increased levels are present in hepatic or liver disease and in hemolytic diseases where the red blood cells are degraded.

Nitrite
Reaction Time: The reaction requires 60 s to completion.
Reactants: Nitrite in the urine reacts with p-arsanilic acid to form a diazonium compound.
Clinical Data: The test for the presence of nitrite is based on the reduction by Gram negative bacteria of nitrate to nitrite. A positive result for nitrite indicates a urinary tract infection but not all bacteria are capable of converting nitrate to nitrite. Some of the organisms that are able to convert nitrate are pathogens *Escherichia coli, Proteus* spp., *Pseudomonas* spp. and *Klebsiella* spp.

Leukocyte Esterase
Reaction Time: Two minutes are required for the reaction to reach completion.
Reactants: LE catalyzes hydrolysis of an acid ester.
Clinical Data: This test requires the longest reaction time, 2 min, and inexperienced or careless laboratorian and practitioners do not adhere to this time period, reporting negative reactions when inadequate reaction time is allowed. An esterase enzyme found in granular WBC's found in bacterial infections reacts to form a purple color, Intensity increases for higher levels of esterase. Normal urine samples should be negative for esterase. An advantage in the use of this test lies in the fact that *non-intact WBCs will provide a positive reaction*, which might not be found during a microscopic evaluation.

10.8   Performance of the Urinalysis

Initially, urine samples will be tested for physical, chemical and microscopic components in a complete urine analysis. Only in cases where indicated will a urinalysis be carried further than the basic components listed. The kidneys basically rid the body of waste products and excess water and in doing so, they regulate many of the vital bodily functions, or physiology of the body. If certain products are unable to be cleared from the body due to various disease processes, levels of some products of metabolism may rise until the patient's life is threatened.

If the functioning units, the nephrons of the kidneys are damaged or malfunctioning, they may be unable to do their job. Then the patient may require dialysis in extreme cases using a machine designed to rid the blood of wastes on a regular basis, sometimes until a kidney is available for transplant. This damage may result from bacterial infection or trauma where an injury may have cut off the blood supply to the kidneys and the tissue became necrotic, a term used for cellular death. The maintenance of a narrow range for pH of the blood is largely controlled by the kidneys. Failure to maintain this pH may also result in quick death. So the importance of a simple test yields vital and quick information.

Examining the three components of a urinalysis (physical, chemical, micro-scopic) was at one time quite cumbersome but is now quick and simple. After the urine sample is examined quickly for volume, color and clarity, the chemical com-ponents are measured if present by a chemically coated dipstick to measure specific analytes of the urine. Some positive results in the chemical results will require con-firmatory tests usually prior to proceeding to the microscopic examination of the properly centrifuged specimen.

10.9   Principle of Urinalysis Procedure

Using the previous theoretical descriptions of the chemistry tests and diseases resulting in the analysis of urine in prior chapters, the complete analysis of the sample is documented in a standardized format. The report form (Urinalysis Report Form 10.1) for the procedure is found following the steps involved in completing the urinalysis and any required confirmatory tests. Urine may undergo a number of changes during states of disease or body dysfunction before blood composition is altered to a significant extent. Again, it is one of the most versatile and useful pro-cedures as an indicator of health or disease, especially in the areas of metabolic and renal disorders. The three steps of a complete urinalysis should enable detection of virtually all abnormalities associated with the urogenital system as well as other systems of the body.

10.9.1   Specimen Requirements

1. A random fresh urine sample is the best sample but at times it is necessary to refrigerate the sample to prevent bacterial growth when immediate testing is not possible.
2. The test should be performed as soon as possible.
3. The urine sample is stable at room temperature for 1 h and refrigerated for 4 h. If sample is refrigerated, *allow it to come to room temperature before testing*.
4. The absolute minimum sample volume is 1 mL. Smaller volumes lead to inac-curate testing.

10.10   Physical and Biochemical Testing of Urine

The physical examination of urine leads to observations that are most often con-firmed by chemical testing. Therefore, the two areas of testing are inextricably inter-woven. Following completion of these first two areas of examination, it follows that the microscopic study will further confirm the results of the physical and chemical findings. In preparation a sample for the microscopic portion of a urinalysis, a prop-erly calibrated centrifuge will optimally operate at 400 RCF's. RPM's (revolutions per minute) and other factors presented in Chap. 9 must be utilized to solve the equation.

10.10.1 Interfering Substances

In preparation for performing a complete urinalysis, abnormal urine color may affect the readability of the reagent areas of the urinalysis reagent test strips. Discolored urine specimens sent to the lab require special attention before completing the chemical analysis. Product inserts included with the various brands of "dipsticks" provide valuable information indicating expected reactions and interfering substances. In particular, biological dyes used in treatment of cystitis typically interfere with some reactions when employing dipstick chemistry.

Initial steps in performing the chemical analysis of a urine sample utilizes reactive pads on a plastic strip to determine the presence of and the qualitative measure of a number of constituents. Early development of these test strips, paper or cardboard was used for affixing the reactive pads. It soon became obvious that colors from the reactions "bled' into the surrounding material and rendered the results inaccurate and even combined with colors from adjoining test pads. Commercial strips are now made of plastic and are impervious to "bleeding over' into adjoining areas provided the test strip edge is blotted to remove excess liquid.

Commercial reagent strips are available with differing numbers of test pads, from single or double pads to more than ten. The number of chemical analytes tested for will vary with the facility and its complexity of testing routine. Although the various brands of strips used include those with differing numbers of tests, the chemical reactions with the indicators and reactive substances in the test pads are similar, regardless of brand used. Major brands used include Multix (Siemens Healthcare Diagnostics Inc., Deerfield, IL), Aution Sticks (Arkray Inc., Kyoto, Japan), Chem Strips (Iris Diagnostics, Chatsworth, CA), and Consult 10 SG (Mckesson Diagnostics, Pittsburg, PA).

10.10.2 Specimen Requirements

1. 10–12 mL fresh urine sample, well mixed.
2. Minimum volume is 1 mL where patient has difficulty obtaining an adequate sample. In this case, it may be necessary to employ the technique used for QC testing by using a pipette to place one drop of urine on each test pad.
3. Perform procedure as soon as possible after collection.
4. Urine sample is stable at room temperature for 1 h or refrigerated for 4 h. If refrigerated, allow urine to sit at room temperature for 15 min before testing.

Reactions are expected on some of the test pads even for 'normal' urine samples. (Table 10.5) lists the basic analytes tested for on the routine chemical tests. Most report forms are annotated for each test product to inform the clinical practitioner that the results are normal or abnormal footnote "a". For automated instruments, abnormal results may be 'flagged.'

Procedure 10.1: Chemical Testing Techniques of Urine Sample
Reagent strips are relatively easy to use, but certain precautions must be observed to insure accuracy in quality control as well as patient results. Package inserts from the manufacturer are provided regarding handling, storage and utilization of the test strips. A well-mixed and uncentrifuged sample is necessary for optimum results. Avoid sunlight and ultraviolet lights for testing urine. The sample must be at room temperature and if refrigerated, must be warmed before testing.

1. Using *uncentrifuged* urine, the sample is mixed well to insure uniformity of the sample.
2. Dip strip containing reactive pads *briefly* into the urine sample, insusring that all pads have been saturated.
3. If performing a manual reading of the strip, a timing device must be used and reaction times for each constituent observed.
4. Remove excess urine by drawing the edge of the strip against the outer rim of the collection container, or by blotting *only the edge* of the strip on absorbent paper such as a paper towel. DO NOT blot the reactive pads themselves!
5. Read the results of each reaction pad at the specified times, using the color chart found on the outside of the strip container.
6. Discard the used strip and record results. Remember that urine does not require handling as is biohazardous waste, as urine is not known to transmit dangerous pathogens.

Table 10.5 Normal values for urine chemistry components

Analyte	Normal
Glucose	Negative to trace
Bilirubin	Negative
Ketone	Negative
Specific gravity	1.005–1.030
Blood	Negative
pH	5.0–6.0
Protein	Negative to trace
Urobilinogen	0.2–1.0 mg/dL
Nitrite	Negative
Leukocytes	Negative

[a]Range that is found in most normal individuals

10.11 Microscopic Examination of Urine

Again, the microscopic analysis of a urine sample should correlate with the physical observations and the clinical status of the patient as well as the chemical evaluations. Care must be taken to obtain an adequate sample where testing has not been delayed, since a number of microscopic elements may be destroyed over time as physical changes occur. Refrigeration is the best course of action when testing is delayed, but other changes may occur even if the sample is refrigerated, such as the formation of amorphous urates or phosphates, depending upon the pH of the sample.

10.11.1 Interfering Substances

1. Hyaline casts and other partially transparent elements may be obscured by excessively bright light and may occasionally yield a positive protein result. Always use subdued light when examining urinary sediment. Experienced microscopists will focus using several levels of light for optimum performance and accuracy.
2. Vaginal secretions may contaminate the urine with epithelial cells, bacteria, or *Trichomonas* (a protozoal parasite).
3. Urine may be contaminated with fecal materials or *Giardia lamblia* (a parasite).
4. Starch granules, oil droplets from lubricants, anti-spermatic preparations, fiber fragments, or bacteria and yeast from contaminated urine containers.

10.11.2 Principle of the Microscopic Examination

Urine solid elements are concentrated by centrifugugation and the sediment examined under the microscope to detect cells and other formed elements such as crystals and casts. Examination of urine sediment is a non-invasive procedure which provides information useful in the diagnosis and prognosis of certain diseases. For example, in renal parenchymal disease, the urine usually contains increased numbers of cells and casts discharged from an organ accessible only by an invasive procedure. A chart may be necessary for identifying various crystals and unidentifiable artifacts. Indices of physical and chemical findings as well as images of the major categories of microscopic elements to aid in the identification of cells, crystals, and artifacts will be found following the simulated urinalysis report form at the end of this chapter (Urinalysis Report Form 10.1).

Procedure 10.2: Microscopic Examination of Urine Sample
Urinalysis procedure

1. Pour urine sample into a disposable 12 mL centrifuge tube. If <1 mL urine is collected, do not centrifuge. Perform microscopic on uncentrifuged urine and note on report.
2. Centrifuge tubes for 5 min at 400 RCF.

3. Pour off the supernatant and resuspend sediment with urine remaining in the tube. Approximately 0.8 mL urine supernatant and 0.1 mL of urine sediment will remain in the bottom of the tube. If graduated tube and pipetter are utilized, follow the instructions provided by manufacturer. In this way, standardization between laboratories, methodology, and correlation with automated urine analyzers.

4. Place a drop of resuspended urine sediment either onto a standard glass microscope slide or on the slide provided by an engineered system such as that by Kova for examining urinary sediment. This allows for consistent volumes of urine and sediment. *When using a standard slide*, place a cover slip over the urine sediment suspension.

5. Adjust the microscope condenser down and close the diaphragm so that light is subdued.

6. Scan ten fields using the low power objective and subdued light. Hyaline casts and other partially transparent solid elements may be obscured by excessively bright light so minute adjustments may be necessary. Count the number of casts seen per low power field and record the average number casts/LPF.

7. Count and record the average range of red blood cells (RBCs) by scanning at least ten fields using the high power objective. If more than one hundred RBCs are present, record >100/HPF.

8. If the field is obscured by more than 100 RBCs/HPF, add a drop of 2% acetic acid to 2 drops of urine sediment to lyse the RBCs. This process enables other cells and elements to be more easily visualized for counting.

9. RBCs may be confused with either yeast, fat droplets, or degenerated epithelial cells. If unable to differentiate the cells, add a drop of 2% acetic acid to 2 drops of urine sediment to lyse the RBCs.

10. Observe and note RBC morphology. Normal, unstained and fresh RBCs in wet preparations sometimes appear as pale yellow-orange discs. They vary in size, but are usually about 8 microns in diameter. With dissolution of hemoglobin in old or hypotonic urine specimens, RBCs may appear as faint, colorless circles or "ghost cells." With hypertonic urine specimens, RBCs may appear crenated with irregular edges and surfaces.

11. Count and record the average number of White Blood cells (WBCs) by scanning at least 10–15 fields using the high power objective. If more than one hundred WBCs are present, record >100/HPF. DO NOT use the oil immersion objective on the urine specimens.

12. If a field is obscured by >100 WBCs/HPF, dilute the sample with saline so all cells and elements are counted. Add two drops saline to one drop mixed urine sediment and place a drop onto the slide. For a one to three dilution, all cells and elements counted using diluted sample must be multiplied by a dilution factor of 3. See following note.

13. Continue scanning using high power objective for crystals, yeast, bacteria, epithelial cells, mucus, and other formed elements. Count and record the elements seen/HPF.

Report test results on appropriate form.
NOTE: Calculations when dilution factor is necessary
If a dilution with saline is required due to extremely high levels, multiply the average number of elements as counted by the dilution factor.
Example: 12 yeast cells seen/LPF × 3 (dilution factor) 36 yeasts/HPF

10.12 Reporting Results

1. Report casts as the average number of casts seen per low power field (Table 10.6). Reference ranges (a) relate to numbers utilized for standard quantification of values observed. Differentiate and quantitate different types of casts as hyaline, cellular, fatty, or waxy. Or instance, ten fields are counted. When three casts are on some fields, four on others, and another with five casts, the average count would be four casts/LPF.
2. Report RBCs as the average number of RBCs seen per high power field. If more than 100 RBCs/HPF are seen, report as >100/HPF, packed or too numerous to count (TNTC). The reporting method is specified by the testing facility.
3. Report WBCs as the average number of WBCs seen per high power field. If more than 100 WBCs/HPF are seen, again report as >100/HPF, packed or TNTC.
4. Report other cellular or formed elements as few, moderate, or many using the following guide as the protocol for estimating microscopic components and enumeration of them (Urinalysis Report Form 10.1).

The experienced technologist can quickly compare the results of the chemical and the microscopic exams, taking into account the physical appearance of the original specimen. Visual interpretation of the chemistry reactions may differ but only slightly between laboratory professionals. Timing is of the essence in evaluating color reaction as a positive reaction, although this is usually only a minor consideration when adequate light and a white background are used to determine whether a reaction has occurred. Color changes only along the edge(s) of the reagent strip and reactions occurring after 2 min are insignificant and should not be reported. An advantage of having a strip reader lies in the fact that timing of reactions require no effort by the testing personnel, but some instruments are unable to take into account specimens that have high levels of pigmentation due to medications and to perhaps specimens with a high bilirubin content. In this case, some subjectivity must be employed to determine presence of a reaction, and the strength of the reaction. Most results will be negative, so testing personnel should not become complacent and overlook significant results (Table 10.7). Reference ranges (*) refer to those found in the average or normal individual.

Table 10.6 Quantification of common microscopic elements

Element	Few	Moderate	Many
Crystals	0–4/HPF	5–10/HPF	>10/HPF
Bacteria	0–25/HPF	25–50/HPF	>50/HPF
Yeast	0–25/HPF	25–50/HPF	>50/HPF
Epithelial cells	0–4/HPF	5–10/HPF	>10/HPF

[a]Reference ranges

Table 10.7 Normal Confirmatory values tests forc positive dipstick urine chemistry components

Analyte	Normal Confirmatory tests
Glucose	Negative to trace Glucose hexokinase
Bilirubin	Negative Diazo tablet (Ictotest)
Ketone	Negative Nitroprusside (Acetest)
Specific gravity	1.005–1.030 Refractometry
Blood	Negative Microscopic presence, hemoglobin
pH	5.0–6.0 pH Meter
Protein	Negative to trace Sulfosalicylic acid
Urobilinogen	0.2–1.0 mg/dL Phenazopyridine
Nitrite	Negative Diazo reagent
Leukocytes	Negative Microscopic examination of cells or fragments

[a]Range that is found in most normal individuals

10.13 Confirmatory Tests for Positive Urinary Chemistry Findings

When positive results are obtained using the dipstick methodology for chemical constituents, environmental factors may be responsible for the values obtained in the absence of disease and will require confirmation of the results. For instance, an elevated pH of the urine sample may cause false positive results for protein when highly buffered specimens or those of patients with cystitis, where bacteria are responsible for the alkaline urine. When significant protein is found by dipstick, further testing may be required. A semi-quantitative test showing grades of turbidity in centrifuged specimens, where blood and mucin is extracted before performing either the screening showing trace to 4+ results may precede a request for a quantitative protein on a 24-h specimen.

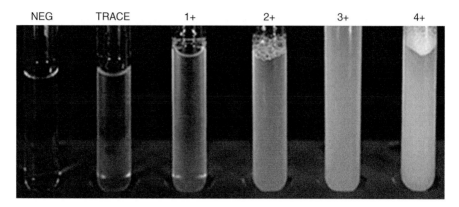

| NEG | TRACE | 1+ | 2+ | 3+ | 4+ |

Fig. 10.4 Confirmatory test for urinary protein by precipitation with acid

10.13.1   Confirmatory Semi-Quantitative Protein by Sulfosalicylic Acid

When the urine sample has been cleared of cells and mucus that may cause a positive reaction when acid is added, the results obtained by the precipitation methods will provide a semi-quantitative value when protein is being excreted by the kidneys due to glomerular damage. Cleaning compounds such as quaternary ammonium solutions or very small amounts of chlorhexidine may also yield false positive results (Fig. 10.4).

10.13.2   Premise for Performance

Protein estimates by a precipitate method using sulfosalicylic acid utilizes a 3% sulfosalicylic acid which precipitates protein in solution, and the presence of protein turns the urine specimen milky with low amounts and forms granules or a solid for higher levels of protein. The degree of turbidity is graded from a trace amount to a 4+ reaction, which causes almost complete coagulation of the test sample when acid is added.

> **Procedure 10.3: Procedure for Semi-Quantitative Determination of Protein**
> Perform a sulfosalicylic acid test for protein on each urine sample showing a positive protein on the dipstick. Some constituents may yield a false-positive result, and it is difficult to perform a quantitative measurement of the urinary protein by use of the dipstick only.
>
> 1. Into a small test tube, pour about 1–2 mL (20–40 drops) of either mixed urine or the supernatant from a centrifuged urine sample. Centrifuging of solid materials provides a more definitive result for the excretion of protein by damaged structures of the kidney.
> 2. Addition an equal amount of 3% sulfosalicylic acid solution to the urine.

3. Mix well by either "flicking" the urine or placing parafilm on the top of the test tube and inverting the test tube 2–3 times for mixing.
4. Grade for cloudiness as follow (Table 10.8).

Report results of test appropriately

Table 10.8   Sulfosalicylic acid (SSA) precipitation test results

SSA results	Description	Protein concentration
Negative	No noticeable turbidity/cloudiness; clear from top to bottom of tube	<or = to 5 mg/dL
Trace	Using bright light, turbidity is barely visible	6–20 mg/dL
1+	Turbidity is considerable, but individual granules not visible	Approximately 30 mg/dL
2+	Granulation of particles are visible but no large clumps (flocculation) are visible	Approximately 100 mg/dL
3+	Considerable turbidity with both granulation and flocculation	200–500 mg/dL
4+	Clumps or solid particulate are present; solution may appear clear when all precipitated protein sinks to bottom of tube Properly report results to appropriate party	>500 mg/dL

Report the graded results to the physician. If glomerular damage is suspected, a creatinine clearance test may be requested and/or a 24-h urine specimen to confirm a diagnosis. Tubular or glomerular damage may be differentiated as follows. The procedure for a total protein based on a 24-h specimen is provided later in this chapter.

10.14   Differentiation Between Principal Urinary Proteins

When the presence of protein has been confirmed by a semi-quantitative method, it may be necessary to determine the source of the excreted protein. The two principal types of protein are *glomerular* or *tubular* and occur for different reasons. When the source of the protein must be ascertained before treatment is initiated, glomerular proteinuria occurs in primary glomerular conditions where the glomeruli are damaged, and sometimes proceeds to a serious clinical condition called the *nepthrotic syndrome*. Typically the protein levels in the urine for this disorder exceed 3.5 g per day, and are accompanied by hypoalbuminemia, hyperlipidemias, lipiduria and generalized edema.

Tubular proteinuria occurs during a disruption of normal reabsorption of protein in the tubules. A third but less serious type of proteinuria is that of orthostatic proteinuria, a functional type as described earlier that should be observed regularly to insure further changes are not in progress. The proteins are identified by their molecular weights and construction and differ between glomerular and tubular disorders. The excretion of proteins may be used to differentiate between the two conditions in the following ratios. Patients with glomerular disorders show a normal to a *slight increase* in the excretion of Beta$_2$ but considerably increased excretion of albumin and total protein. Most of the patients with tubular dysfunction excreted *large amounts* of Beta$_2$ microglobulin, although they both excrete normal or only slightly increased amounts of albumin but somewhat increased quantities of total protein.

10.15   Acetest: Semi-Quantitative Test for Acetone

As is the case for the finding of glucose in the urine, the presence of ketone bodies is related to a metabolic function rather than to renal physiology. Ketone bodies are comprised of compounds similar to each other and include acetoacetic or diacetic acid, Beta-hydroxybutyric acid, and acetone. The presence of ketones should correlate with the metabolism of fat for energy, when an impairment prevents the body from using dietary glucose normally, as found in diabetes mellitus and in starvation. In cases of serious liver damage, the liver is unable to store glycogen, which is the form of glucose that is stored for energy. In this case, ketones may also be elevated, since body fat is being used for energy rather than glucose due to the lack of availability of glycogen. Ketone bodies are found in low levels normally and are not detected in the urine.

10.15.1   Premise for Performance

Acetone is an example of a simple ketone. This test is based on the development of a purple color when acetoacetic acid or acetone reacts with nitroprusside. The determination for the presence of ketones by Acetest reagent tablets may be performed on urine or plasma, the liquid portion of blood (Fig. 10.5). Acetoacetic acid or acetone in urine or blood will form a purple colored complex with nitroprusside in the presence of glycine.

Fig. 10.5 Confirmation test for presence of urinary ketones

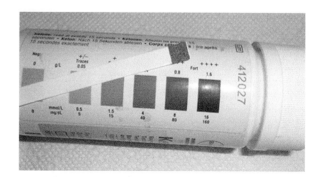

Procedure 10.4: Confirmation of Presence of Ketones

Procedural steps

Perform an Acetest on each specimen showing a positive ketone on the dip-stick using the

Following procedure

1. Place an Acetest table on a white paper
2. Add one (1) drop of urine directly on the tablet
3. At 30 s, compare the color of the tablet with the color chart provided by the manufacturer
4. Report as negative, 1 + (for small amount), 2+ (for moderate amount), or 3+ (for large amount)
5. Serial dilutions may be performed if required to obtain a better estimate of ketone presence

Properly report results to appropriate office

10.16   Ictotest: Semi-Quantitative Test for Bilirubin

The presence of bilirubin may be related to a diseased liver or an obstructive condition of the bile duct. An increased level of hemoglobin due to the lysis of red blood cells will also result in the finding of increased levels of bilirubin in the urine.

10.16.1   Premise for Performance

Bilirubin by Ictotest reagent tablets is a reaction is based on the coupling of a unique solid diazonium salt with bilirubin in acid medium giving a blue or purple reaction product (Fig. 10.6).

Fig. 10.6 Bilirubin presence confirmed by Ictotest

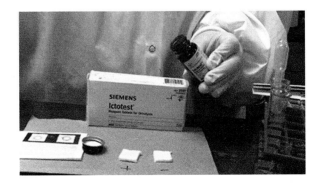

10.16.2   Performance

Perform an Ictotest on each specimen showing a positive bilirubin by the dipstick method using the following procedure.

Procedure 10.5: Semi-Quantitative Test for Bilirubin
1. Place a square of the absorbent test mat (provided by manufacturer) onto a white paper
2. Place ten (10) drops of urine onto the center of the test mat
3. Place one (1) Ictotest tablet on the moistened mat
4. Carefully place one (1) drop of distilled/deionized water onto the top of the tablet. Wait five (5) seconds. Add a second drop of water to the tablet so that the water runs off the tablet onto the mat
5. The presence of a blue or purple color on the mat indicates a positive test for bilirubin. (slight pink or red color should be ignored)
6. The test is subjectively graded as negative or trace to 4+. See manufacturer's product insert for example of positive results. Properly report results

---

10.17   Glucose: Semi-Quantitative

The presence of glucose may be related to large amounts of glucose in IV solutions, or a more serious onset of diabetes. Diabetes mellitus is the most common disorder found with a positive glucose level and perhaps half the cases of diabetes are discovered during a routine urinalysis. When a positive glucose is found in the urine, a blood test for glucose follows to determine if the blood glucose is affected.

10.17.1   Premise for Performance

Glucose and other reducing substances may be measured by Clinitest reagent tablets for reducing sugars. This test is based on the classic Benedict's copper reduction reaction. Copper sulfate react with reducing substances in urine, converting cupric sulfate to cuprous oxide. Colors range from blue through green to orange. This test is used to detect sugars other than glucose (Fig. 10.7).

Performance
Perform a Clinitest (five drop method) on each specimen giving a positive glucose on the dipstick, as well as all at-risk children using the following procedure:

Procedure 10.6: Clinitest: Semi-Quantitative Test for Glucose and Other Reducing Substances

1. Place five (5) drops of urine into a clean glass test tube
2. With the same size dropper, add ten (10) drops of deionized water
3. Drop one (1) Clinitest table into the test tube. Watch while boiling reaction takes place. Do not shake tube during the reaction or for 15 s after the boiling (care should be exercised as the tube becomes HOT) has stopped. Remember to observe for the "pass through phenomenon"
4. Determine results from the chart provided with the kit by the manufacturer and report results

Fig. 10.7 Confirmation of reducing substances other than glucose by Clinitest

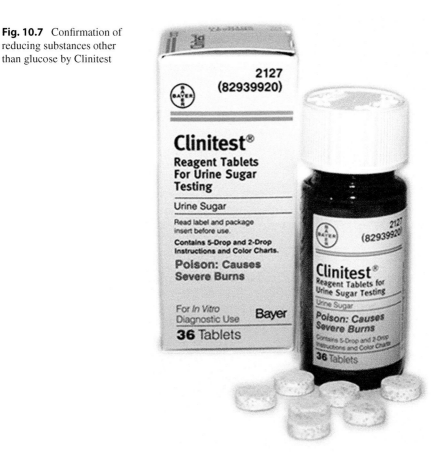

10.18   Tests for Quantitated Protein by Dye-Binding and Turbidimetric Method

The following procedures are used for determining protein in urine and cerebrospinal fluid.

CSF protein is reported only as mg/dl as a total protein for the entire volume of cerebrospinal fluid would be difficult to measure and would not be a reasonable procedure. On the other hand, it is often necessary to determine the entire protein output through the kidneys for a 24-h period. The procedure is the same for both fluids, and two methods may be employed. One is that of the turbidity of a sulfosalicylic acid and protein in solution, while the other is a simple dye-binding process. The process for blood protein determination as well as albumin also may use a dye-binding procedure, and these blood products are reported in g/dL. This is reasonable as the protein in urine and arguably in CSF as ultrafiltrates where the amount measured should be much less than that found in blood.

10.19   Summary and Principle

Although this section outlined the performance of total protein using the urine as a sample, the method for performing total protein for cerebrospinal fluid is the same. Both fluids are reported in mg/dL while blood from which these fluids (urine and CSF) may obtain their protein, is reported in grams/dL although the source of protein in CSF is arguable. In addition, if required, protein may be measured for other body fluids using one of the methods of either a turbidimetric or dye-binding method. There is some controversy as to whether the cerebral spinal fluid is produced by the ependymal cells and includes fluid containing protein, or is an ultrafiltrate of plasma, same as other body fluids.

Measurement of urinary proteins is becoming increasingly important in the detection of renal pathology. Proteinuria, an increased amount of protein in urine, can occur in increased glomerular permeability, defective tubular reabsorption and abnormal secretion of protein into the urinary tract. Albuminuria (increased albumin in urine) has been implicated as an early indicator of renal damage in conditions of diabetes that can be reversed if detected and treated sufficiently and early in the disease course. It would be advantageous to remember the significance of microalbumin, which might precede the presence of larger amounts of protein in the urine. There are normally low amounts of microalbumin in the urine, but when it reaches the measurable level, damage has begun in the kidneys of diabetics. Measurement of CSF total protein as well as other specific proteins is used to detect increased permeability of the blood brain barrier.

This technique may be used with urine, where specimen blanks due to color must be used to negate the effects of urine color on the absorbance readings of the spectrophotometer. CSF should be crystal clear so not specimen blank would be needed unless the specimen were xanthochromic (yellow from blood products). Proteins in CSF and urine are precipitated in a finely dispersed form by trichloroacetic acid. Absorbance of the sample is read at 600 nm. The dye-binding procedure is now preferred by most, as it is simpler to read a color difference than the degree of precipitation. A protein standard is similarly treated and is used as comparison between the optical density of a known standard and an unknown specimen.

Both fluids are reported in mg/dL while blood serum from which these fluids (urine and CSF) may obtain their protein, is reported in grams/dL. Measurement of urinary proteins is becoming increasingly important in the detection of renal pathology. Proteinuria, an increased amount of protein in urine, can occur in increased glomerular permeability, defective tubular reabsorption and abnormal secretion of protein into the urinary tract. Albuminuria (increased albumin in urine) has been implicated as an early indicator of renal damage in conditions of diabetes that can be reversed if detected and treated sufficiently and early in the disease course. It would be wise to remember the significance of microalbumin, which might precede the presence of larger amounts of protein in urine. There are low levels of microalbumin normally in the urine, but when it reaches the measurable level, damage has begun in the kidneys of diabetics. Measurement of CSF total protein as well as other specific proteins is used to detect increased permeability of the blood brain barrier.

Specimen Collection and Preparation
Urine: Random or 24-h specimens may be used.

Spinal Fluid: Great care must be exercised in handling CSF samples. They are difficult to collect, and some are highly infectious. CSF should be free from hemolysis. Centrifuge all specimen containing red blood cells or particulate matter.

Procedure 10.7: Total Protein Procedure (Turbidimetric): Total 24-h Urinary/CSF Protein

Reagents needed
   Total protein reagent (aqueous solution of trichloroacetic acid, 5% w/v)

Protein standard	166 mg
Precautions:	For in vitro diagnostic use
Reagent caustic:	Do not pipet by mouth
Reagent preparation:	Reagent and standard are supplied ready to use

Specimen collection and preparation
Urine: Random or 24-h specimens may be used as described in earlier chapters

1. Pipet the following volumes into cuvettes labeled U (unknown), RB (reagent blank) and S (standard), and SB (sample blank—for all urines) and mix well
2. Incubate all cuvettes for 5–10 min at room temperature
3. After incubation, mix each covet well and read absorbance (A) of U, S and SB when applicable, vs RB at 420 nm

Quality control:	A commercial set of controls, along with standards are available
Results:	Calculated using the following equation:

Absorbance of unknown/absorbance of standard × calculated value of standard

Example calculation:

Abs Standard (166 mg/dL)	0.221	Calculated Results
Abs #1	0.112	84

Using the calculations equation above, the following results are obtained

$$0.112/0.221 \times 166 \text{ (value of the standard)} = 84 \text{ mg/dL}$$

Value to be reported = 84 mg/dL

For a 24-h urine sample with a volume of 1440 mL, the calculation for the total protein excreted would be as follows (1 dL = 100 mL):

1440 mL/100 dL = 14.4 dL
14.4 dL × 84 mg/dL = 1210 mg (dL's would cancel each other)
Convert 1210 mg to grams by dividing mg by 1000 (1000 mg in 1 g)
Calculated value of protein excreted = *1.21 g excreted in 24 hs*

Total Protein for CSF, Urine, Miscellaneous Body Fluids

This method is a quantitative dye-binding method for proteins in all body fluids. This procedure is similar to the Turbidimetric method presented in Table 10.8. Reagents are available commercially as a generic dye-binding method. Settings and volumes of sample and reagent are as follows. The procedure is also adaptable for automated and semi-automated instruments.

Procedure 10.8: Total Protein Procedure, Dye Binding

1. Pipet the following volumes into cuvettes labeled U (unknown), RB (reagent blank) and S (standard), and SB (sample blank—for all urines) and mix well

	Unknown(s) (U)	Standard (S)	Reagent blank (RB)
Reagent	2.0 mL	2.0 mL	2.0 mL
Sample	20 μL	–	–
Standard	–	20 μL	–
Water			20 μL

2. Incubate all cuvettes for 5–10 min at room temperature
3. After incubation, mix each covet well and read absorbance (A) of U, S and SB when applicable, vs RB at 600 nm

> Quality control: A commercial set of controls, along with standards are available
>
> Results: Calculated using the following equation:
>
> Absorbance of unknown/absorbance of standard × calculated value of standard
>
> Example calculation:
>
> | Abs standard (166 mg/dL) | 0.221 | Calculated results |
> |---|---|---|
> | Abs #1 | 0.112 | 84 |
>
> *Using the calculations equation above, the following results are obtained*
>
> $$0.112/0.221 \times 166 \text{ (value of the standard)} = 84 \text{ mg/dL}$$
>
> *Value to be reported = 84 mg/dL*
> *For a 24-h urine sample with a volume of 1440 mL, the calculation for the total protein excreted would be as follows (1 dL = 100 mL):*
>
> 1440 mL/100 dL = 14.4 dL
> 14.4 dL × 84 mg/dL = 1210 mg (dL's would cancel each other)
> Convert 1210 mg to grams by dividing mg by 1000 (1000 mg in 1 g)
> Calculated value of protein excreted = *1.21 g excreted in 24 h*
>
> *Note*: Quantitative values should correlate with screening methods used to confirm the presence of protein in urine in Chaps. 8 and 10

10.20   Microscopic Elements of Urine and Body Fluids

Blood Cells

Blood and epithelial cells may be found in specimens that are of a neutral, acid and alkaline pH. However, some environmental conditions such as pH extremes may serve to cause deterioration and disintegration of cells. Many of these images are of elements that are often found in urine sediment prepared using the steps provided in Procedure 10.2) (Figs. 10.8, 10.9, 10.10, 10.11, 10.12, 10.13, and 10.14).

Casts

Casts may be associated with remnants of cells or comprised of whole blood cells. Often the matrix is a proteinaceous material in which cells and debris from destroyed cells are embedded. Hyaline casts in themselves may not be pathogenic but may include either white or red blood cells from a pathologic condition (Figs. 10.15, 10.16, 10.17, 10.18, 10.19, 10.20, and 10.21).

Fig. 10.8 Mixed
squamous epithelial, rbc's
and wbc's

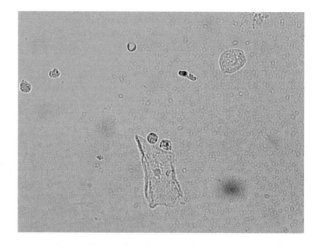

Fig. 10.9 White blood
cells

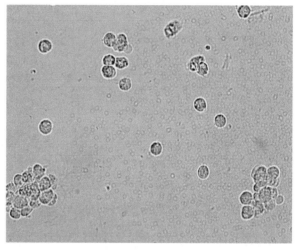

Fig. 10.10 Renal tubular
cells

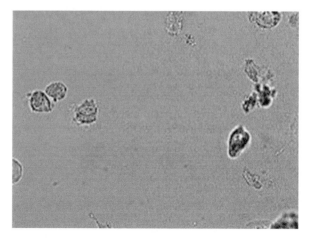

Fig. 10.11 Transitional
epithelial cells

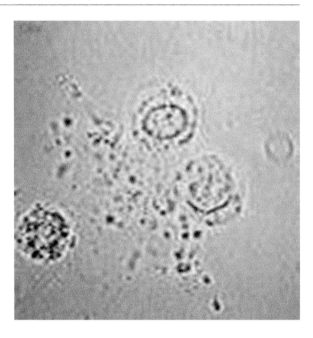

Fig. 10.12 Squamous
epithelial cell and budding
yeast

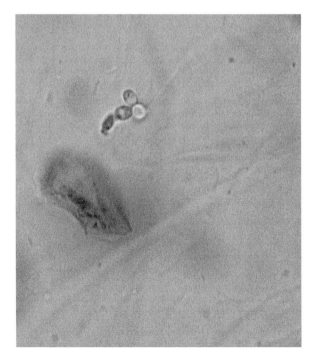

Fig. 10.13 Miscellaneous bacterial organisms

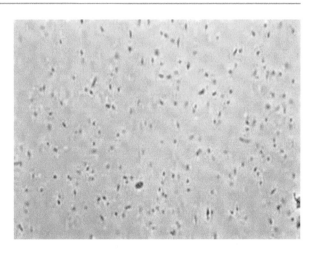

Fig. 10.14 Spermatozoa and miscellaneous cells

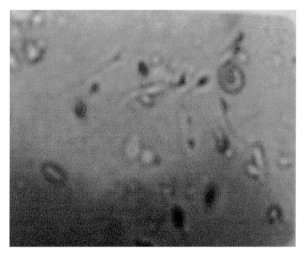

Fig. 10.15 Hyaline cast (center of field)

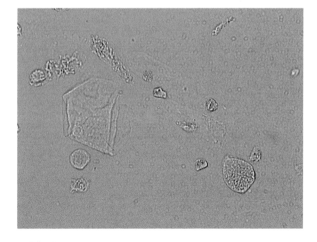

Fig. 10.16 Cellular and
granular casts with cellular
inclusions

Fig. 10.17 Stained
granular cast

Fig. 10.18 Waxy cast

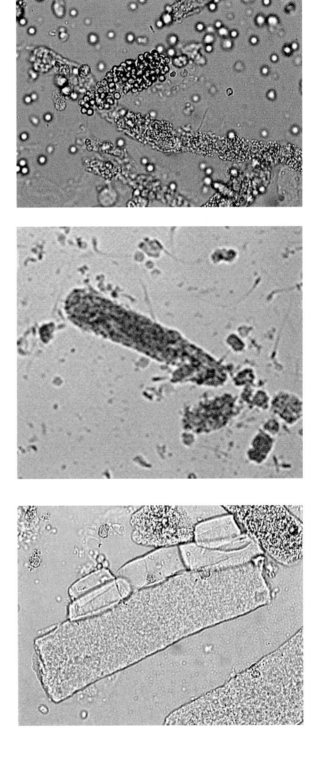

Fig. 10.19 WBC casts

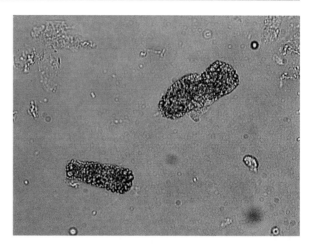

Fig. 10.20 RBC cast

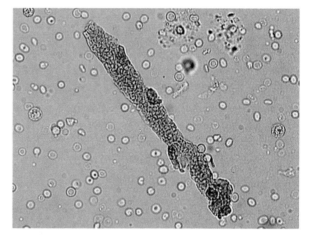

Fig. 10.21 Cellular cast

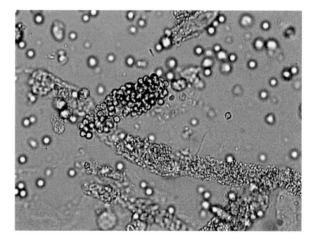

Protozoa

The *Trichomonas* sp., of which there are several, although the *T. vaginalis* is the most virulent and is transmitted sexually, is the chief parasite found in the urine of the human. The cyst form, which is practically indistinguishable from the WBC, is found in older urine samples. The active form, the trophozoite, is quite active in fresh, warm urine and is easy to visualize. In rare cases, parasite eggs such as those of *Enterobius vermicularis*, found around the rectal opening, may contaminated the urine of infected individuals. In fecally contaminated specimens from those with *Giardia intestinalis* infections, both intestinal parasites and their eggs may be found in the urine. The eggs of a parasitic organisms called *Schistosoma. hematobium* may be found in the urine of individuals from Mideastern countries where a disease called schistosomiasis is endemic (Fig. 10.22).

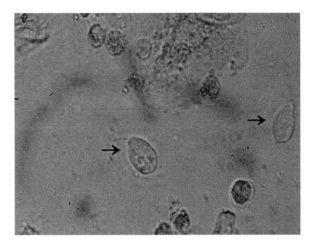

Fig. 10.22 Pear-shaped *Trichomonas* sp.

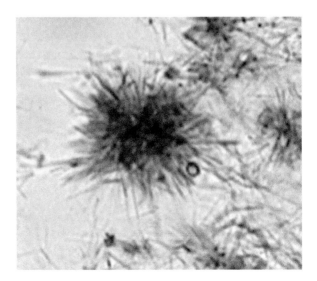

Fig. 10.23 Tyrosine crystals

Fig. 10.24 Leucine
crystals

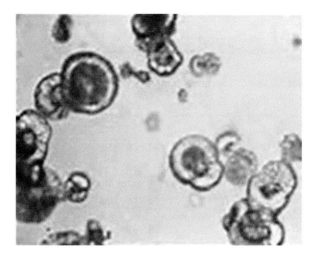

Fig. 10.25 Cystine
crystals

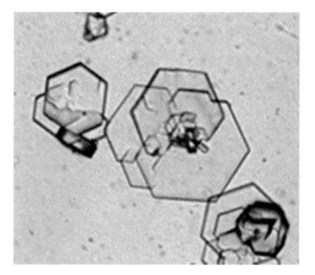

Crystals

Crystals form due to a variety of reasons and causes. Some relate to environmental conditions and increased concentrations of solutes that are normally present in urine and even other body fluids. However, some are due to metabolic diseases and to the administration of certain medications.

Abnormal Crystals

Figures 10.23, 10.24, and 10.25

Acid Urine Crystals
Figures 10.26, 10.27, and 10.28.

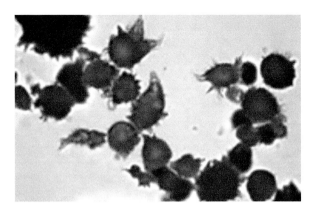

Fig. 10.26 Ammonium urates, Bright-field

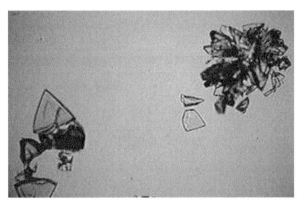

Fig. 10.27 Uric acid crystals, Bright-field

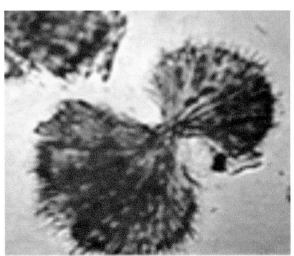

Fig. 10.28 Sulfonamide crystal (sheaf of wheat)

Acidic, Neutral or Alkaline Urine Crystals

Figures 10.29 and 10.30.

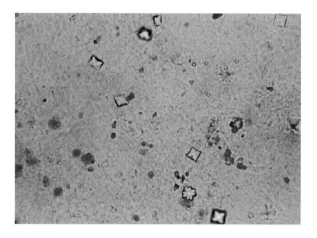

Fig. 10.29 Calcium oxalate crystals

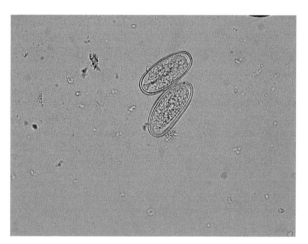

Fig. 10.30 Pinworm eggs (*Enterobius vermicularis*) sometimes found in urine

Alkaline Urine Crystals
Figures 10.31 and 10.32.

Bacteria and Yeast
Bacteria may be a result of a contaminated urine sample, and is usually accompanied by increased numbers of squamous epithelial cells when this occurs. It is sometimes possible to distinguish between rod-shaped organisms and round (coccal-shaped) organisms by Bright-field microscopy. The presence of yeast in the urine sample may be a result of heavy antibiotic usage, or of vaginitis, where yeast has contaminated the specimen (Fig. 10.33).

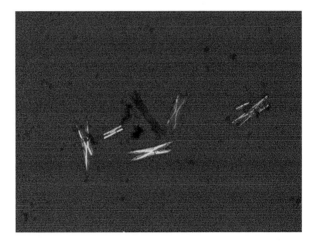

Fig. 10.31 Triple phosphate crystals, polarized

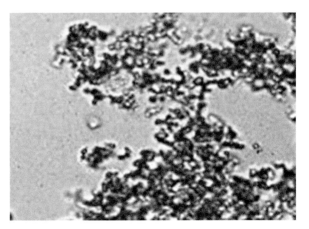

Fig. 10.32 Amorphous phosphate crystals

Fig. 10.33 Groups of
budding yeast

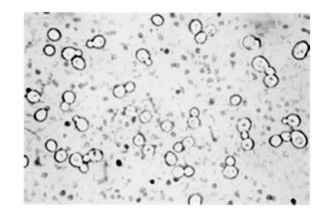

Case Study 10.1

A middle-aged and obese female visited an outpatient clinic that had a clinical laboratory on the premises. She had complained of upper right quadrant pain for several
weeks, her husband revealed. A urine sample and a blood sample for a complete
blood count were obtained. The blood cell count showed normal results, but upon
standing, the plasma appeared to be dark yellow. The results of the urinalysis
revealed the following findings in Urinalysis Results Report, Case 10.1). The following questions should be answered from the report.

1. What are the abnormal values found in this report?

_____

2. If the urine were shaken, what would the laboratory technician expect to see?

_____

3. Explain the differences between high levels of urobilinogen and of bilirubin.

_____

_____

4. What is the probable diagnosis for the condition from which this woman is
   suffering?

_____

_____

Urinalysis Results Report, Case 10.1

Physical appearance		
Color	Dark amber	
Character	Clear	
Chemical screening		
Leukocyte esterase	Negative	
Nitrite	Negative	
Urobilinogen	Normal amount	

Protein (test strip)	Negative	
pH	5.5	
Blood	Negative	
Specific gravity	1.015	Repeat testing by refractometer for confirmation
Ketone	Negative	
Bilirubin	Positive—3+	Confirmed by Ictotest
Glucose	Negative	
Sediment evaluation		
Squamous Epithelials	Occasional	
Renal Epithelials	0	
Erythrocytes	0	
Leukocytes	1–2	
Casts	0	
Crystals	0	
Bacteria	0	
Other (specify)	0	

Urinalysis Report Form 10.1

Patient Name _____ Patient ID # _____ Date _____

Age _____ Gender (Circle One) M or F Physician _____

Time Requested _____ Time Performed _____ Time Reported _____

Examination Requested ☐UA With Microscopic ☐ Dipstick UA Only

☐ Culture & Sensitivity ☐ Other

Physical Examination

Color ☐ Colorless ☐ Straw ☐ Yellow ☐Amber ☐Red ☐Brown

Character ☐ Clear ☐ Hazy ☐ Cloudy ☐Turbid ☐Other

Chemical Examination by Manual Dipstick [Multistix 10 SG (Bayer)]

(Circle the appropriate responses)

Glucose (mg/dL) Negative 100 250 500 1000 >2000

Bilirubin Negative + Small ++ (Mod) +++ (Large)

Ketones Negative Trace Small Mod Large

Specific Gravity 1.000 1.005 1.015 1.020 1.025 1.030

	Non-hemolyzed	Hemolyzed
Blood (please check)	☐ Negative	☐ Negative
	☐ Trace	☐ Trace
	☐ Small	☐ Small
	☐ Moderate	☐ Moderate
	☐ Large	☐ Large

pH (please circle)   5.0   6.0   6.5   7.0   7.5   8.0   8.5

Protein   Neg   Trace   +/30 (1+)   ++/100 (2+)   +++/500 (3+)   ++++/2000 (4+)

Urobilinogen   Normal   2   4   6

Nitrites   Negative   Positive

Leukocytes   Negative   Trace   SmallModerate   Large

Confirmatory Tests   Protein____   Bilirubin _____   Urobilinogen Acetone _____

Microscopic Examination

Constituent	Reported Values	Reference Values
White Blood Cells	_____	0-4 / high-power field (HPF)*

High power (HPF) refers to 40 x microscopic objective or higher; Low power or LPF refers to 10 or 20 x objective

Red Blood Cells	_____	0-4 / high-power field (HPF)
Squamous Epithelial Cells	_____	Occasional; higher in females
Renal/tubular Epithelial Cells	_____	0
Casts [Identify Type(s)]	_____	0 / low-power field (LPF)**
Yeasts (1 – 4+)	_____	Negative
Bacteria (1– 4+)	_____	Negative
Mucus (1– 4+)	_____	Negative

Constituent	Reported Values	Reference Values
Crystals (Identify)	_____	Negative
Amorphous Sediment	_____	Negative
Miscellaneous (Identify)	_____	
Comments (Unusual Findings)	_____	

Performed by: _____   Date: _____

Review Questions

1. Where would tests be sent for further evaluation that are not routinely performed in a routine hospital laboratory?
   a. To a senior technologist
   b. To the pathologist
   c. To another department of the lab
   d. To a reference lab
2. One of the contraindications of using a urine preservative is:
   a. Some analytes may be destroyed
   b. The materials may be too expensive
   c. The specimen would become dilute
   d. Urine should never be preserved

3. Urine screening tests except for microscopy can legally be performed by:
   a. Only trained lab professionals
   b. Certified nurse assistants
   c. Medical assistants
   d. All of the previous responses
4. A urine sample is comprised primarily of:
   a. Blood plasma
   b. Hormones and ultrafiltrates
   c. Electrolytes and food products
   d. Water
5. The most important component of the following list in the evaluation of urine is:
   a. Chemical constituents
   b. Viscosity
   c. Color
   d. Odor
6. Which of the following would not require a confirmatory test when a positive result was obtained by dipstick chemistry?
   a. Protein
   b. Leukocyte esterase
   c. Bilirubin
   d. Acetone (ketones)
7. Urinary sediment would be used to determine the presence of:
   a. Glucose
   b. Acetone
   c. Bilirubin
   d. Yeasts
8. Which of the following findings would not be particularly important in diagnosing an illness related to the urinary tract?
   a. Color
   b. Urine chemistry results
   c. Specific gravity
   d. All of the above would
9. High levels of metabolism of fats for energy would give a positive result of:
   a. Glucose
   b. Leukocyte esterase
   c. Urobilinogen
   d. Ketones
10. Musty odors of the urine may sometimes be attributed to:
    a. Diabetes
    b. Phenylketonuria
    c. Maple Syrup Disease
    d. Alkaptonuria

11. The clarity of urine is referred to as:
    a. Turbidity
    b. Viscosity
    c. Mucosity
    d. Concentration
12. The specific gravity of urine using the refractometer compares the sample with:
    a. Water
    b. Air
    c. Other urine samples
    d. Standard solutions
13. Urobilinogen is formed directly from:
    a. Urochrome
    b. White blood cells
    c. Bilirubin
    d. Hemoglobin
14. The chemistry test performed on urine that is most sensitive to sunlight is:
    a. Complete urinalysis
    b. Glucose
    c. Ketones
    d. Bilirubin
15. The chemistry test performed on urine that is most sensitive to high alkalinity is:
    a. Glucose
    b. Protein
    c. Ketones
    d. Bilirubin
16. A species of bacteria that is able to convert nitrates to nitrites is:
    a. *Staphylococcus aureus*
    b. *Clostridium perfringens*
    c. *Escherichia coli*
    d. *Streptococcus pyogenes*
17. The best type of specimen for a complete urinalysis is:
    a. Fresh
    b. Preserved
    c. Refrigerated
    d. Stored at room temperature
18. Most test results provided by urinary dipstick are:
    a. Quantitative
    b. Semi-quantitative
    c. Direct
    d. Direct
19. The purpose of centrifuging a urine sample is to:
    a. Dilute the sample results
    b. Concentrate the sample results
    c. Make the results more specific
    d. Make the tests easier to perform

20. The Clinitest is used to:
   a. Give a true value for glucose
   b. Give an accurate bilirubin level
   c. Detect reducing sugars
   d. Determine the presence of acetone

Answers Found in Appendix C

Cerebrospinal Fluid Analysis

11

Objectives

Understand the proper collection of cerebrospinal fluid

List the tests performed on each of the three tubes in which CSF is transported to the laboratory

Relate the formation of cerebrospinal fluid and its role in the maintenance of the central nervous system

Correlate clinical laboratory results with pathological conditions

11.1 Introduction to the Testing of Cerebrospinal Fluid

Body fluids with a possible exception of CSF all originate from the blood plasma that circulates throughout the body, providing nutrients and oxygen to every area of all the systems of the body. Arguably, cerebrospinal fluid does not arise from plasma, but recent evidence attributes the formation of the fluid to its origin as components of blood plasma, although the *blood-brain barrier* (*BBB*) prohibits the free exchange of blood fluids across this barrier. Approximately 20 mL of CSF are produced each hour by the choroid plexuses of the brain's ventricles through the ultrafiltration of blood plasma as a function of active secretion and perhaps transport. The fluid is reabsorbed by the *arachnoid villi* of the three membranes called meninges that cover the central nervous system which is comprised chiefly of the brain and the spinal cord (Fig. 11.1). The three meningeal membranes are called the *pia mater*, the *dura mater* and the arachnoid mater. If no abnormal conditions such as hydrocephalus occurs, where excessive CSF is found in the ventricles of the brain, the production of CSF is sufficient to maintain an approximate total volume of 100–170 mL in adults, and 10–60 mL in newborns.

The purpose of cerebrospinal fluid is to protect the underlying nerve tissues of the brain and spinal cord from mechanical trauma as well as to circulate nutrients such as glucose to the tissues and to remove waste products generated as a process of the metabolism of the central nervous system. Another important component of

© Springer International Publishing AG, part of Springer Nature 2018
J. W. Ridley, *Fundamentals of the Study of Urine and Body Fluids*,
https://doi.org/10.1007/978-3-319-78417-5_11

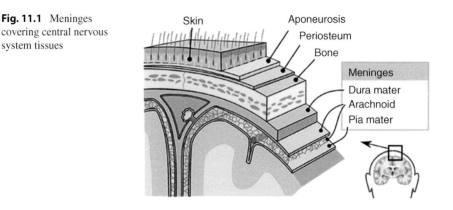

Fig. 11.1 Meninges covering central nervous system tissues

the protective mechanisms for the brain is that of the blood–brain barrier. The arrangement of capillaries with a tightly knit junction surrounding the capillaries that provide a separation of circulating blood and the *extracellular fluid* of the brain is not found in membranes or other structures of the body. The epithelium of the *choroid plexus* in addition provides added protection of the brain from certain elements found in the blood. Except for the brain, materials are freely exchanged between the capillaries and the various tissues of the body. This barrier also extends to the diffusion of certain medications which may be injurious to the central nervous system. Due to this protective system, the exclusion of certain drugs from the brain poses a challenge when medications designed to affect the brain must be bioengineered to penetrate this barrier.

Endothelial cells around the choroid plexus also restrict the diffusion of microscopic organisms such as bacteria and large hydrophilic molecules capable of attaching to water molecules into the CSF. Small hydrophobic molecules that repel water molecules are allowed to diffuse into the CSF, and these include oxygen, hormones and carbon dioxide. But cells of the barrier are capable of actively transporting necessary nutrient products such as glucose across the barrier along with specific proteins. Neurons or nerve cells gain practically all of their nutritional needs from aerobic metabolism of glucose, unlike other types of body cells that need additional nutrients such as protein. The nervous system requires large amounts of oxygen, therefore the blood flow in the brain of approximately 15 mL for each 100 g/min. If this flow is interrupted or falls below this level, nerve tissue begins to malfunction and to die.

In addition, the blood-brain barrier includes a thick basement membrane and *astrocytes* as added protection against invasive organisms and materials (Fig. 11.2). These specialized cells are known as astroglia or simply glial cells, although there are several types of these cells. They perform many functions that include biochemical support of the endothelial lining of the blood-brain barrier. They aid in providing nutrients, ion balance required to enable propagation of nerve impulses, and have a part in the repair and scarring process of the brain and spinal cord following traumatic injuries or infections.

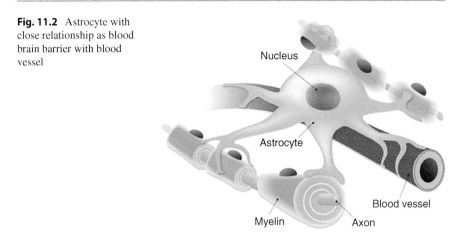

Fig. 11.2 Astrocyte with close relationship as blood brain barrier with blood vessel

Constituents of the CSF that are analyzed for evidence of illness related to the central nervous system differ greatly in concentration from similar elements found in blood. Active transport accounts for movement of materials into and out of the blood, with a particular emphasis on glucose as a nutrient, urea as a waste product and bicarbonate as a buffer to maintain an optimum pH. Some clinical components are normally found at higher levels in cerebrospinal fluid than the levels that are normally present in the blood, but other constituents are found in diminished levels when compared with those in the blood, particularly protein.

The testing of cerebrospinal fluid offers more challenges than do those from other anatomical sites, including that of blood. The collection of CSF is a difficult procedure that is potentially fraught with complications for the patient, and the handling requirements for the fluid present additional challenges. Specimens are small in comparison with those from most other body fluids. It is not a simple matter to request recollection of spinal fluid due to errors and accidents. In addition, since the procedures using CSF are done relatively infrequently in most clinical sites, the written protocol for collection, handling and testing of the material must be strictly adhered to in order to provide valid results. Most facilities do not have a department or specialized workers who primarily work with cerebrospinal fluid or for that matter, with all the basic body fluids. Quality control data may provide a broader range of results (large standard deviation figures) when the target values are drawn from a smaller number of results, so averages may be widely skewed by a few aberrant results.

11.2   Infection Control

Infection control when collecting and testing CSF is necessary to prevent infecting the patient as well as protecting the medical professionals who collect and handle the clinical material. Standard Precautions that were formerly known as Universal Precautions require protective steps for all persons who may be exposed to the fluid. These precautions are especially of importance when handling cerebrospinal fluid,

Fig. 11.3 Procedures
require face shield and
mask along with protective
gown and apron

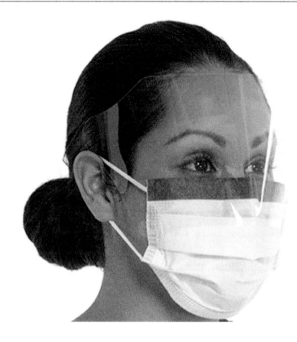

since a substantial number of pathogens capable of causing meningitis are likely. Many of these organisms are quite contagious and the prognosis for those suffering from certain strains of bacterial meningitis is poor.

Care must be exercised when involved with specimen collection, handling of and transporting the specimen, as well as precautionary measures necessary to avoid contraction of an infection by the testing personnel. All body fluids are capable of harboring infectious organisms, so avoiding direct contact with the specimens and items that come in contact with the clinical materials must be prevented. This is accomplished by scrupulous maintenance of a clean work space, the wearing of personal protective equipment, and washing of the hands and proper disposal of protective over garments such as gowns, protective eyewear and masks (Fig. 11.3).

Infection Control Flash
Cerebrospinal fluid is capable of harboring a number of virulent organisms, statistically more so than other fluids. Other than blood, it is perhaps the body fluid sample which would require the highest level of personal protection. CSF from patients with meningitis may contain a variety of classes of organisms other than bacteria, including fungi, viruses and even parasitic entities.

11.3   Routine Laboratory Tests for Cerebrospinal Fluid

Testing of cerebrospinal fluid is not only important in diagnosing infectious diseases such as meningitis. Other clinical findings other than viral or bacterial infections may relate to demyelinating diseases such as *multiple sclerosis*, in which the

Fig. 11.4 Gram stain kit
used for bacterial staining,
to enhance identification of
bacterial organisms

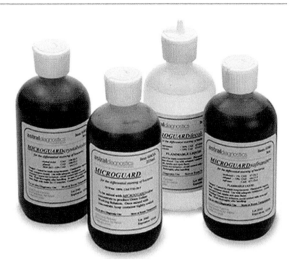

myelin sheath surrounding nerve tracts has been damaged or destroyed, hemorrhages that reveal the presence of blood within the subarachnoid spaces, and certain
malignancies affecting the central nervous system. Specimens from CSF are evaluated for the presence of red blood cells indicating a traumatic injury to the head or
back, and white cells are counted and then stained for differentiation as to the predominant type present. The type of white blood cells will indicate the type of infection, whether viral or bacterial or otherwise.

In addition to tests called *Gram stains*, which provide visual evidence of the
presence of bacterial and other rarer cases of meningitis by fungi or parasites, blood
cell counts and differentiation of the types of white blood cells present that require
specialized staining will be performed (Fig. 11.4). Chemistry tests for glucose will
be performed, along with those for protein, where normal values will be significantly lower than that found in the serum, measured by milligrams versus grams for
serum. It may be necessary to perform both blood and CSF protein determinations
for comparison so the presence of disease can be determined. Fractionations of
protein may also be necessary through a procedure called protein electrophoresis, a
process where various weights of protein fractions migrate at different rates and
distances. When combined with a specific gel, these proteins are placed in an electric field and results may result in a pattern that is indicative of a significant number
of specific diseases.

11.3.1 Specimen Collection for Cerebrospinal Fluid

A physical examination of the candidate for collection of cerebrospinal fluid must
be carefully conducted to insure the patient is physically capable of enduring the
procedure. Localized infections of an intended puncture site will contraindicate the
procedure of a *lumbar puncture*. Some newer diagnostic procedures such as *computerized tomography* (CT scans) and magnetic resonance imaging (MRI) have

minimized the numbers of invasive lumbar puncture and the side effects of such a process. But for confirmation of meningitis, the organism itself must be recovered from the CSF and tests for identification of the species, as well as antibiotic sensitivity tests must be performed from the fluid itself. Requirements for collecting CSF include rather extensive patient orientation and preparation. There are as well specific requirements for identification of the samples, types of containers required and the order of collection of the first through the last portion of the sample, as those samples used in the various tests are specific.

Specimens of cerebrospinal fluid are obtained by a procedure called lumbar puncture, where a sterile needle is used to withdraw samples of fluid from spaces between the third and fourth, or the fourth and fifth vertebrae (Fig. 11.5). The location where the puncture is performed is a requirement since some areas of the spine are quite vulnerable to damage to the sensitive spinal cord encased within the vertebrae. Complications following the procedure include headaches in many cases. Another problem area includes excessive bleeding, although a small amount of blood will almost always be present in the specimen, a condition called a *traumatic tap* or bloody tap. A sudden change in the intracranial regions due to sudden withdrawal of fluids is responsible for the potential to develop a headache and increased intracranial pressure can actually cause a *cerebral herniation* or tearing of the brain tissue that may result in paralysis or even death.

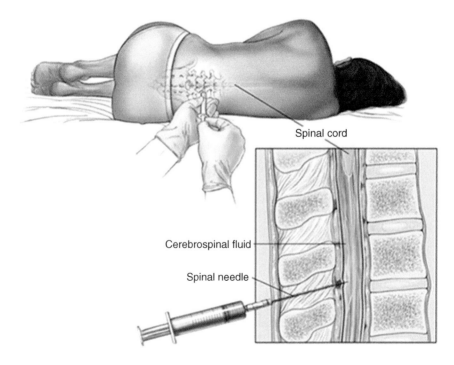

Spinal cord

Cerebrospinal fluid

Spinal needle

Fig. 11.5 Vertebrae containing spaces where cerebrospinal fluid is located

Extreme care must be exercised in the collection of cerebrospinal fluid due to the possibility of exacerbating medical conditions already present as well as those previously outlined. The skin where the puncture will be performed must be carefully disinfected, often by povidone-iodine, a general purpose iodophor that is used as a dilute solution for surgical scrubs and other medical procedures. This iodine must be removed prior to performing the spinal tap, however, since contamination by the solution may act as a bactericidal agent that will destroy any causative organisms that may have contributed to meningitis, giving erroneous information. A sterile surgical drape is placed over the site to further insure protection of the patient against environmental contamination before the puncture is initiated. The resulting fluid of as much as 10–20 mL will be divided into three or four specially numbered tubes for laboratory testing. If the cerebrospinal fluid is sterile and no disease conditions are present, the fluid will be crystal clear and sterile, with an appearance likened unto that of water.

The skin preparation for the lumbar puncture will most often include at least two 30-s scrubs with the povidone-iodine. Scrubbing is performed in a pattern of ever widening concentric circles beginning at the site where the needle will penetrate the skin, and the iodine solution may be left on the skin for several minutes to insure the destruction of skin contaminants. All residual iodine should be cleansed from the site by swabbing the area with 70% *isopropyl alcohol* before the puncture is performed. Allergies to certain preparations used for surgical scrubs may require the use of substitute cleansers such as chlorhexidine instead of iodine.

To avoid the development of serious medical complications resulting from the lowering of intracranial pressure during the withdrawal of the samples, the physician should measure the intracranial pressure following the insertion of the needle and before aspirating any fluid from the spinal column. This is accomplished by allowing some of the initial fluid to rise into a manometer tube, a sterile and slender cylinder that contains graduated markings. The patient is placed in a right or left lateral position, lying on his or her side and with the neck fully flexed that is called a fetal position. When certain conditions of the patient require alternate positioning, it may be necessary to seat the patient on a stool with his or her head and shoulders bent forward. Most normal adults will normally present an initial pressure of an equivalent value between 70 and 190 mm in comparison with water.

The pressure may also be accomplished by comparing the pressure with the weight of mercury and varies with the presence of certain conditions. Newborns may indicate a pressure of 50 mm of H_2O, 80 mm of H_2O for young children or up to 250 mm of H_2O for obese, adult patients. The pressure will vary by as much as 10 mm of pressure when the patient moves, strains or coughs, along with slight changes caused by breathing. Medical conditions that produce a marked rise or fall in the pressure exerted by the cerebrospinal fluid should be observed for and monitored during the procedure. For pressures exceeding 200 mm, only 1–2 mL of fluid should be removed. When only 1–2 mL is aspirated from a person with elevated pressure, the pressure may drop significantly. This occurs with either a spinal compression above the puncture site or a cerebral herniation is present, both of which are serious complicating factors. If only a small variation in pressure is noted after aspirating 1–2 mL, then the normal process of removing 10–20 mL of CSF can proceed.

After determining that the fluid pressure is normal, the normal aspiration of fluid begins, and the resulting fluid is dispensed into a three or four tube system, whichever is being utilized. The fluid is slowly forced from the syringe sequentially into the sterile, numbered and screw-capped tubes in 3–5 mL aliquots. The first 3–5 mL of CSF removed will be placed into tube #1, the second 3–5 mL will be placed into tube #2, and so forth. After collecting the fluid, and before the needle is withdrawn, the initial pressure before the aspiration began, the closing pressure following completion of the fluid aspiration, and the volume of fluid extracted are recorded. All three tubes or four are examined for the presence of visible blood and is noted for possible treatment based on the presence of blood that may be present in all three or more tubes.

Tube #1 is used for chemistry tests such as glucose and proteins, following centrifugation to remove any red blood cells occurring as a result of the needle puncture that may have produced minimal bleeding. The second tube is used for Gram stain for any type of microorganism, and bacterial cultures are performed from this tube. The third tube is used for enumerating red and white blood cells, as well as preparation of a slide for staining in order to differentiate the percentages of the various types of white cells in the fluid. The number of tubes collected may vary by medical facility and might include up to 5 tubes.

11.3.2 Physical Appearance of Cerebrospinal Fluid

Although the initial appearance of a normal sample of CSF is of a crystal and clear solution and the physical appearance of CSF can provide valuable diagnostic information. The appearance of CSF will include the following characteristics, a situation that is not unlike the initial examination of urine and other body fluids. Although a grossly bloody CSF can be indication of intracranial hemorrhage or puncture of blood vessel when collecting specimens, the presence of red blood cells in only one of the three to five collection tubes (Table 11.1), or blood in all three or four, will yield information based on the origin of the blood, shown in the following information.

Standard Process for Collection of CSF

a. CSF is collected aseptically and divided into 3–5 sealable sterile tubes (Table 11.1)
b. Properly label tubes, preferably before the collection is initiated. As with any laboratory procedure, improperly labeled sample containers will impact quality and interpretation of test results.
c. Samples are divided into 3 or 4 tubes, and procedures are performed in the following sequence to avoid errors of interpretation. Some facilities require a fifth tube for special tests such as cytology, and identification of fastidious

Table 11.1 Division of CSF sample for applicable testing

Tube #1	A white blood cell count is performed on tube #1. The presence of great numbers of erythrocytes may require lysing of the RBCs in order to count the leukocytes
Tube #2	A Gram stain and bacterial culture for identification and microbial antibiotic sensitivity determination are critical
Tube #3	Glucose and protein determinations which would aid in differentiation between a viral or bacterial infection as well as the presence of abnormal proteins characteristic of certain diseases
Tube #4	If performed, a second cell count is compared for comparison to Tube 1
Tube #5 (optional)	Cytological studies may be performed to determine the presence of malignancies; cellular cultures for viral agents as well as special culture techniques for mycological agents (yeasts, molds, fungi) may be necessary

microorganisms where quick identification may be critical for timely treatment, but the 3-tube method is most often used.

d. For inpatients, a minimum of 1 mL of CSF is required to complete the following procedures. The sample is transported to the laboratory on ice at 2–8 °C. In the event that a sample is too small (QNS—quantity not sufficient), the cell count and the culture for microorganisms based on the results of the cell count will be performed. A Gram stain when high levels of white blood cells are found would also be a critical procedure, where timely results may greatly benefit the patient.

Initial Assessment for Clarity and Presence of Blood

1. Blood will be distributed evenly between three CSF specimen tubes when a cerebral hemorrhage has occurred

2. Blood collected from traumatic tap will reveal blood in the first tube may form clots due to the introduction of plasma fibrinogen into the specimen, since the origin of the blood is from the circulatory system of the body where clotting factors are found.

3. When blood is present in all three tubes, a cerebral hemorrhage may have occurred where blood is present in the ventricles of the brain.

4. RBC's must remain in CSF for approximately 2 h before noticeable hemolysis begins to take place. A *xanthochromic* (yellowish) supernatant would be result of blood that has been present longer than that introduced by traumatic taps, having originated in the brain or in the spinal column. The distribution of color between tubes, and the colors exhibited by each of the tubes, will be the first physical measurement performed in the testing of cerebrospinal fluid (Table 11.2). This is a process that is similarly used for urine samples and any other body fluid that is tested for a disease process. When assisting with the collection of CSF, it is important to provide the specimen tubes in the correct order as the specimens are obtained.

Table 11.2 Physical appearance of cerebrospinal fluid

Crystal clear	Cloudy, turbid	Hemolyzed, bloody	Xanthochromic
Normal and free of lipids and blood cells	Presence of lipids, infection causing increase of WBCs	Traumatic puncture, cerebral herniation, subdural hematoma, spinal injury	Describes supernatant that is either pink, orange, or yellow Presence of red blood cell degradation products dependent upon amount of blood and the length of time present May also be caused by elevated serum bilirubin, carotene, markedly increased protein concentrations, and melanoma pigment, immature liver function in infants (especially premature)

11.3.3 Laboratory Analysis of Cerebrospinal Fluid

Clinical findings as well as attendant medical conditions that are correlated with clinical laboratory results from the examination of cerebrospinal fluid will often provide a definitive diagnosis and treatment plan for the patient. Most of the examinations of CSF are for the purpose of establishing the presence of bacterial meningitis, and to a lesser extent, the presence of mycobacterial infections of the central nervous system, comprised chiefly of infection by the organism causing tubercular infections. Less frequent reasons for the testing of the fluid is to determine the presence of fungal or parasitic cases of meningitis.

The routine laboratory examination of CSF is initially divided into several components. Following the physical examination of the fluid for clarity and the presence of blood, counts for both red and white blood cells are performed. This is sometimes performed through the use of sophisticated automated cell counters, but most commonly are done manually using a microscope and a specially designed volumetric slide called a hemocytometer. Some automated cell counters are not sensitive enough to enumerate the low counts of both red and white blood cells that may be found in significant numbers through the manual count. Chemistry tests and bacterial cultures comprise the bulk of tests typically performed in hospital laboratories.

Other more sophisticated procedures may be performed in larger medical centers, teaching and research laboratories and in commercial reference laboratories. The procedures may include cytological examinations for abnormal tissue cells, and this may be done by pathologists who are specialized physicians that serve in hospital laboratories. Immunophenotypic or genetic studies, biochemical tumor markers for certain malignancies and those found in conditions where the myelin sheath of the nerve fibers are damaged or destroyed are performed in some advanced laboratories. Immunological studies such as those designed to find specific classes of *immunoglobulin* of which antibodies are formed such as *IgG* to aid in the diagnosis of *multiple myeloma*. It should be noted for completeness that while no clinical test is currently in existence for diagnosing Alzheimer's Disease, the presence of three specific proteins in the spinal fluid of those with mild cognitive disabilities may predict with some confidence the impending development of this dread disease that robs so many of their ability to function normally in their daily lives.

Some tests on CSF are done routinely on all CSF samples but others are done only when they are indicated by other abnormalities discovered during routine examinations. The routine tests most often performed on all samples are those of white and red blood cell counts, differentiation of white blood cells, glucose and protein, and bacterial cultures if indicated by elevated white blood cell counts. Glucose and protein results from CSF should be compared with those found in the blood plasma in order to determine ratios for the values. Some clinicians believe that if the initial intracranial pressure is normal, and if the chemistry levels and differential counts for white blood cells are within normal ranges, then no further testing is warranted.

Differentiation between a subarachnoid hemorrhage and from a traumatic puncture is important and is an initial step in the evaluation of CSF fluid. Pathological bleeding from trauma to areas of and around the central nervous system with respect to the brain and the spinal cord are relatively simple to determine. When the sequentially collected tubes show an even red color in all the tubes, whether cloudy or clear, a subarchnoid hemorrhage below the meninges of the brain has most likely occurred. A subsequent clear condition of the tubes following the #1 tube is most likely a clue that a traumatic puncture while aspirating the CSF caused the presence of the blood cells. In addition, upon centrifugation, a subarachnoid hemorrhage will show a xanthrochromic color ranging from pink, orange or yellow color due to the presence of hemoglobin that has been freed from the red blood cells as the red cells become *lysed* or deteriorate.

In a specimen obtained by a traumatic spinal tap, the blood cells may be centrifuged from the sample and the supernatant will be clear. It may be helpful if the specimen in question is compared with a tube of clear water with both held against a white and unblemished sheet of white paper. Lysis of red blood cells in CSF from the victim of a subarachnoid hemorrhage will normally begin within 2 h of the onset of bleeding. It should be noted that the supernatant from such a hemorrhage will appear clear if the determination is made less than 2 h following the hemorrhage when the number of red cells is minimal. Cells resulting from a traumatic tap will begin within an hour, so it is necessary to do an immediate evaluation of the specimen following collection. The evidence of bleeding, if successful *hemostasis* or cessation of bleeding has occurred within a short time following the hemorrhage, will disappear within a few weeks but a yellow color (xanthochromasia) will be seen due to bilirubin remaining from the destruction of red blood cells.

Normal cerebrospinal fluid does not contain clotting factors, but when blood is present in the fluid from a traumatic tap, fibrinogen may be found. The origin of blood found in CSF can be determined by a very sensitive test for *D-Dimer Fibrin*, which is present in the cerebrospinal fluid of those suffering from a subarachnoid hemorrhage. But in some cases, blood from a traumatic tap may also be accompanied by a subarachnoid hemorrhage, so other techniques may be necessary to deduce the source of the blood. Cases of meningitis known as suppurative or pus forming and tubercular meningitis where the levels of protein are significantly increased may result in the formation of clots. But it could readily be assumed that in most cases there is no clotting in the case of subarachnoid hemorrhages.

Another helpful phenomenon in the recovery of patients who have endured a subarachnoid hemorrhage is the presence of *phagocytes* that are cells that eat organisms and even cells called astroglia. These cells are involved in the maintenance of the nerve tissues of the central nervous system. The process that occurs in subarachnoid hemorrhage is called *erythrophagia*, which is a process of ingestion of red cells. Ingestion of the red blood cells leaves a residue of hemoglobin, an iron-containing pigment that is released from the blood cells. Within two days of the hemorrhage, these macrophages may be seen in the fluid, and will contain granules of iron, called hemosiderin. This process is also present only in subarachnoid hemorrhage but is not found in fluid from a traumatic tap. These granules may be found as much as four or more months after the hemorrhagic episode, and may be identified as being hemosiderin by staining them with a stain called *Prussian blue*, which is also useful in other laboratory procedures where the presence of iron is suspected.

11.3.4 Microscopic Cell Counts and WBC Differentiation

Since automated cell counters are usually not standardized for the capability of counting blood cells from cerebrospinal fluid, except in cases of extremely bloody samples, a counting chamber called a hemocytometer is used for this purpose. Cells may arise from conditions other than bacterial or viral meningitis, which might be either lymphocytes in a viral infection, and neutrophils when a bacterial infection is present. Remember that a yeast-like organism, *Cryptococcus neoformans*, the causative agent for cryptococcal meningitis, has similar morphology to that of lymphocytes. An India ink prep should be used to confirm immunological testing to more specifically identify the yeast-like organism. Red blood cells may indicate either a traumatic injury or a subdural bleed from a blood vessel rupture. Other cells may be present and the laboratory technical personnel must understand that it is vital to look for abnormalities and to properly identify and report them. Malignant tumor cells can appear as single cells or in clumps, and differentiation between cells of the nervous system that may normally be observed, those of the choroid plexus and ependymal calls that line the ventricles where CSF is found.

For differentiation, a process called *cytocentrifugation* in which a specialized centrifuge called a *cytofuge* (Fig. 11.6) is frequently used for preparing smears to stain with a hematological stain, usually that of *Wright's* or *Wright's-Giemsa*, for white blood cell differentiation. This method of concentrating the white blood cells makes the process more efficient and less time-consuming, since the cells may be quite few in number. Two types of white blood cells are extremely important in differentiating a viral from a bacterial type of meningitis. The predominance of white cells called *neutrophils* or *polymorphonuclear cells* most often indicates a bacterial infection. An increase in the percentage of mononuclear cells called *lymphocytes*

Fig. 11.6 Centrifuge (cytofuge) used for preparing concentrations of stained cells

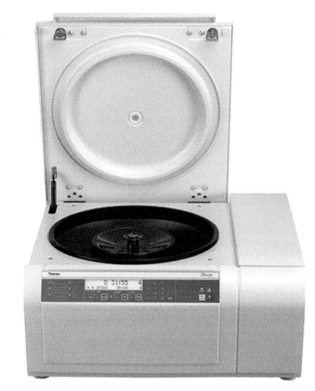

may indicate a viral infection of the central nervous system. Units of measurement known as international units (IU) are used on a global basis with the exception of the United States, where two types of units of measurement may be used to accommodate other nationalities and make it easier to transfer medical reports and records to other countries.

11.4   Red Blood Cell Count

Normally there will be few or no red blood cells present in cerebrospinal fluid. The presence of large numbers of RBCs would indicate the possibility of a subarachnoid cerebral hemorrhage, in the tissue beneath the meningeal lining of the central nervous system. Traumatic punctures with a small amount of bleeding will yield negligible numbers of cells unless severe localized bleeding was induced by the procedure. Therefore, RBC counts are seldom performed since the presence of RBC's should be negative normally but may be performed on undiluted samples under most circumstances. Cellular and chemical components (Table 11.3) may be quickly performed to determine whether meningitis is present and to aid in rapid and definitive treatment based on deviations of results obtained from established normal ranges.

Table 11.3 Normal CSF values derived from procedures utilizing English and SI units

Constituent of CSF	English units	SI units
RBC (Erythrocyte) count	0	0
WBC (Leukocyte) count Adults Newborns, small children	0–5 mononuclear cells/µL 0–35 mononuclear cells/µL	0–0.0005×10^9/L 0–0.0003×10^9/L
WBC (Leukocyte) differential, adults Lymphocytes Neutrophils Monocytes	40–80% 15–45% 0–4%	0.40–0.80 0.15–0.45 0.0–0.4
WBC (Leukocyte) differential, newborns, small children Lymphocytes Neutrophils Monocytes	5–35% 50–90% 0–4%	0.05–0.35 0.50–0.90 0.0–0.4
Total protein Adults <60 years of age Adults >60 years of age Newborns, small children	15–45 mg/dL 15–60 mg/dL 15–100 mg/dL	150–450 mg/L 150–600 mg/L 150–1000 mg/L
Glucose	50–80 mg/dL	2.75–4.40 mmol/L

NOTE: Procedure 11.1: The presence of RBC's may indicate a true rupture of a blood vessel or be present as the result of a traumatic puncture for obtaining the fluid. The condition of the red blood cells and the color if the remaining tubes (there should be four or five containing fluid) is the most important aspect of examining cerebrospinal fluid

Procedure 11.1: Red Blood Cell Count, Cerebrospinal Fluid

1. After mixing the cerebrospinal fluid sample carefully by twirling and inverting, use a Pasteur pipette or other disposable pipette to carefully deliver a small amount of CSF under the cover glass of the hemocytometer on both sides. If a V-shaped depression is present, this step is much simpler. Do not overfill the chamber, as it may take longer for the slide to equilibrate to the correct level. Allow equilibration of the depth in the chamber by placing the hemocytometer in a Petri dish for at least 5 min. The Petri dish should contain water-soaked bibulous paper to provide humidity, which serves to prevent evaporation of the sample from the hemocytometer, resulting in an erroneous count.

2. Use the low-power objective (10×) to scan both gridded sides of the hemocytometer to determine the presence of blood cells and to insure consistency of the solution, insuring that no clumps and heavy areas of concentration are present. Each major square and both sides of the slide should have roughly equal distributions of red blood cells.

3. Under the 40× objective, count the red blood cells using a manual hand-held "clicker" in the five squares found in the center (Fig. 11.7) of the ruled area, on each side of the slide.

    The four corner squares and the center square that are most closely gridded are counted.

4. The RBCs will be round and small and may appear to be a yellowish color. Sometimes a biconcave morphology, with a central area of pallor, may be observed. Normally the surfaces of the cells will be smooth with no aberrations on their surfaces.

5. When the numbers of red cells for the 10 squares on the 2 sides of the chamber exceed 200, fewer squares may be counted and then multiplied by a factor to equal the numbers that would have been counted had all 10 squares been used. For example, if 3 squares are counted on one side of the chamber and 2 are counted on the other for a total of 5 squares, the number of cells counted should be multiplied by 2.

6. Extremely bloody samples may require dilution with an isotonic solution such as normal saline that will not disrupt the cell membranes of the red blood cells. In the circulation of red blood cells, the count is measured in millions, while white blood cells are measured in thousands per unit of diluent, such as the number of cells per mL. Except in extremely bloody CSF, red blood cells would not reach a count equivalent to that found in the circulating blood supply. When the specimen is particularly bloody, it is necessary to dilute the sample volumetrically with an isotonic diluent. It may also be necessary to count fewer squares and adjust the calculations as appropriate to obtain an accurate count.

7. For calculating the number of red blood cells per volume of CSF, 10 squares on the two sides of the hemocytometer are counted. The calculation of the count is achieved by multiplying the count obtained by the dilution. No dilution is required normally unless the sample is visibly bloody, so the actual count for an undiluted specimen would contain no dilution factor. The volume factor is obtained by performing the following function.

    The actual count for an undiluted specimen would contain no dilution factor. The volume factor is obtained by performing the following function:

---

1 µL (10 mm² × 0.1 mm)

Total cells counted × dilution factor (if applicable) × volume factor = cells per µL (mm³)

Example
When 10 squares are counted, a volume of one microliter (1 µL) is counted. Assuming 210 cells were counted, the results would be calculated as follows:

    210 (number of RBCs counted in 10 small squares) × volume factor = 210/µL

8. The hemocytometer should be disinfected by using bleach or a commercial disinfectant by soaking the instrument for at least 5 min in the solution. The slide is then rinsed with deionized or distilled water or with 70% alcohol and is then dried using lens paper.

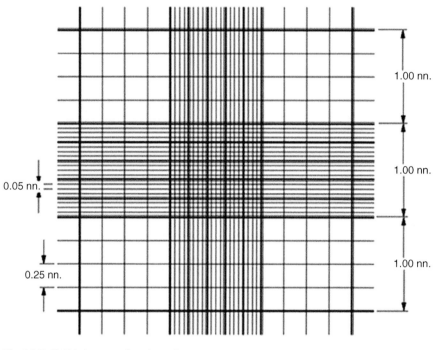

Fig. 11.7 Gridded square of neubauer hemocytometer

11.5   White Blood Cell Count

Under normal circumstances, only a few (0–5) white blood cells per µL will be found in CSF in adults. These will chiefly be mononuclear cells that include lymphocytes and monocytes. The numbers normally found in newborns are slightly higher (0–35) per µL. Any red blood cells must be lysed (destroyed) by the use of acetic acid or other lysing solution. The use of glacial acetic acid produces dual benefits of clearing the sample of all but the white cells, and also gives some distinction to the nuclei of the white cells, enabling an estimate of the presence of mononuclear cells or those categorized as polymorphonuclear. A prepared smear is made and then stained to provide a definitive percentage of the types of white blood cells present. Steps required to perform a quantitative white blood cell count are found in Procedure 11.2, as follows.

Procedure 11.2: White Blood Cell Count, Cerebrospinal Fluid

1. Insure mixing of the cerebrospinal fluid sample carefully by twirling and inverting the tube containing the specimen. Rinse a Pasteur pipette or other disposable pipette with glacial acetic or other appropriate solution

such as a stain. Using an absorbent sponge, wipe the outside of the pipette including the tip to remove any excess acid that would dilute the specimen as well as serve as a contaminant to the remaining sample when the pipette is inserted into the specimen.

2. Tilt the tube containing the CSF sample and place the tip of the pipette into the solution. Tilting the pipette enables sample to flow by capillary action into the pipette. Allow the pipette to fill at least half its length. Place a gloved finger over the large end of the pipette to prevent the sample from spilling.

3. Holding the pipette in a horizontal position, carefully tilt and turn the pipette to achieve complete mixing of sample with the small amount of acetic acid remaining in the pipette.

4. Carefully deliver a small amount of CSF under the cover glass on both sides of the hemocytometer. If a V-shaped depression is present, this step is much simpler. Allow several minutes for the slide to equilibrate to the correct level and to enable complete lysis of any red blood cells present.

5. Use the low-power objective (10×) to scan both gridded sides of the hemocytometer to determine the presence of white blood cells and to insure consistency of the solution, insuring that no clumps or inconsistently heavy areas of concentration are present. Each major square and both sides of the slide should have roughly an equal distribution of cells.

6. Using the 10× objective, count white blood cells using a manual hand-held counting device in the four corner squares, and large center square on each side of the slide. The four corner squares and the entire center square that is the most closely gridded are to be counted.

7. The WBCs can be tentatively classified as mononuclear or polymorphonuclear, but a stained smear for differentiation is preferable.

8. When the numbers of white cells for each of the 10 squares on the 2 sides of the chamber exceed 200, fewer squares may be counted and multiplied by a factor to adjust for the numbers that would have been counted in the 10 squares. For example, if 3 squares are counted on one side of the chamber and 2 are counted on the other, add the numbers and multiply the sum of the two sides by 2.

9. For calculating the number of white blood cells per volume of CSF, *10 large squares on the two sides* (Fig. 11.7) of the hemocytometer with gridded squares are counted. The calculation of the count is achieved by multiplying the count obtained by the dilution.

10. The hemocytometer should be disinfected by using bleach or a commercial disinfectant by soaking the instrument for at least 5 min. The slide is then rinsed with deionized or distilled water or with 70% alcohol, and dried using lens paper.

Calculating Cells Per Microliter

When 10 squares are counted, five larger squares which would include both sides of the Neubauer counting chamber, a volume of one microliter (1 μL) is counted. Assuming 210 cells were counted, the results would be calculated as follows:

Calculations for CSF Cell Count

First, the volume factor is obtained by the following function:

$$1\,\mu L\left(10\;mm^2 \times 0.1\;mm\right) = 10$$

Secondly, the equation for conducting the cell count is:

$$\text{Cells}\,/\,\mu L = \#\,\text{Cells counted} \times \text{Dilution}\,(1)\,/\,\#\,\text{Squares Counted}\,(9) \times$$
$$\text{Volume of 1 square}\,(0.1)\,\mu L$$

Simplified Version, No Need for Volume Correction

Count four large squares and the large center square, using a Neubauer hemacytometer

Four squares (0.4 μL) and large center square is (0.1 μL)

Example

$$\frac{Cells}{\mu L} = \frac{1\;\mu L}{1\;\mu L\;(0.1 \times (10)}= cells/\mu L\,(\text{volume counted})$$

$$\text{Total cells counted} \times \text{dilution factor}\,\left(\text{if applicable}\right) \times$$
$$\text{volume factor} = \text{cells per}\,\mu L\left(mm^3\right)$$

Calculation

For 10 squares (five from each side) a volume of one microliter (1 μL) is counted.

Assume that 210 cells were counted on the two sides

Example Calculation

$$210 \ (\text{number of WBCs counted in 10 small squares}) \times$$
$$\text{volume factor} \ (1) = 210/\mu L$$

11.6 Miscellaneous Procedures for Cerebrospinal Fluid

A number of tests are routinely performed upon cerebrospinal fluids for the diagnosis of various disorders. Most of the tests for CSF relate to meningitis, but other procedures are designed to diagnose a variety of medical conditions. Some of these sophisticated tests are normally not performed in a general laboratory, but the following are categories of procedures are performed routinely in most clinical laboratories.

11.6.1 Cellular Differentiation and Morphology

Cellular differentiation for distinguishing percentages of white blood cells and evaluating the morphology of red blood cells will require a concentration procedure as well as a staining procedure. Concentrations are routinely performed with the use of a *Cytospin* (Shandon Corp., Pittsburgh, PA., but other methodologies are available. The sample is rotated slowly for up to 10 min during which time the liquid from the specimen is absorbed by filter paper, and the cells are concentrated in a small circle on a microscope slide. This area of concentration can be stained with Wright's stain or another hematological or cytological stain and evaluated microscopically. It should be noted here and will be mentioned in another section of this book, that the presence of an unusual yeast-like organism, *Cryptococcus neoformans*, may be mistaken for lymphocytic white blood cells. This is reemphasized from earlier references, since this mistake could lead to dire consequences.

11.6.2 Bacterial and Viral Infections Differentiations

For the determination of the presence of bacteria, it is also necessary to concentrate any bacteria present in the sample, since the fluid should be in a sterile condition so the presence of *any* bacteria is of medical interest. Bacterial meningitis results in fatal consequences if not quickly treated adequately and accurately, sometimes within hours, or may result in sensory loss of hearing and of motor functions of a permanent nature. Therefore, a Gram stain procedure used for identification of the morphology of bacteria should be performed, particularly when large numbers of polymorphological white blood cells are present. Bacterial organisms that are commonly experienced in cases of bacterial meningitis include *Hemophilus influenza, Streptococcus pneumoniae, Neisseria meningitidis*, and *Group B streptococci*, an organism that causes "strep throat." It is paramount that the causative organism be presumptively identified, as adequate antibiotics must be administered quickly and antibiotic sensitivity testing should be performed to insure the appropriate therapy has been initiated. Cases of meningitis due to fungi are frequently detected microscopically with use of certain stains and dyes.

Viral infections of the central nervous system may be as lethal as those of bacterial origin. Since viruses will not reproduce on bacterial media, cultures of viruses are done on cell cultures, as viruses reproduce intracellularly. Even though an increase in mononuclear lymphocytes is often seen in viral infection, during the early stages of the infection, there may be an increase in the level of polymorphonuclear white blood cells (segmented neutrophils). Some rapid tests for the diagnosis of viruses are available for a quick diagnosis, many of which are generally the type considered to be *indirect testing*. In this type of testing, the actual causative organism is not detected visually or by chemical means but by the reaction of the body's immune system against the invading organism. The procedure utilizes antibodies produced by the body against specific viruses, and reactions between these antibodies and antigens of the actual organism are observed for reactions between them, where antibodies form complexes with the antigen and antibody linked together. Another useful procedure is the use of the presence of C-reactive protein (CRP) in CSF.

But this procedure is not definitive for differentiating between bacterial and viral cases of meningitis. Elevated levels of CRP, an acute phase reactant that occurs in various inflammatory reactions, in the fluid is used by some to identify bacterial meningitis. A protein called myelin basic protein (MBP) is useful in diagnosing 90% of those suffering from multiple sclerosis, a disease of the central nervous system, where the nerve sheaths are demyelinated. MBP is also increased for a number of other medical conditions, so the presence of elevated levels of MBP are used only as an adjunct to clinical signs and other clinical tests for the definitive diagnosis of MS.

Most CSF protein comes from the transport of plasma proteins through the capillary endothelium located in the choroid plexus and the meninges (a small amount of protein is synthesized). To analyze protein from CSF, the sample must be concentrated multiple times over in order to have enough concentration for performing a protein electrophoresis. Remember, CSF proteins are measured in mg/dL while plasma proteins are measured in grams/dL (1000 mg in 1 g). Contamination with peripheral blood during the spinal puncture will result in faulty measurements. Changes in the permeability of the capillaries may occur due to various forms of meningitis, hemorrhage, death of cerebral tissue (strokes) and trauma. Some hormonal imbalances may also be contributing factors.

11.6.3 Chemical Analysis for Cerebrospinal Fluid

The blood-brain barrier described previously described, enables selective passage through the membranes from the blood to the brain. These structures result in differing concentrations or even the absence of certain components found in the blood when compared with those that are found in the cerebrospinal fluid. Duplicate testing of both the blood plasma and the CSF are usually performed to compare the results, since high levels of a constituent in the blood may also produce high normal levels in the CSF. The most common chemistry procedures performed for CSF are glucose and protein, along with certain enzymes as appropriate, lactate, and tumor markers.

A decreased glucose level is often indicative of a bacterial meningitis and increased activities of the brain cells which utilize glucose for energy. In bacterial forms of meningitis, along with more rarely tubercular and fungal cases, CSF lactate levels may be needed. Lactate levels of more than 25 mg/dL occur in bacterial meningitis along with tubercular and fungal infections. Levels of more than 35 mg/dL occur most often with bacterial meningitis. Difficult cases where a definitive diagnosis is preferable, lactate levels rather than glucose levels are preferred for accuracy.

Protein determinations are used to diagnose a number of medical conditions in addition to meningitis (Table 11.4). It is often necessary to perform an electrophoresis to determine the fractions of certain proteins that are present in cerebrospinal fluid. Of course, the level of total protein in the CSF is much lower than that found in the blood plasma. For instance, the protein level of plasma is measured in grams per deciliter (dL) and in CSF is measured as milligrams per deciliter (100 mL). When a traumatic puncture occurs, the protein levels may be elevated due to

Table 11.4 Factors impacting CSF protein values

Decreased CSF protein	Increased CSF protein
Leakage of CSF from tears of the lining of the brain or spine	Traumatic puncture with plasma contamination
Diagnostic procedures such as pneumoencephalography (air is inserted into the cranial space for radiographical images) and increases intracranial pressure	Increased permeability of blood-brain barrier from alterations resulting from inflammation
Hyperthyroidism	Infectious or toxic conditions where the arachnoid villi are affected
	Blockages from tumors, scar tissue, etc
	Increase in white blood cells (lymphocytes), where increased levels of immunoglobulins (a protein) are formed as a reaction to an infectious process

Table 11.5 Conditions affecting CSF glucose values

Decreased CSF glucose	Elevated CSF glucose
Delay in testing following specimen collection—increased glycolysis	Diabetic coma due to *hyperglycemia*
Meningitis of organisms including bacteria, mycobacteria (TB), fungi, amoebae, and other parasites	Bloody or traumatic spinal tap
Low glucose levels in the blood (hypoglycemia)	
Subarachnoid hemorrhage	
Tumors (*neoplasms*) of the meninges	
Utilization of glucose by leukocytes and bacteria (this assumption is controversial)	
Insulin shock in diabetics	

contamination with blood plasma protein, and only a small amount will dramatically increase that found in CSF. In general, protein levels for cerebrospinal fluid are used as follows:

Glucose determinations are also important in differentiating the potential for a viral versus a bacterial meningitis (Table 11.5). Tests for the level of glucose should be done as quickly as possible following the collection of CSF. Glycolysis, a process where glucose is converted to pyruvic acid for energy, occurs quickly and will artificially produce a lower level of glucose than the levels originally contained in the sample of CSF (Table 11.5). Normally, the glucose level in CSF, which is the sole energy source for the nerve cells of the central nervous system, are about 60% of the levels found in the blood. Therefore, an increase in glucose of the CSF can be sometimes attributed to a high level in the blood. Normal levels of glucose will usually be the case in viral meningitis. These differences between the two types of samples can be important in completing the clinical picture for diagnosis of medical conditions. In general, glucose levels in the CSF are used as follows:

11.6.4 Other Tests for Diagnosis of Meningitis

In brain injuries, where *hypoxia* or low levels of oxygen often occur, the *lactate* level in the spinal fluid may be elevated. In the first day following a severe head injury, the lactate level will rise, and a return to normal signals improvement in the medical condition of the patient. Sustained high levels of lactate signal a poor prognosis for the victim of a head injury. Lactate levels are also used in differentiating between viral meningitis which yields low levels, as opposed to those of bacterial, mycobacterial, and fungal cases of meningitis, where high levels are frequently encountered.

Tissue enzymes are used to diagnose a number of medical disorders where specific tissue been damaged by infectious processes or by injury or lack of oxygen. Increased levels of lactic *dehydrogenase* (LD) are increased in cases of brain injury, as are those of *creatine kinase* (CK) and *aspartate aminotransferase* (AST) is frequently found in some cases where brain injury has occurred. However, these do not identify the cause of the disease, but merely serve to confirm that the organs of the central nervous system are most likely involved.

11.7   Summary

Cerebrospinal fluid (CSF) bathes the areas of the central nervous system and serves to protect and to nourish the vital tissues such as the brain. No one specific test will pinpoint the absolute diagnosis of meningitis, to include the causative organism, but requires a variety of tests that are correlated with clinical findings and physical examinations to extend confidence to the diagnosis. The most important component of providing adequate treatment is to perform immediate screening tests on the CSF to guide the rapid treatment before the condition deteriorates and death ensues.

Laboratory tests such as WBC counts, can establish the absolute presence of RBCs in the central nervous system, and other microscopic procedures which serve to provide visualization of causative organisms. Bacteria, fungi, mycobacteria and perhaps parasites may be observed microscopically, sometimes with the use of stains and dyes, but might not provide speciation of the organisms. This is done by bacterial culture, tests for antibodies specific for certain viruses. Other tests, particularly those of glucose and protein determinations, are used jointly to provide clues as to the origin of the meningeal inflammation, whether bacterial, viral, or as a result of other infectious agents.

Case Study 11.1

A 3-year-old boy awakes with a fever of 102.8. He grows increasingly lethargic during the day and by evening his face is flushed and he is extremely dehydrated. He has refused to eat or drink. When his father takes him to the pediatrician's office, the child complains of a headache and constantly grasps at the back of his neck. Blood is obtained and a complete blood count and the white blood cell count is elevated. The child is immediately transported to the hospital for further treatment.

Blood cell count:	$13 \times 10^9/L$
Leukocyte differential:	71% lymphocytes and 17% neutrophils; the remainder of the cells included 1% eosinophils and 11% monocytes
Reference values:	WBC's $0.15 \times 10^9/L$ and more than 25% neutrophils

1. What would be the following procedure most probably performed upon this child?

2. What would be the significance of increased lymphocytes?

3. Upon microscopic examination of the CSF from this patient, cells resembling lymphocytes were seen in great numbers. In addition to being white cells called lymphocytes, what is the other possibility for a causative organism?

4. What is the next step to confirm the organism suggested in the previous question?

_____

5. What would be the most likely diagnosis for this patient?

_____

Review Questions

1. The most common condition for which a lumbar puncture is performed is for the diagnosis of:
   a. Subarachnoid hemorrhage
   b. Streptococcal pharyngitis
   c. Malignancy of the CNS
   d. Meningitis
2. The centrifuged supernatant from cerebrospinal fluid is pink to yellowish. The most likely cause is:
   a. Clear
   b. Traumatic lumbar puncture
   c. Subarachnoid hemorrhage
   d. Viral meningitis
3. As a result of a traumatic spinal tap, which of the following patterns would be observed from a sequential collection of CSF?
   a. More red color in tube #1
   b. Even redness though all tubes
   c. More red in tube #3 than in tube #1
   d. Red color increases from #1 to #4 tubes
4. When polymorphonuclear cells are increased in a CSF sample, the likely cause is:
   a. Viral meningitis
   b. Bacterial meningitis
   c. Allergic reaction to povidone-iodine
   d. None of the above
5. Viral meningitis is usually diagnosed by:
   a. Increase in lymphocytes
   b. Positive antibody level for specific virus
   c. Increase in neutrophils
   d. a & b
6. Excess cerebrospinal fluid is retained in the ventricles of the brain in which of the following?
   a. Hypoglycemia
   b. Hydrocephalus
   c. Acute viral meningitis
   d. Leakage of CSF, cerebral herniation

7. Under normal conditions, glucose and protein levels in the CSF would be:
   a. Higher than that found in blood
   b. Same as that found and blood
   c. Lower than that found in blood
   d. Will vary, even in normal individuals

8. Which of the following is used to prevent infection of the CNS during lumbar puncture?
   a. Creatine kinase
   b. Sodium hypochlorite
   c. Povidone-iodine
   d. 70% isopropyl alcohol

9. The most commonly diagnosed demyelinating disease of the CNS is:
   a. Multiple myeloma
   b. Multiple sclerosis
   c. Multisequential antibody titers
   d. Viral meningitis

10. Intracranial pressure is monitored during a lumbar puncture. When the pressure drops significantly following aspiration of a small amount of CSF, the likely reason is:
    a. Spinal compression above puncture
    b. Too much fluid was withdrawn
    c. Presence of a cerebral herniation
    d. This is a normal occurrence
    e. a & c

11. The origin of blood found in CSF can be determined by:
    a. The fact that the blood clotted
    b. Test for D-Dimer Fibrin
    c. Presence of C-reactive protein
    d. Pus in the fluid

12. Cytocentrifugation is chiefly used for:
    a. WBC cellular differentiation
    b. RBC cellular differentiation
    c. Separation of viruses from bacteria
    d. None of the above

13. When doing a *preliminary* differentiation of leukocytes while using a hemocytometer, which of the following would be used to enable an estimate of the types of cells present?
    a. Wright's stain
    b. Povidone-iodine
    c. Glacial acetic acid
    d. Cytological stain

14. Which of the following would be elevated following hypoxia with an impact on the brain?
    a. Glucose
    b. Creatine kinase
    c. Lactic dehydrogenase
    d. Lactate

15. A decreased CSF protein might result from:
    a. Plasma contamination
    b. Tears of the lining of the brain
    c. Traumatic puncture
    d. Blockages by tumors and scars
16. An increased CSF protein might result from:
    a. Plasma contamination
    b. Tears of the lining of the brain
    c. Traumatic puncture
    d. Blockages by tumors and scars
    e. a & c
17. A decreased CSF glucose may be the result of which of the following:
    a. Delay in testing
    b. Bloody or traumatic spinal tap
    c. Diabetic coma
    d. All of the above
18. An increased CSF glucose may be the result of which of the following:
    a. Delay in testing
    b. Bloody or traumatic spinal tap
    c. Diabetic coma
    d. All of the above

Answers Found in Appendix C

Semen Evaluation

12

Objectives

Understand the need for proper protocol in the collection of sperm samples to provide consistent and meaningful reports

Relate the reasons for observing Standard Precautions when transporting and handling sperm samples

Recognize the correlations of screening tests and the actual procedures that result in clinical reports

Classify the characteristics of semen that may indicate the presence of factors that might negatively influence the ability to contribute to pregnancy

List the important factors that must be accounted for to insure proper testing of semen (ie., temperature of sample, mixing, etc.)

12.1 Introduction to the Testing of Semen and Seminal Fluid

As a miscellaneous body fluid, the testing of semen is one of the most frequently ordered laboratory examinations and most often the first for determining the causes of infertility as well as to assess the effectiveness of a *vasectomy*, a surgical procedure performed for birth control purposes. For some inexplicable reason, perhaps dictated by lifestyle changes, statistics show that over the last 50 years, the average total sperm count for an American male has decreased from levels of approximately 120 million sperm per milliliter of fluid to slightly over 50 million per mL. This effectively changes the average or normal range for an acceptable count dramatically from just five decades ago. Available data also shows changes in the normal range for residents of a number of countries. Some researchers have postulated that geographical differences and an average decline in sperm counts for some countries may be due to endocrine disruptors present during *in utero* development of the fetus. Environmental contamination and the availability of widespread medications and their use may be causative factors but no proof exists of such.

© Springer International Publishing AG, part of Springer Nature 2018
J. W. Ridley, *Fundamentals of the Study of Urine and Body Fluids*,
https://doi.org/10.1007/978-3-319-78417-5_12

So the debate continues in the search to understand a precipitous decline in numbers and quality of *spermatozoa*. The logical assumption could be made that certain environmental chemicals, both naturally occurring and those produced by humans, have potentially altered sperm counts. Incidentally, the development of new chemicals occurs on almost a daily basis and recent governmental restrictions have been relaxed, allowing more chemicals to reach the market. This factor could result in the variations seen in the results of semen analyses that are seen in diverse geographic locations. But in addition to lower total sperm counts, some researchers have reported concurrent losses in the quality of sperm in the average North American male over the past several decades. Today, a normal average sperm count is 20 million, and this would have been considered significantly decreased even during the 1960s and 1970s. The semen analysis is designed to provide assessments of a sample of *ejaculate* for both quantity and quality. In spite of these changes in total counts, the population is still rising and it is estimated that up to 40% of the cases of infertility can be traced to inadequate sperm counts or quality of sperm, or both.

In some legal cases, semen samples are increasing in use when conducting studies during forensic procedures. Paternity cases may be confirmed or disproven by using genetic studies of semen along with accompanying skin cells that may be analyzed and compared to determine criminal culpability. Some enzymes released in semen are also valuable in forensic cases, where rape is charged, to prove sexual contact was made. These enzymes are present even when the male has undergone a vasectomy, as the seminal fluid even with no sperm cells will still provide proof of coitus.

12.2   Infection Control

A number of sexually transmitted diseases are transmitted by exchange of body fluids including semen. This fluid is a medium capable of harboring large numbers of infectious pathogens that cause serious consequences for others. An organism that is quite prevalent and that is widely spread through semen and vaginal fluids is the HIV-1 virus that causes AIDS. On a global basis and in the majority of these infections, much of the transmission of HIV-1 is via sexual contact between men. But early in the history of a growing knowledge of HIV-1, dental procedures also contributed to a significant number of infections. So Universal Precautions evolved into Standard Precautions with measures developed by governmental agencies to protect the health of employees and others who may come in contact with semen.

Training and education are now mandated by state and federal legislation as a component of a healthcare facility's policies and must be adhered to conscientiously. The extreme danger of being exposed to the human immunodeficiency virus (HIV) has required more stringent monitoring of procedures recommended by the Center for Disease Control and Prevention (CDCP). It is unlawful in many jurisdictions for a person knowingly infected with HIV to engage in sex with a partner without informing the partner of his or her medical status.

It is important that the person handling semen exercise extreme protective measures to avoid self-contamination or to others who may later come in contact with semen products unwittingly, such as custodians. When equipment used for semen analysis is not disposable, it should be thoroughly cleaned in accordance with the manufacturer's recommendations. Disposable supplies and equipment should be used if possible and disposed of properly in biohazardous receptacles before transport to an approved disposal facility.

Infection Control Alert
The most common body fluids from which HIV is transmitted are those of semen and vaginal fluids. Blood is also a body fluid that is highly involved in the transmission of HIV, most often from the sharing of needles by IV drug users

12.3 Routine Tests for the Analysis of Semen

Spermatozoa or sperm cells are chiefly evaluated with respect to numbers present, the quality of the morphology of the cells, and the motility of the sample. While these tests are the major measures of male fertility, other factors are evaluated and observed as a part of the total analysis of semen. Some of these additional analytes include cells other than spermatozoa that are present in the semen, and the presence of some of these chemical analytes contribute to the maintenance and viability of sperm cells. When additional components are evaluated in a coordinated manner, they can give a clear idea of a semen sample's viability and quality or deficits related to sperm cells.

The freshly-collected semen sample is kept at room temperature in strictly clean containers to avoid contamination prior to testing. For the post-vasectomy sample, a representative sample of a well-mixed specimen is examined microscopically for the presence of any spermatozoa. It is not unusual to find a few non-viable sperm cells even in a post-vasectomy sample for several weeks following the surgical procedure. After a 30-min wait following sample collection, semen will normally completely liquefy when certain factors are present. Then the motility of the individual sperm cells may be observed as well as the morphology of a representative number of the cells. The following characteristics are observed during a complete semen analysis.

12.3.1 Volume

The volume of the ejaculate is the first characteristic that is observed, after insuring the sample was properly collected in the appropriate container and the time of transport is acceptable. Samples should be received in the laboratory within minutes of collection, and in some facilities, a private area is provided for collection of the sample. This latter provision would be invaluable for those who are having problems conceiving.

The normal volume of ejaculate from a healthy man ranges from 2 to 6 mL (Fig. 12.1). A low volume of less than 1 mL may be the result of an incomplete

Fig. 12.1 Cylindrical
measuring device for
quantitation of volume

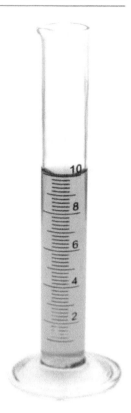

ejaculation or spilling of the sample rather than that of a medical condition. The donor should be questioned as to whether specimen loss may have been a factor if a low volume sample is submitted. The major portion of the fluid is produced in structures of the urogenital system, primarily from the seminal vesicles. Low volumes may be due to problems with seminal vesicle function while an extremely high volume of seminal fluid may present a problem with achieving pregnancy due to a low sperm count per mL. This issue is due to a dilutional factor where a count may be artificially lowered by a higher volume of fluid. The specimen is most easily measured after complete liquefaction. Smaller versions of the following measuring devices are used for measuring semen.

12.3.2 Semen Viscosity

Initial ejaculate may be highly viscous and appear as a gelatinous mass. When the soluble factors of seminal fluid are normal, the semen should liquefy in 30 min or fewer. This allows the sperm free motility. If the semen does not liquefy or if it is very thick in consistency after liquefaction, an infection of the seminal vesicles and perhaps of the *prostate gland* may be a factor in fertility.

12.3.3 Semen pH

The pH of semen is normally somewhat alkaline due to the secretions of the seminal vesicle. Vaginal fluid and the surface mucosa of the vagina are quite acid, and an alkaline pH for the seminal fluid serves to protect the sperm from the acidity. An acidic pH of the semen would result from medical problems with seminal vesicle function. This is usually found in association with a low volume of ejaculate with an absence of *fructose*. Fructose, a sugar produced in the seminal vesicles, provides energy for cell motility, and if fructose is absent in the seminal fluids, the flow of sperm through the ejaculatory duct may be disrupted.

12.3.4 Microscopic Examination

Visual examination by microscope of a semen sample is an important component of a complete analysis of semen. The total sperm count is the number of cells found in 1 mL of the sample. Fewer than 20 million cells per mL is considered a low count, and may result in failure to achieve pregnancy easily. Some men may have no sperm for a variety of reasons and are said to be *aspermatic*.

12.3.5 Quality of Spermatozoa

The quality of sperm cells is measured chiefly by its percentage of motile cells and whether organized progression is present, which may be more significant than the actual count itself. Large numbers of non-motile sperm would negatively impact on a resulting pregnancy. In addition, the morphology of sperm cells is a factor in determining if pregnancy may ensue. Since sperm counts have become lower in the majority of the world, motility are both graded by the World Health Organization (WHO) on a scale ranging from A to D. Cells graded C and D (Fig. 12.1) are considered poor and incapable of fertilizing an ovum.

12.3.6 Clumping of Spermatozoa

Sperm tend to clump (also called *agglutination*), where large numbers of spermatozoa adhere to each other in small groups. This phenomenon inhibits sperm motility and prevents the movement of the sperm toward the egg.

12.3.7 Leukocyte Presence

A few white blood cells (leukocytes) are normally present in seminal fluid. When a significant number of leukocytes are found in the seminal fluid, this would indicate that a potential bacterial infection may be present. An infection of the genitourinary tract may negatively affect the viability of the spermatozoa.

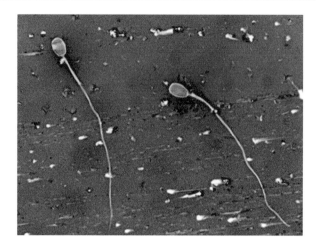

Fig. 12.2 Image of normal spermatozoa

12.3.8 Microscopic Examination

Visual microscopic examination of the sample is perhaps the most important and initial component of a complete sperm analysis. Sperm count means the number of sperm present per mL of semen. Again, if the sample has fewer than 20 million sperm per mL, this is judged to be a low sperm count. Fewer than 10 million is extremely low. Some men may have no sperm at all for various reasons and in these cases they are said to be *aspermatic*.

12.3.9 Morphology of Sperm

A small number of abnormally formed sperm cells are found in all semen samples and are not capable of fertilizing an ovum. A sperm with normal morphology will have an oval and regularly shaped head (Fig. 12.2). A mid-section that connects the head to the tail is slightly smaller in width than the head, and the normal sperm will have a single long and straight tail. Abnormally-shaped sperm are distorted in shape or size and may exhibit other abnormalities. When large numbers of sperm are abnormally shaped with completely round heads, small heads called pin heads, double heads, or those with two tails or no tail, the sperm are incapable of fertilizing the egg. A normal semen sample will have at a minimum 15% of the total number that are of a completely normal form.

12.3.10   Additional Fertility Factors

In some cases of infertility, the routine analytical examination of semen will result in normal findings for numbers, morphology and progression. In this scenario, other somewhat common issues also lead to the inability to become pregnant. Frequently the cervix is convoluted in the female, posing barriers to the sperm for reaching the uterus and into the Fallopian tubes. Structural barriers related to scar tissue from infections of the female may effectively prevent fertilization of eggs and may require dilation of the cervix or surgery to correct the condition.

There are sometimes immunological problems related to infertility for both male and female. Antibodies to the sperm may affect the motility and viability of fusing the sperm and egg to form a zygote. Antibodies may be present in the male's semen or on the surface of the sperm, or the blood plasma of either the male or female and may even contain antibodies that make it difficult to achieve a viable pregnancy. Fertility specialists might take steps to circumvent these immunological problems, but a number of options are available that lead to pregnancy when abnormalities in either partner are present.

For instance, when the semen volume is low, with little likelihood of pregnancy, the sperm sample may be concentrated and artificially introduced into the cervix. Again, structural defects of the cervix may pose a barrier for the sperm cells in traversing a timely path to the Fallopian tubes. Artificial insemination is then a possibility if adequate sperm cells are available. Another tactic is that of in vitro fertilization, where egg and sperm are introduced in a special tube and enables a zygote through merging of the egg and sperm. After a period of growth by division, the zygote is then implanted into the uterus.

Other biochemical tests may be required to determine if the absence or decreased levels of the various nutritive components are present. Chemistry evaluations are used to measure levels of several different biological components normally present in semen. Low or diminished concentrations of fructose, citric acid and *acid phosphatase* may be involved in problems of achieving pregnancy. Sometimes mineral deficiencies such as zinc and biochemical components called transferrin and lactoferrin may be implicated.

Points to Remember

The simplest set of laboratory procedures for determining causes of infertility involves the testing of the semen. This procedure is less invasive and much less expensive and time consuming than others involving the female and should be tested initially. The complete analysis of a semen sample includes a number of tests that may provide a clue as to infertility and the causes of the problem, as well as treatment modalities available

12.3.11   Specimen Collection for Semen

Seminal fluid is a commonly tested body fluid that is analyzed chiefly for two reasons. The purposes relate to fertility studies and increasingly to insure that a successful vasectomy was the result of surgery, both of which require microscopic examinations to observe numbers and quality as well as for the presence of any sperm. In the case of post-vasectomy studies, the microscopic evaluation is the only test performed. It is not uncommon following a vasectomy to require a repeat procedure when sperm are present in the sample presented to the lab. Additionally, reverse surgery is sometimes requested when one has undergone a vasectomy and wishes to have children.

The sample should be kept from significant temperature changes, so a container into which the sample is ejaculated should be pre-warmed to prevent shock to the fresh sperm cells. Using a condom is not acceptable due to difficulty in quickly extracting the sample. Also, some condoms possess a slightly *spermicidal* effect on the sperm. *Coitus interruptus* is a technique where sexual intercourse is halted prematurely before ejaculation, then collecting the product. But an early portion of the sample may be lost or contaminated by vaginal flora and normal fluids, providing inaccurate results. Some find it psychologically difficult to produce semen on demand but other techniques are available where fertility specialists may employ a number of methods of collection.

Semen is composed of four fractions produced by accessory organs of the genitourinary system that must be taken into consideration when examining seminal fluids. A number of accessory glands are responsible for the production and nourishing of sperm cells during preparation for fertilization of the ovum. Millions of spermatozoa are normally produced during each ejaculation, but only one normal sperm cell is required for fertilization of the egg.

One of the glands useful in this complex process of producing viable spermatozoa is the Cowper's or bulbourethral gland. These glands are pea-sized and is located behind and to each side of the urethra and are responsible for discharging a component of the seminal fluid into the urethra. The urethra, an opening leading to the outside of the genitourinary systems, serves to discharge semen by ejaculation, a forceful function of the nervous system. During sexual arousal, each bulbourethral gland produces clear, viscous secretions called pre-ejaculate and function in a similar way to the Bartholin glands of the female, located near the vagina. This fluid lubricates the urethra to allow passage of the spermatozoa and aids in flushing any matter such as residual urine material. It is a common occurrence for this fluid to pick up sperm, which is then eliminated as drainage.

The male *gonads* or *testes* are *normally* paired organs which function jointly with an associated structure called the epididymis (Fig. 12.3). The female gonads are called *ovaries* (Fig. 12.4). The spermatozoa are initially produced in the testicles and are nurtured and mature in the *epididymis* and infections of these structures can pose grave medical danger. Each epididymis is a small oblong organ found on the posterior surface of each testicle, formed by a system of small ducts simulating a coiled mass of up to 6 m in length. The ducts are tightly convoluted and appear as a tangled mass before ending in the *vas deferens*. A *vasectomy*, the method for sterilizing males, is clipped and ligated to prevent sperm from leaving the vas deferens while sperm cells formed there are reabsorbed by the body.

The prostate organ in the male is a gland composed of a median lobe and two lobes to each side that surround the neck of the bladder and the urethra. A slightly alkaline, milky fluid from these glands forms the majority of the seminal fluid. Prostatic fluid is extremely important in the coagulation and liquefaction of semen, factors that are determined when fertility studies are performed. Any disruption of

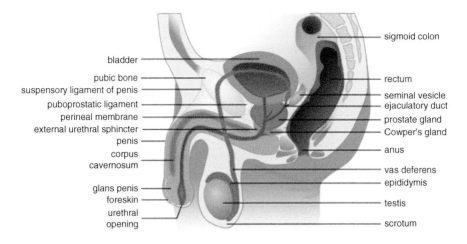

Fig. 12.3 Male reproductive organs and accessory glands

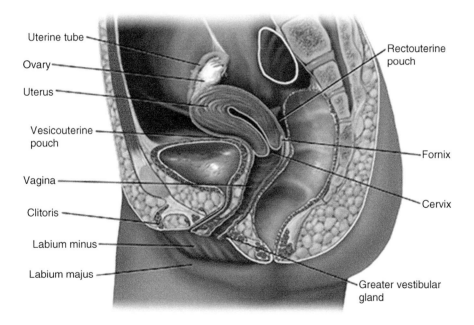

Fig. 12.4 Female reproductive organs and accessory glands

the liquefaction will prevent the sperm from being freed to travel to the *Fallopian tubes* where the egg is fertilized. Seminal vesicles nourish the sperm during maturation, and these organs provide the majority of the fluid of which semen is comprised. This sticky fluid provides fructose and additional nutrients necessary for enabling the sperm to mature normally.

In addition to these organs as chiefly responsible for nourishing the sperm during maturation, the seminal vesicles produce the majority of the fluid of which semen is comprised. The fluid is a viscous or sticky liquid that furnishes fructose and other nutrients for spermatozoal maturation. For a semen analysis, a fresh semen sample, no more than a half hour old, is needed in order to determine whether normal liquefaction is occurring within a reasonable time. The person being tested will normally abstain from sexual activities for at least 2–4 days, a practice that helps to produce a normal volume and concentration of sperm. The donor will be asked to provide a sample into a clean, wide mouthed bottle for quick delivery to the laboratory.

12.3.12 Physical Appearance of Semen

After 30 min and no more than an hour, the semen sample should be liquefied and the initial viscosity diminished or eliminated. At this point, the initial examination should begin immediately. The observation is done at *ambient* or room temperature and is an important component of the evaluation. The gross appearance of the sample should be a homogeneous material normally of a white to gray color. If blood cells are present, the condition is described as *hematospermic* and unless a sample is quite opaque, a low sperm cell count may be indicated. If a sample appears dense or concentrated with a high level of whitish turbidity, an inflammation related to a bacterial pathogen organism may result in an elevated white blood cell count.

Volumes of total semen vary greatly when measured in a 10 mL graduated cylinder or volumetric centrifuge tube. Other methods of volume measurement involve aspiration of the sample into a large-bore pipette, using an aspirating bulb or a plunger type mechanism. Disposable plastic pipettes and other systems for measuring the sample should be free of detergents, contaminants or chemicals that could alter test results. The entire sample is measured to the nearest tenth of an mL, and normal samples will range from 2 to 6 mL if proper collection techniques are employed.

The consistency of the sample is described by its viscosity and this consistency changes gradually over a 30-min time period in most cases. Liquefaction should never require more than 60 min, and an extremely viscous sample will form long threads of mucoid material when dropped from a pipette as the drops to fall from the tip of the pipette or other device. Samples with increased viscosity will form longer threads extending an inch or more from the pipette tip. In addition, considerably viscous samples are more difficult to aspirate from the collection container holding the sample. After complete liquefaction, drops from the pipette tip will fall as discrete beads of liquid with no mucoid threads between the drops and the pipette tip (Fig. 12.5). When liquefaction is partial or does not occur, motility of the sperm cells is impeded, leaving the cells may flounder helplessly in the solution with little or no forward progress. In this case, a uniform mixture of sperm and diluent must be prepared in order to gain an accurate count of the cells. But the dilution factor must not be forgotten when the count is calculated!

Fig. 12.5 Normally
liquefied semen sample

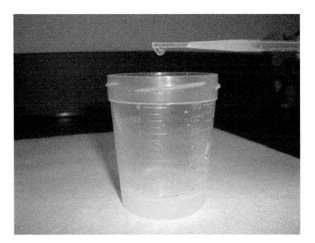

12.3.13   Laboratory Analysis of Semen

When the numerical number of spermatozoa in the seminal fluid has been established as normal, several other factors must next be considered when performing other components of a complete fertility study. In routine studies it is sometimes necessary to evaluate more than one semen sample to rule out any causative factor that is semen related. Two or more samples may be required, with the timing of the multiple collections on a varied schedule, since semen output varies diurnally. *Samples should be collected at least a week apart.* But collection and examination would optimally be accomplished over a 2-week schedule, while not exceeding a period of more than a few months. Averaging of the duplicate samples provides a baseline figure to establish meaningful values and serves to rule out any variations between samples. It may be necessary to separate sperm cells from seminal secretions after liquefaction, particularly if medications are suspected as a factor in preventing impregnation attributed to either the male or female partner.

12.4   Microscopic Cell Counts and WBC Differentiation

Again, it is *mandatory* to delay the evaluation of semen for fertility studies until after complete liquefaction. Procedures may vary based on the needs relative to patient history information, taking into account any circumstances related to infertility, prior vasectomy procedures (particularly if a vasectomy was reversed), and for forensic studies. Routine reference values used include only the procedures commonly performed in routine analytical examinations. Other related factors such as biochemical values are considered on an individual basis, and are correlated with other parameters (Table 12.2).

As alluded to previously, the microscopic determinations routinely evaluated for semen specimens are both quantitative and qualitative.

Since the vitality, a term for living, and the motility or normal progression of sperm cells may diminish over time, observations should be initiated as quickly as possible following collection and completion of liquefaction. Some laboratories maintain samples at 37 °C prior to beginning an examination of the sample but many perform the procedures at room temperature. As the sample cools or if encountering sudden room temperature changes, results may be substantially altered, particularly when evaluating motility. Light microscopes are most commonly used in a clinical laboratory and can be used for unstained specimens. A type of microscope called a *phase contrast microscope* provides a dark background with illuminated cells and organisms, and is preferred by some when performing microscopic examinations for both fresh semen and washed sperm cells that may be useful for immunoassays, based on tests where the reaction of antibodies against antigens is measured. Either type of microscope however does require skill gained from experience in viewing a variety of samples.

A "*wet mount*" procedure involves a process where a liquefied and thoroughly mixed semen sample is placed on a microscope slide and is not used for a quantitative measure, but for a qualitative analysis. A single drop is needed and is covered by a 22 × 22 millimeter (mm) cover glass (Fig. 12.6). The preparation that is made from fresh sperm will be allowed to sit for at least a minute on the slide, but not so long as to begin a drying out process, in order to stabilize the depth of the preparation following placement of the cover glass. The wet mount is then examined for sperm cells and is the only observation necessary for a post vasectomy specimen. A sample that is too thick or the sample has not completely liquefied or is extremely concentrated will pose difficulties in observing single spermatozoa for accurate assessment leading to an effective evaluation. The microscopic examination of a specimen by wet mount enables visualization regarding approximate numbers of sperm, and are reported as rare, few, several, many sperm cells per high power field. The estimate derived from a wet mount examination should correlate with a systematic count performed by using a diluted sample and a hemocytometer. The presence

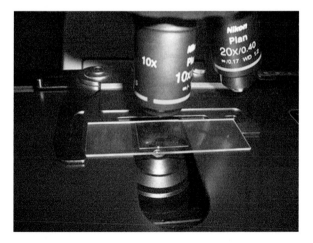

Fig. 12.6 Wet mount uses standard microscope slide and 22 mm cover slide

of agglutination of sperm, the motility of the sperm as Grade A, B, C or D (Table 12.1) and the percentage of live forms (viability) and morphology (normal appearing forms) are reported using this methodology.

When examining normal semen preparations for numbers of sperm cells, other than those for post vasectomy evaluations, mature sperm cells should comprise a majority of the cells seen. Cells other than sperm cells that are routinely found in semen samples include *squamous epithelial cells* often found in the male reproductive tract. These cells may be increased in men with urethritis due to shedding of these cell cases into the sample during ejaculation. Some white cells and immature forms of sperm cells may be routinely found in semen samples. When variations between numbers of sperm seen from one microscopic field to another are considerable, the sample might not be completely liquefied or completely mixed before pipetting onto the microscope slide. The preparation should be repeated in the event large variations are seen in the various fields. Sperm agglutination resulting from the aggregation where clumps of cells present inconsistent distribution of cells, leading to erroneous conclusions in the wet mount evaluation.

Motility is also referred to as mobility and is the ability of individual sperm cells to move effectively in the seminal fluid and is also determined from a wet mount preparation. The percentage of sperm cells that are either Grade A or B is calculated by determining the percentage of motile forms and dividing it by the total sperm count, before converting the figure to a percentage form. Only sperm counts from an unstained specimen can be evaluated for motility, since most stains may be spermicidal or will at least retard the movement of the cells. In a normal sperm evaluation for motility, 50% or more should be motile, while less than 50% motility may increase the possibility of infertility. A rather accurate method of determining motility is derived by counting 200 sperm cells from at least five fields and dividing the results by 2. The percentage of the motile forms is calculated as follows (See Box 12.1):

Table 12.1 Microscopic evaluation for motility of sperm

Grade A sperm	Sperm can progress swiftly in a straight line
Grade B sperm	Sperm are capable of moving forward, and may normally progress either in a curved or crooked line, or at a slow pace
Grade C sperm	Spermatozoa move their tails, but lack progress from one area to another
Grade D sperm	The cells are immobile and appear to be dead

Table 12.2 Normal values, routine semen analysis

Test component	Normal range
Total volume	2.0–6.0 mL
Sample pH	7.2–7.8 (slightly alkaline)
Sperm count	Greater than 20 million/mL
Morphology	At least 70% as normal forms
Viability	75% will be motile
White blood cells/mL	Fewer than 1 million WBC's per mL
Red blood cells	None to rare

> **Box 12.1: Calculation of Motile Sperm Count**
> % motility of sperm cells = 200 (total counted) − non-motile sperm/total sperm/200 × 100 or % Motility = # of motile sperm/total # of sperm counted

Fig. 12.7 Uniting of sperm and ovum

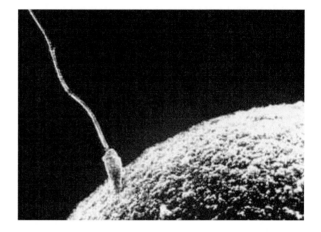

Artificial insemination as described previously may sometimes be required in cases of infertility related to the male, where a semen sample is collected and concentrated to increase the relative count per volume of diluent. The concentrated sample is then injected into the *cervix* or neck of the female's uterus. In addition, a variation of in vitro fertilization may be performed, where eggs are harvested and the washed and concentrated sperm cells are incubated with the egg to enable penetration of the sperm into the ovum (Fig. 12.7). The resulting fertilized egg is implanted into the uterus of the female, where it might attach and begin to grow into a fetus. This procedure has provided hope of having children in large numbers of infertile couples.

Agglutination is a phenomenon observed in some individuals, where motile sperm adhere to each other in a consistent manner and not just as a few isolated clumps. Adherence with head to head or tail to head, etc. is common. Only motile sperm are reported as clumped or agglutinated, and in the event an indefinite pattern of clumping is observed, a report detailing agglutination is not made. But when agglutination in a definite pattern is observed on a consistent basis where multiple testing has occurred, there is often an accompanying immunological reason for infertility based on the presence of antibodies. It is important to note the agglutination on a number of high power microscopic fields, rather than merely a few fields or a single field.

Viability refers to the presence of life as the ability to fertilize a female's ovum (single egg). This procedure requires staining of the sperm cells using a supravital staining method. A number of stains or combination of stains may be used, but a simple preparation of eosin or eosin with other stains provide for adequate evaluations of the viability of sperm cells. The color reaction between dead and live cells can be readily observed, as *dead cells do not absorb the stain*, while live sperm cells do retain the stain. Live cells that are non-motile will also take up the stain as will those that are motile, so no distinction between motile and non-motile sperm cells can be made by this procedure. Estimates of viable and motile cells in a sperm sample is important since the numerical values of dead or nonviable cells should not be significantly greater than those of non-motile cells.

Morphology of the sperm cells is another important feature when evaluating an individual or a couple for infertility. This procedure also requires staining of the sample, which may require the uses of several different stains, and does not indicate differences between the rates of motility or non-motility. It merely provides a classification of cells and whether they are normal or abnormal in shape or level of maturity. In the event that more than a third of the sperm cells are abnormal or immature, there is an increased rate of infertility.

Preparation of the smear and staining require diligence in order to provide a specimen that can be readily evaluated. A smear of the semen is made on a slide but must not be too thick, since inconsistent staining will cause difficulty in evaluating the maturity and morphology of the sperm cells. The slides are made in the same manner as that prepared for evaluating red and white blood cell morphology, with a "feathered" edge, where the smear is thin enough to visualize individual cells. This is accomplished by drawing out a drop of semen along a slide by using the edge of a second slide that is held at an angle, while smearing the sample along the length of the slide. This procedure requires skill and practice before one becomes accomplished at quickly making an acceptable smear.

A second method is that of pressing down a second slide on the first slide containing a drop of semen, and then prying the slides apart. This accomplishes the making of two smears simultaneously, both of which will be extremely thin when the sample is completely liquefied. Several stains may be used for sperm cell studies that are similar to those used in histology labs such as that for surgical tissue samples are stained, where *hematoxylin* and eosin (H & E) stains are employed. *Papanicolaou stains* used for cervical "Paps" smears along with *Wright's stain* are similarly utilized for sperm evaluation, applying similar techniques for preparing and enabling a better image staining of blood smears and of the basic parts of a sperm cell.

The outline of sperm cells may be the only features seen, depending on the stain used and quality of the smear. Some sperm cells that exhibit abnormal forms that are impossible to recognize easily will be discounted, particularly when overlaid by other structures present in the semen. It is necessary to count at least 200 cells in order to obtain a representative number for accuracy. Morphological features of sperm cells include the head and tail, separated by the midpiece and then the endpiece. Abnormalities may be noted in the head or the tail, as abnormalities of the midpiece and the endpiece are not readily interpreted. In most instances, abnormalities will refer to a double-headed sperm cell or one that has an enlarged or an extremely small head (pinhead). As described earlier, tail abnormalities may include double tails, kinked or coiled tailpieces, or by an abnormally lengthened tail.

Bacteria, blood cells and other extraneous materials may be found in semen. Since semen is collected in a clean or sterile container, no bacteria should be observed. But bacterial infections of the urethra, the prostate glands, and epididymis may reveal microscopic bacteria when examined by microscope. In addition, where infectious processes may be at play, increased levels of white blood cells, sometimes accompanied by red blood cells, may be noted. No red blood cells should be seen in a normal semen sample. The presence of bacteria or increased numbers of white cells will indicate the need for a bacterial culture. Sometimes other sexually transmitted microorganisms such as *Trichomonas vaginalis*, a protozoan that can infect both men and women, may be noted, especially in fresh semen (Fig. 12.8). The *Chlamydia trachomatis* bacterium has also apparently been a growing cause of male infertility; but its role is not as clear as in female infertility but has been blamed for an increasingly important cause of infertility for decades. *Candida albicans*, a species of yeast that may be transmitted sexually, is also visible by microscope in the semen sample.

Immunological disorders, while a rare cause of infertility, are frustrating to couples desiring children. After sperm cells are noted that adhere to each other in a distinct pattern through a wet mount examination, the clumping together reflects the possibility of an immunological disorder. Definitive testing is required to confirm the presence of these antibodies existing in sperm, circulating blood plasma, and vaginal fluids, so either of the sexes might contribute to an immunological cause for infertility. In preparation for these tests, sperm cells are washed to remove any extraneous proteins present in the seminal fluid, and then the cells are tested using commercially available antibodies. An antisperm antibody test is available to detect special antibody proteins that fight against the sperm cells. This test basically uses a sample of sperm and adds a substance that binds only to the affected sperm that may be coated with antibodies, a process found also in blood banks, where RBC's are coated with antibodies (direct Coomb's test).

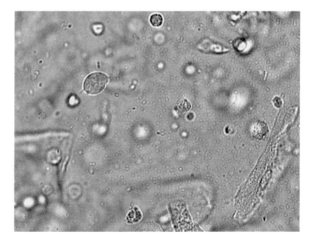

Fig. 12.8 *T. vaginalis*, a pear-shaped protozoan transmitted sexually

Semen can cause an immune system response, called immunologic infertility, in either the man's body, which would be an autoimmune condition by making antibodies against one's self, or in the woman's body, where she produces antibodies against her mate's sperm. Immunoglobulins are comprised of four different classes, all of which may produce antibodies. These proteins are called IgG (immunoglobulin G), IgA, IgM, and perhaps IgE, which produce allergic reactions. The antibodies can damage or kill the sperm cells, incapacitating them so they are unable to fertilize the egg. This occurs when large numbers of sperm antibodies adhere to the surface of the man's sperm cells, making it difficult for the sperm to fertilize an egg.

In autoimmune cases, where a man makes antibodies against his own sperm is due to malfunctions of his immune system which recognizes his sperm as foreign objects. This may occur following injury to the testicles or after surgical procedures affecting the urogenital system, such as removal of a surgical tissue sample called a biopsy or following a vasectomy procedure. Infections of the accessory organs of the genitourinary system such as that which affects the prostate gland may also initiate an autoimmune reaction. The testicles serve to keep the sperm separate from the other tissue cells of the body and the immune system, serving as a preventive measure against this type of reaction. Due to genetic differences between the male's sperm cells and the inability of the female to tolerate these differences may result in an allergic reaction by the female to her partner's semen, resulting in the formation of antibodies to the sperm. This kind of immune response is a rare cause of infertility that is not fully understood but may affect fertility.

12.5 Performing the Total Sperm Count

Insufficient numbers of spermatozoa often result in infertility, but certain causes for low numbers may be revealed for correction during a complete analysis of semen. The sperm count is frequently done by use of the Neubauer hemocytometer, although other counting chambers are available. Another counting chamber that is specifically designed for the enumeration of sperm cells is called the Makler Counting Chamber, which does not require dilution of a sample of sperm but a pretreatment process is required for use with this system. Another advantage of the Makler system lies in the fact that the depth is consistent and allows the sperm cells to be counted on a single plane without the focusing up and down of the stage of the microscope once it is focused to provide a clear view. Automated counters may be used and are referred to as Computer Assisted Semen Analysis (CASA) instruments, a general term used for any automatic or semi-automatic method for semen analysis. Some of these systems perform tracking of sperm motility as they move across a digital table. Some of these instruments are also capable of determining velocity or speed of the cells. Although these instruments may provide good results, most institutions perform only a handful of semen analyses per month or even year. Therefore, these sophisticated instruments are not cost effective.

In preparing the sample for counting using the Neubauer hemocytometer, a liquefied sample that has been thoroughly mixed is paramount in importance. The sample is diluted at a 1:20 ratio using a staining solution of sodium bicarbonate with dilute formalin and a tryptan blue or gentian violet as a representative stain, although other stains are available. Note that staining the sample is not necessary when a phase contrast microscope is employed for the count rather than the brightfield microscope. A drop of the diluted and stained semen sample is placed on the Neubauer hemocytometer which has been scrupulously cleaned, followed by placing a standard cover glass on the counting chamber. This diluent is toxic to sperm cells so motility will be non-existent but will result in an easier counting experience.

When using the Improved Neubauer hemocytometer, the diluted sample is placed on both sides of the hemocytometer and is allowed several minutes for the cover glass to settle to the proper depth. Sperm counts are done using the central and closely gridded square in the middle of the slide. There are 25 smaller squares within the larger square, and 5 of these squares that comprise the 25 total squares in this area are counted. The five squares to be counted are the four corner squares and the center square. Care should be taken not to count the same sperm cell more than once. When the sperm count is low and fewer than 10 sperm are counted per square, all 25 squares are counted. Allowances are made for any differences in the number of squares counted when performing the calculations for the total count. For example, when more than 10 cells per square but up to 40 cells per square are observed, 10 squares should be counted. But for a normal count, where more than 40 spermatozoa are found in each square, only 5 squares as described are counted. A systematic procedure where all the cells that are touching the line on the top and left side of the counter may be counted, while those on the lower and right margins are not counted.

Procedure 12.1 Total Sperm Cell Count

1. A thoroughly mixed semen sample is diluted at a 1:20 ratio with diluents containing a preservative and dye with staining capabilities. As an example, 25 μL (0.025 mL) is diluted with 475 μL (0 0.475 mL) of the reagent. Larger volumes of each at the same proportions may be used since larger volumes used of the semen and the diluent discount any slight errors in measurement since with small samples, a small error is magnified

2. Mix the diluent and sample adequately and using a pipette, allow a small amount of the sample to flow under the cover glass on both sides of the hemocytometer

3. Prepare a humidifying cover by use of a petri dish or similar container with a lid, where a slightly moist filter paper pad has been placed in the dish. Too much water will wet the bottom of the hemocytometer and make it difficult to pick up the slide, and may cause the slide to 'stick' or adhere to the stage of the microscope. Place the hemocytometer in the petri dish and allow approximately 5 min for the cover glass to adjust to the desired depth

4. Following the settling of the cells and the cover glass, place the slide on the stage of a microscope. Again, a phase contrast microscope is best suited for enumeration

5. Using the 40× objective, count spermatozoa in the five squares in the larger center square on both sides of the slide. Divide the total count for both sides by 2, providing an average of the two sides, leading to greater accuracy. A disparity of more than 5–10% between the two sides necessitates recharging the sample onto a clean hemocytometer slide, repeating the count on both sides. DO NOT count extremely abnormal forms of spermatozoa

6. If the dilution factor described in step #1 differs from a 1:20 dilution, allow for the different ratio of semen to diluent and calculate the number of sperm cells per mL of specimen. Convert the total sperm count using the total volume of the ejaculated sample, if required by the medical facility where the count is performed

12.5.1 Calculation of Total Sperm Count

For calculations of the total sperm count per milliliter (mL) of a diluted sample, a conversion is required to obtain the result. The calculation is similar to the steps when performing blood cell counts. The area counted, the dilution factor of the sample, depth of the counting chamber, and an average of the counts for sperm cells from BOTH sides of the hemocytometer are used, dividing the counts from the two sides by two in order to determine a mean average of the two sides. The depth factor for the Neubauer hemocytometer is a constant 0.1 mm, which simplifies the process (Fig. 12.9). Differences will be factored into the equation for deviations from the dilution factor and the areas counted are changed. When a 1:20 dilution is performed and the sperm cells are counted on the five squares of the large center square of the hemocytometer, the results in millions of cells per mL, the count is relatively simple to complete by merely *adding 6 zeros to the average number of cells counted*.

Diagram indicating Depth of Counting Chamber of a Hemocytometer Slide

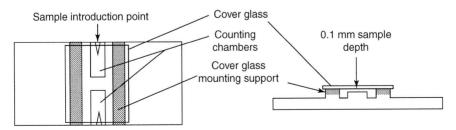

An example calculation is as follows:

If 47 spermatozoa are counted on one side, and 51 on the other, the average count would be 49. It would only be necessary to add 6 zeros to the count, making a count

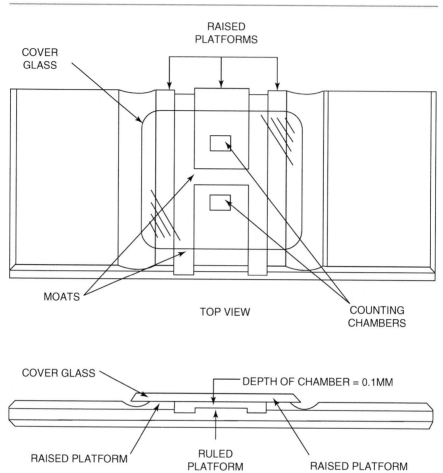

Fig. 12.9 Diagram indicating depth of counting chamber of a hemocytometer slide

of 49,000,000. If a 1:10 dilution is used, based on the lower number of sperm cells (fewer than 40 per square), 10 squares are counted, and for a 1:50 dilution, only 2 of the center squares are counted.

12.5.2 Miscellaneous Observations

A number of areas now involved in the testing of sperm cells were not available to patients until the past few years. Clinical genetic counseling prior to attempting pregnancy refers to the laboratory analysis of either of both the DNA and RNA to aid in the diagnosis of disease. Clinical genetic testing varies greatly from other types of laboratory tests as it may be applied as a definitive diagnosis of genetic predispositions that could perhaps predict the likelihood of developing a particular disease before symptoms even appear. In addition, if any genetic expression would likely be transmitted to any resultant children are critical related to the health of offspring, choices can be made as to the wisdom of fathering offspring. In these cases, treatment or options for alternative methods of reproduction should be considered. Family history where various diseases are prevalent over the generations should be explained by a genetic counselor regarding the statistical likelihood of parenting children with genetic defects.

Other new and exciting possibilities in reproductive health are now available. One such procedure is that of cases where an infant or small child may require treatment for diseases such as cancer who have undergone radiation treatment that limits or eliminates the possible of becoming parent. When there is a likelihood that reproductive organs may be damaged, the possibility of preserving the ability to become a parent a number of years or even decades later is possible. Harvested tissues from the testicles or ovaries may be preserved for the future, and the tissues could be grown and might be coaxed to produce spermatozoa or ova.

Microbial tests are available that include the culturing of semen samples to determine if an infectious process may be responsible for infertility such as a low sperm count or the complete absence of sperm cells. More extensive testing for the presence of fastidious and unusual microbes capable of causing sterility in an individual is available that goes beyond the routine culturing of samples for the presence of routine strains of bacteria.

12.5.3 Post-Vasectomy Evaluation

Repeat post-vasectomy specimens may be performed to prevent pregnancy even years after the surgical procedure as these procedures may have resulted in an incomplete block to the ejaculation of sperm from the vas deferens. Reversal of a surgical vasectomy may be desirable by some, in the event a couple wishes to again become a parent or become a first time parent. In legal proceedings, an assault by one who has undergone a vasectomy can still produce seminal fluids for DNA evidence.

12.5.4 Post-Rape Analysis

Seminal fluid in an individual who is incapable of producing sperm might contain high levels of an enzyme called acid phosphatase in the seminal fluid, indicating the occurrence of a sexual contact. A small amount of leakage when a condom has been used result in minute amounts of leakage and result in substantial levels of acid phosphatase in vaginal washings. Blood groups (ABO) and types (Rh factor) may narrow the number of those suspected of committing a sexual assault. Forensic testing may require that specific body fluids gathering of data for analysis that can be used in legal proceedings, according to the laws of various jurisdictions.

The clinical laboratory professional may be required to aid in collecting and storing of specific body fluids where a legal process known as "chain of custody" is followed, verifying that a sample was properly collected, identified, and transported to be used as evidence if needed later for legal proceedings. Documentation of storage procedures and the manner of handling the sample and placement in an environment to prevent alteration of the sample is vital for future prosecution by legal authorities.

12.6   Summary

A number of tests may be performed on semen specimens to determine the cause of infertility. In addition, certain biochemical tests as well as microscopic tests may be performed for legal processes where paternity or sexual assault may have occurred. Seminal fluid exists as a fluid containing vital components for nourishing and sustaining the sperm cells called spermatozoa as they mature and are ready for fertilizing the female egg.

As in other body fluids, sperm cells and their fluid require a visual, macroscopic evaluation which includes volume, color, consistency, and any other observations that cause an abnormal appearance. Infertility studies may include chemical analysis as is done for urine samples where testing is done for the presence of and levels of certain enzymes, but energy sources for the sperm cells such as fructose and citric acid used in the energy cycle. And as in urine and other body fluids, a microscopic evaluation includes a total count and the presence of blood cells and other elements that may be important in the evaluation of the semen sample. It should be remembered that both quality and quantity may be important in the evaluation of semen, and even esoteric tests involving the immune system may be rarely necessary to determining the causes of infertility.

Case Study
A 27-year-old man and his 25-year-old wife visited a family practitioner. They report that they had hoped to have two children by the wife's thirtieth birthday but had been unsuccessful during their 2-year marriage. The physician told the couple that the first step would be to analyze the semen of the husband, and if the tests proved to be normal, then the couple would be referred to a fertility specialist. The couple was given instructions to abstain from having sex for a period of time and then to collect a sample that could be transported to a nearby hospital laboratory within a few minutes of collection. The following results were obtained:

Total volume	3.7 mL
Liquefaction	58 min
Sample pH	7.2
Sperm count	28.2 million/mL
Morphology	78% are normal forms

Viability	77% are motile
White blood cells/mL	0.8×10^6/mL
Red blood cells	Rare

1. What is/are the abnormality(ies) found in this semen evaluation, if any?
2. What would be the most likely solution to the problem(s) if any are present?

Review Questions

1. What is the most common test performed to determine causes of infertility in a couple?
   a. Marital counseling
   b. Evaluation of the ova of the female
   c. Performing chemistry tests on semen
   d. Complete sperm count
2. Which of the following is most cost effective in determining causes of infertility?
   a. In vitro fertilization
   b. In vivo fertilization
   c. Complete sperm count
   d. X-rays of female reproductive organs
3. Which of the following would not be a factor in determining sperm motility?
   a. Infection of the prostate glands
   b. Epididymitis
   c. Vasectomy
   d. Antibodies against the sperm
4. Which of the following is the best way for collecting sperm samples?
   a. Coitus interruptus
   b. Collection from a condom
   c. Masturbation
   d. None of the above
5. The most important component to be considered in determining a male's fertility status is:
   a. pH of the semen
   b. Volume of the semen
   c. Sperm count
   d. Wife's monthly hormone changes
6. The semen should be collected on which of the following schedules to detect a man's fertility status that is based on a semen analysis:
   a. At least 2 samples are analyzed
   b. Specimens are collected 7 days apart
   c. Analysis spans 2–3 months
   d. All of the above

7. Sperm counts are performed based on the following units of measurement:
   a. Count per liter
   b. Count per microliter (µL)
   c. Count per deciliter (dL)
   d. Count per milliliter (mL)
8. Sperm cells that are for the most part aligned head to tail is exhibiting which of the following?
   a. Immunological response
   b. Agglutination
   c. Normal liquefaction
   d. Molecular attraction
9. Semen should liquefy within:
   a. Ten minutes
   b. Not at all normally
   c. Within thirty minutes
   d. After one hour
10. A more dilute semen sample would most likely show:
   a. Increased count per unit
   b. Decreased count per unit
   c. Same as a less dilute sample
   d. Impedance of sperm motility

Answers Found in Appendix C

Serous Fluids Analysis

13

Objectives

Differentiate between the sites from which serous fluids are collected

Discuss the origin of body fluids in body cavities, their respective purposes, and how they are formed

Describe the reasons for collecting certain body fluids using an anticoagulant to prevent fibrin clots

Understand the requirements for employing consistent protocol for the collection and transport of each of the serous fluids

Discuss the need for observing Standard Precautions when collecting, transporting, storage, and testing of samples

Describe patterns of infection and their impact on glucose and protein concentrations

Compare the gross appearance of serous fluids with those of the physical properties of urine

Differentiate between exudates and transudates

Understand use of compensated polarized microscopy for differentiating between the various birefringent crystals found in fluids

Describe disease conditions where mononuclear and polymorphonuclear white cells are predominant

Discuss procedures where amniotic fluids provide information based on the condition and maturity of the fetus

13.1 Introduction to the Testing of Serous Fluids

The basic definition of serous fluids, regardless of origin and where they accumulate, refers to the fact that each fluid is the product of constituents of the blood serum. There are three serous cavities in the human body, which include the *pericardial* or heart cavity, the *pleural* or lung cavity, and the peritoneal or abdominal

© Springer International Publishing AG, part of Springer Nature 2018
J. W. Ridley, *Fundamentals of the Study of Urine and Body Fluids*,
https://doi.org/10.1007/978-3-319-78417-5_13

cavity, to which it is sometimes referred. The fluids associated with these cavities are normally pale and perhaps yellow in color, and may originate from glands located within the body cavities. Some of the fluids contain specialized cells that are associated with the functions of the organs which are nourished and enriched by the serous fluids found in these areas.

These cavities are lined with serous membranes which maintain a lubricant to *prevent friction* from occurring between organs and the walls of the cavity. In the pleural cavity, the serous membranes also function in other ways in providing for the respiratory functions required to maintain life and health. Cavities of the body from which samples may be collected include pleural, pericardial, amniotic and peritoneal fluids. These cavities are also sometimes referred to as somatic cavities and consist specifically of two large cavities (pleural and abdominoperineal) and a smaller cavity (pericardial), all of which are covered with a mesothelium. A membrane of visceral mesothelium coats the organs and parietal mesothelium coats the somatic walls lining each of the cavities.

Serous cavities are formed during the early development of the embryo, where a structure called the *blastoderm* provides for the development of the cavities and the linings for them and for the organs. The blastoderm is comprised of a disk of cells that develops between the yolk sac and the egg, and the amniotic cavity that leads to development of the embryo. Three cavities develop from the blastoderm, and invagination (folding) into the coelom, a cavity between the split layers of *mesoderm*, leads to the formation in mammals to pleural, peritoneal and pericardial cavities. These three body cavities are then lined with two thin, mesothelial membranes into what is known as serous membranes. The first of these two membranes line the cavity in which the organ or organs are found, and the second surrounds the organs themselves. The lining that is in contact with the body wall of the cavity is called the *parietal layer* or membrane, and the layer surrounding the organs is called the visceral membrane.

Only sufficient serous fluid is provided to prevent inflammation resulting from the organs in contact with the body cavities. This contact occurs during breathing during which the lungs expand and contract, circulation involving beating of the heart and expansion of the arteries, digestion, and gross movements of the body during various activities required during daily life. The fluid produced as a lubricant for this purpose is derived from ultrafiltrates from the blood that comes in contact with the organs and cavities that are filled with blood capillaries. The fluid that lubricates the organs and the cavity linings is known as a *transudate*, since it is normally continuously produced and reabsorbed. This fluid does not accumulate to any significant extend except in injuries or certain infectious diseases involving the organs or cavity linings. All the body cavities are subject to accumulation of fluids, and when they do aggregate inside body cavities, they are then referred to as *effusions*. The fluids may be found in excessive amounts in the pleural, pericardial and peritoneal cavities due to various diseases.

Transudates are protective materials that are formed as an ultrafiltrate of blood plasma and are distinguished from exudates by their physical properties. Volumes of transudates that exceed the small amount needed to prevent friction between organs and serous membranes may arise. They form most often due to a systemic disorder that disrupts the balance in the regulation of fluid filtration and reabsorption. There are numbers of examples of diseases causing changes in transudates exist that occur due to conditions involving changes in hydrostatic pressure that may lead to serious illness. Some of the more frequent conditions include *congestive heart failure* and others include certain liver diseases and those found in a kidney disease known as the nephrotic syndrome. Exudates are produced by an inflammatory condition that directly involves membranes of the particular cavity or organ and not by malfunctions of organs themselves. Some of these conditions include infections that may be a result of bacteria and viruses and less frequently by fungi and parasites. Malignancies are known to produce *exudates*, where an accumulation of fluid around an organ with a neoplasm occurs. Although similarities exist between, certain physical factors are used to differentiate between transudates and exudates.

Points to Remember
Normal amounts of fluids in low volumes are maintained in all body cavities. When these fluids increase in volume, it is usually a result of inflammation, infection, or mechanical failure of a movable part, such as a joint or other location where friction occurs

Several procedures are available to differentiate between a transudate or exudate, an important distinction for diagnosis of a number of medical processes. Baseline levels from the blood system should be performed as a means of determining abnormal results from exudates and transudates. This is not always done routinely and must be requested by the physician if he or she feels this would be pertinent clinical information. Some facilities provide significant numbers of tests related to fluid accumulation. One of these routinely includes lactate dehydrogenase or LD that aids in determining if necrosis of an organ is occurring. Another chemistry procedure that is not routinely ordered is that of amylase, a digestive enzyme that is increased in malignancies of the esophagus or pancreas, as well as when acute inflammation of the pancreas is present. An explanation of routine examinations to determine differences and commonalities between these normal transudates and those that accumulate as the result of physical damage to the organs or membranes surrounding them are characterized as follows (Table 13.1).

13.2 Infection Control

Since all body fluids carry an inherent risk of contracting an infection, Standard Precautions should be observed in the collection, transport and processing of these specimens. Since both exudates and transudates are derived from components of the blood, and exudates generally occur due to an infectious process by a microbiological organism, extreme precautions are necessary. The use of protective equipment should be employed when centrifuging or mixing the sample with other fluids. Precautions should be observed in disposing of samples and containers in which the

Table 13.1 Differentiation of transudates and exudates

Characteristics	Transudate	Exudate
General results, origin	Increased hydrostatic pressure; low colloid osmotic pressure	Inflammation (may be infectious) changes in capillary permeability resulting from acute inflammatory reaction
Physical appearance	Clear or pale yellow	Variety of colors ranging from yellow, greenish, and reddish (bloody)
White blood cells	<1000/mL	>1000/mL
Red blood cells	Undetectable unless traumatic aspiration occurs	Extremely elevated, particularly when resulting from a malignancy
Glucose	Correlates with plasma level	Lower than that found in plasma, especially in infectious processes and if high cell counts are present
Total protein	<3.0 g/dL	Usually greater than plasma level
Lactic dehydrogenase (LDH)	Low in comparison with serum or plasma levels	<200 SI/L (elevations due to amount of cellular elements from damaged red blood cells
Physical appearance	Clear or pale yellow	Variety of colors from yellow, brown, greenish, and reddish (bloody)

specimens were collected, stored or used in a laboratory procedure are required, as well as cleaning of the work areas following the collection and processing of the materials.

Infection Control Flash

Body fluids for the most part exist as ultrafiltrates of blood plasma. Blood is a major fluid for harboring infectious organisms and transmitting the infections to others, as well as contamination of equipment. Body fluids should be treated with the utmost respect, and protective wear and equipment should be consistent with the risk level posed by the procedure being performed. For example, during cauterization, centrifugation and any procedure that might result in the generation of splatter or aerosolization, eyewear including a shield should be employed

13.3   Routine Laboratory Tests for Analysis of Serous Fluids

Testing of miscellaneous serous fluids other than those treated separately is based on the differences of fluids originating in the various body cavities. While the types of tests are common among all body fluids, the normal values for specific types of fluids will vary greatly. As is the case in the examination of both urine and cerebrospinal fluid, the samples are evaluated *macroscopically* for physical properties and appearance, as well as for the chemical components where low or high levels may be equally important in the diagnosis of disease conditions. For normal levels of chemicals and even those that are specific to a particular fluid and of no importance in other fluids, the normal ranges are compared with the values obtained by chemistry tests.

In addition to the major body fluids, some body fluids are extremely specialized in their functions and are limited in the number of tests required for analysis of the fluids for the detection of a certain disease. One of these is that of nasal secretions, a fluid that may indicate both allergic reactions and other inflammatory conditions of the respiratory system. The collection of nasal secretions that are stained with a hematological stain are examined to confirm the presence of *eosinophils*, a type of white blood cell that is often increased during an allergic attack, and is the most common test performed on nasal secretions. Perspiration can also be analyzed for elevated levels of sweat chloride, as levels of chloride in the perspiration of infants may be up to five times higher than in normal infants when a disease called *cystic fibrosis* is present. Sometimes saliva is used as a clinical sample for the testing of digestive enzymes as well.

Perhaps arguably, the third important component of the testing of serous body fluids includes the microscopic component. Differentiating between an exudate and a transudate is often necessary to determine adequate treatment. One way of differentiating between the two requires testing for the presence of white blood cells. If increased, the type of predominant cells is differentiated to provide a valuable clue as to the type of causative organism may be involved in an infection of the body site from which the fluid is collected. The presence of red blood cells must be evaluated as to the cause, such as a traumatic injury or bleeding during the collection of the specimen. Some microscopic organisms ranging from bacteria to parasites, fungi, yeasts and parasites may be determined from stained preparations of the fluid.

13.3.1 Specimen Collection of Serous Fluids

The collection of any serous fluid should be accompanied by careful attention to antiseptic procedures. Samples are collected both for laboratory analysis as well as for relieving pressure and discomfort from accumulated fluids around vital organs, in particular those of the heart and lungs. Specimens are generally collected by aspiration, as a minimal amount of fluid must be available for procedures leading to the diagnosis of a disease condition. Samples must be collected based on the needs relative to an individual body site and appropriately handled during the collection of samples. Only valid results for diagnosis can be relied upon when the sample is properly collected and placed in appropriate containers before transport to the collection site using thoughtfully established protocols. When storage of the sample is necessary, a preservative for maintaining cell morphology may be required when testing is not immediately available. To collect a sample in a most efficacious manner, coordination between testing personnel and the clinician collecting the sample must be accomplished, as well as preparation and transport for testing.

To avoid contamination of the samples and a nosocomial infection of the patient from which the sample is being collected, sterile procedures must be followed throughout the collection. In addition, the clinical personnel collecting and

Table 13.2   Samples for analysis of serous fluids

Tube #1	EDTA anticoagulated tubes are used for study of the physical properties of the sample, for cell counts and morphology of the cells, and the differentiation of the white cells for diagnostic purposes
Tube #2	An anticoagulated tube containing heparin is centrifuged to separate any cells present from the sample before chemistry tests are performed, in order to avoid erroneous test results. Heparin does not interfere with most laboratory tests
Tube #3	A sterile heparinized tube (anticoagulated) is recommended for microbiological tests, such as the Gram stain for bacterial morphology and culturing of the sample for bacterial growth

testing the sample must protect themselves against infection during the procedure. Avoiding mechanical injury to organs and tissues should be paramount to prevent dire and perhaps lifelong consequences for the patient. When fluids are removed from the body for testing, therapeutic advantages may accrue to the patient by relieving pressure on the organs and impacting the area where the organ is located. For instance, fluid removal from the chest that made breathing difficult, or for cases of congestive heart failure with fluid accumulation or bleeding around the heart from injury may provide immediate relief for the patient. Even peritoneal effusions can cause difficulty in the movements of the diaphragm, as well as compressing abdominal organs resulting from a condition called *ascites*. As in the collection of cerebrospinal fluid, the fluid aspirated may be divided into several numbered tubes to determine if blood is the result of a *traumatic puncture*. An important fact to remember is that some fluids will clot due to the presence of blood clotting factors, so anticoagulated samples are necessary for a majority of the laboratory tests. Regardless of the type of fluid being collected, it is often necessary to obtain at least three anticoagulated tubes (Table 13.2) of fluid for the various tests required.

13.3.2   Physical Appearance of Serous Fluids

The amount of fluid from each of the major body cavities described in this section will vary greatly, and in some cases the amount may be too small to accurately describe the physical appearance. Frequently there is only sufficient fluid in a specific site to lubricate the area to prevent friction and mechanical inflammation. Differentiation between a transudate and an exudate should be the primary focus initially, and the use of the data as seen in Table 13.1 will enable the distinction between the two types of fluids, which depends basically upon the concentration of the sample. The turbidity, odor, and color of the fluid will provide an initial estimation related to abnormalities that may exist in the areas of the body from which the fluids are obtained, as do the body fluids of cerebrospinal and synovial fluid.

In cases where the osmotic pressure is decreased, due to a low level of plasma protein, the condition enables more fluid to move into the body cavities. When fluid levels increase in the serous spaces in the cavity, a *serous effusion* is said to have occurred. Decreases in hydrostatic pressure, increases in hydrostatic pressure, increased capillary permeability which occurs in acute inflammatory reactions, a decrease in lymphatic reabsorption, or obstructions that prevent reabsorption of water in the cavity, can all lead to an increase in the volume of the body fluid found in the affected site.

13.3.3 Laboratory Analysis of Serous Fluids

The routine examination of serous fluids, regardless of source, will include a description of the gross appearance of the sample. Besides the crystalline clear appearance of normal cerebrospinal fluid, most serous fluids are clear but are often pale yellow (Fig. 13.1). Turbidity of the various fluids often indicate the presence of large number of white blood cells or bacteria, but elevated levels of proteins or fat (lipid) components are also capable of imparting turbidity to the fluid. Bloody fluid will indicate either a hemorrhage from vascular injury or from an accident, or a traumatic puncture in the collection of the fluid. Following the macroscopic evaluation of the sample of body fluid, other laboratory tests that include chemistry procedures appropriate for the given body fluid are performed. This includes quantitative cell counts and microbiological stains and bacterial cultures that facilitate the diagnosis of the medical condition of the patient. Quantitative cell counts and evaluation of cellular morphology require that samples be collected with anticoagulants that will preserve the integrity of the red and white blood cells. EDTA is

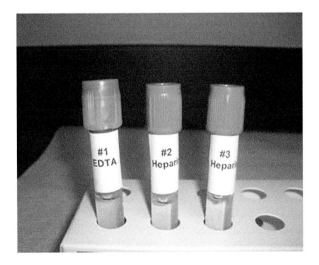

Fig. 13.1 Samples collected with anticoagulants to preserve cell morphology and chemistry results

the preservative of choice, and chemistry exams must be performed using a lithium anticoagulant to avoid alterations of the test results by using EDTA-preserved samples.

Several chemistry tests are available for determinations on various body fluids. Some of these constituents are more applicable for certain types of body fluids. Protein values and differentiation of the types of protein represented in the total protein level are possible by sophisticated testing. Glucose values for body fluids are generally lower than those found in the blood, usually at a level of 60–80% that of blood, as discussed previously. The levels should be correlated with those of the blood in order to make an accurate assessment of the levels. Both elevated and decreased levels are clinically significant in certain medical conditions. Bacterial infections of the fluid will reduce the glucose levels of the fluid as bacteria utilize glucose, but viral infections will not affect the glucose level. Low levels are also found in tumors that are *metastatic* growths as increased metabolism of growing tissue may utilize large amounts of glucose, and in diabetic coma. Lactate dehydrogenase (LD) levels are valuable in determining the presence of white blood cells, where intact cells may not be present for a number of reasons including delays in testing of the fluids.

Bacterial and serological procedures are also appropriate for some fluids, particularly in cerebrospinal fluid, but may be valuable when conditions such as tubercular infections of organs of the body where effusions are produced. Bacterial identification may be determined by using a Gram stain that differentiates between groups of bacteria, and the use of an acid fast stain for tubercular infection that occurs not only in the lungs but in other organs of the body. An *encapsulated yeast* called *Cryptococcus neoformans* may be detected by an *India ink prep.* This procedure aids in the rapid presumptive identification of a causative organism (Fig. 13.2). Rapid treatment may be necessary to prevent the rapid deterioration of the patient, particularly when it is found in cerebrospinal fluid, a potentially serious condition that may have fatal consequences.

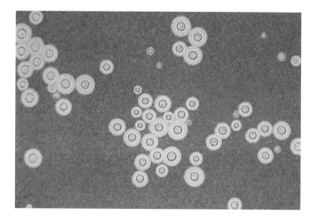

Fig. 13.2 India ink prep depicting the presence of *C. neoformans*

13.3.4 Microscopic Cell Counts and Cell Differentiation for Miscellaneous Body Fluids

For miscellaneous body fluids which include those that are rarely tested when compared with cerebrospinal fluid, urine, semen and synovial fluid, test procedures for cell counts and differentiation of the white blood cells are similar. Red and white blood cell counts are generally performed by manual procedures, since automated cell counters used for whole blood counts are not sufficiently sensitive for counting low numbers of cells with any reasonable degree of accuracy. For counting blood cells, the procedure is performed on the specialized slide called a hemocytometer as is the practice when analyzing cerebrospinal fluid. When white blood cells exceed an established low number, a stained smear is used to obtain a differentiation between polymorphonuclear cells and those that are mononuclear.

As previously mentioned in this publication, a specialized cytocentrifuge (cell centrifuge) may again be used for preparing a smear from an aliquot of the CSF sample. In some cases, this sample may be obtained from a centrifuged sample containing an increased number of cells. This is desirable since an actual count is not being performed which would be artificially elevated but does provide for efficiency in differentiating the white cells. The cytocentrifuge, such as the brand called the Cytospin, uses a slow spinning of the sample and provides an adequate yield of cells from an extremely small amount of fluid.

By using this instrument, the fluid is slowly centrifuged for approximately 200 revolutions per minute for 5–10 min, and a filter paper accompanying the slide absorbs the liquid portion of the sample, leaving only cells. The small circle on the slide is where the solid components composed mostly of blood cells and organisms from the total volume of sample is concentrated. The result is the formation of a small 6-mm circle which is then stained for microscopic identification. This procedure may be used for isolating tumor cells when necessary, a process where a histological or cytological stain may be employed for identification of malignant cells. Other concentration methods are available but are more expensive and time consuming than the one described here. In addition, some methods tend to distort the morphology of the cells and organisms, making it more difficult to evaluate the components from the fluid.

The differential count is performed by physically counting the white blood cells, using a differential counter for enumeration. As few as 100 cells may be counted and the percentages of each reported, but a 200-cell count provides a more accurate evaluation. When the method for concentration and staining allows for more specific identification, such as is possible with the Cytospin instrument, white cells called neutrophils (polymorphonuclear), lymphocytes (mononuclear), monocytes, eosinophils and basophils may be identified if required (Fig. 13.3a–c). Unusual cells from tissue types representative of the body site from which the sample is obtained as well as tumor cells may be referred to anatomic pathologists for evaluation.

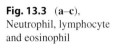

Fig. 13.3 (a–c),
Neutrophil, lymphocyte
and eosinophil

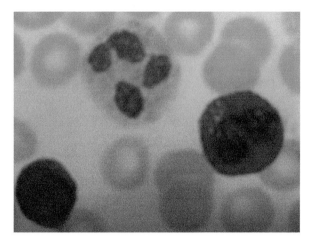

13.4 Performing Total Cell Counts for the Serous Fluids

As was previously stressed, the major reason for performing both the red and the white blood cell counts is to differentiate between the fluids, identifying them as either exudates or transudates, the latter of which will primarily have the lowest count of both red and white blood cells. During collection, it is important to determine if a traumatic tap, in which blood has been introduced into the specimen during the aspiration of the fluid, has occurred. Once this is determined, the presence of large numbers of red blood cells would indicate injury or hemorrhage into the body cavity. The sample is collected in sequentially numbered tubes where the initial tube may reveal the presence of blood that again indicates a traumatic tap. The specimen used for cell counts and morphology of the cells must be collected in an EDTA (purple stoppered) tube, as it contains an anticoagulant that preserves the morphology of the cells. Both red and white blood cell counts may be performed in the same manner. Cell counts cannot be performed accurately on clotted or partially clotted samples. In critical cases where a repeat collection cannot be obtained, cell counts performed on blood that is clotted or has clumps of cells must be noted for the physician to interpret.

The total count of white blood cells is used to aid in differentiating between a transudate with a simple effusion, or from an acute bacterial infection of the membranes surrounding the body cavity. In some cases an infection of the blood itself (septicemia) may infect a number of cavities, including that of the *myocardial* (heart) sac surrounding the organ. It is important to note that unlike the process employed in the examination of cerebrospinal fluid and blood, *other serous fluids cannot be mixed with acetic acid since the fluids contain extremely elevated levels of protein, and the acetic acid will clump the white blood cells and perhaps cause clumps in the fluid.* When large numbers of red blood cells are present, it is necessary to lyse (destroy) the red blood cells in order to visualize the white blood cells in the sample. A solution called Turk's solution will stain the white blood cells and lyse the red blood cells, greatly enhancing the ability to obtain accurate white blood cell counts. Merely diluting the sample may prevent the sample that has a tendency to clot from clotting in some instances. When cytologic examinations are needed due to morphology of the cells found, or the known presence of a tumor, clotted fluids will yield the quality of cells needed for the special stains used by the anatomic pathologists. But the clots will need to be broken up before the sample is submitted for pathological procedures.

NOTE: This procedure, enumerating cells of a serous fluid is applicable to all types of serous fluids.

Procedure 13.1: Manual Cell Counts for Serous Fluid

1. After mixing the serous fluid sample carefully by twirling and inverting the capped sample for several minutes, use a Pasteur pipette or other disposable pipette to carefully deliver a small amount of the anticoagulated fluid at the point of the V-shaped cut in the hemocytometer slide. The cover glass of the hemocytometer on both sides should be carefully filled, taking precautions to avoid overfilling, where the fluid leaks from under the cover slip and into the moats around the polished surface of the two sides. Overfilling the chamber may take longer for the slide to equilibrate to the correct level. Allow equilibration of the depth in the chamber by placing the hemocytometer for 5 min in a petri dish with water-soaked bibulous paper. This prevents evaporation of the liquid sample placed on the hemocytometer, which might result in an erroneous count

2. Use the low-power objective (10×) to scan both gridded sides of the hemocytometer to determine the presence of blood cells and to insure consistency of the solution. This process would insure that no clumps and heavy areas of concentration are present. Each major square and both sides of the slide should have roughly equal distributions of white and red blood cells if the slide is properly charged

3. Under the 40× objective, count the red blood cells using a manual handheld "clicker" in the five squares found in the center of the ruled area, on each side of the slide. If the cells are so numerous as to touch each other or to overlap, a dilution of the preparation using an isotonic solution that will not destroy or distort the cells should be performed and the slide should be recharged. The four corner squares and the center square of the most closely gridded part of the slide is to be counted

4. The RBCs will be round and small and may appear to be a yellowish color. Sometimes the *biconcave* morphology, with a central area of pallor and no irregular surfaces when properly anticoagulated and diluted. White blood cells will be slightly larger and may appear granular when compared with the cytoplasm of the red cells. Nuclei may be visible in the white cells but will not be seen in RBCs unless they are very young cells

5. Five square millimeters on both sides of the slide are counted. When the numbers of red cells per the 10 squares on the 2 sides of the chamber exceed 200, fewer squares may be counted. The count should then be adjusted by a factor to equal the numbers that would have been counted in the 10 squares. For example, if 3 squares are counted on one side of the chamber and 2 are counted on the other, add the numbers and multiply by 2
6. Extremely bloody samples may require dilution with an *isotonic* solution such as "normal" saline in order to avoid disruption of the cell membranes of the red blood cells. Except in extremely bloody fluid, red blood cells should be quite low in number. When a specimen is particularly bloody, it is necessary to dilute the sample volumetrically with an *isotonic* diluent. It may be necessary to count fewer squares and to adjust the calculations as appropriate to obtain an accurate count when excessive numbers of cells are encountered
7. When calculating the number of blood cells per volume of fluid, the total number of cells for the 10 squares on the two sides of the hemocytometer are used. The calculation of the count must be multiplied by the dilution factor. No dilution is required normally unless the sample is visibly bloody, so the actual count for an undiluted specimen would contain no dilution factor

Values used in the calculation are:
Number of cells counted
Dilution factor if necessary
Volume counted is determined by the equation and depth of chamber (0.1 mm × area counted)
8. The calculation formula is as follows:

Box 13.1: Calculating the number of blood cells per volume of fluid

Number of cells counted X dilution / Area counted X dilution = cell count / uL

Example: The fluid is turbid and is diluted 1:20. A total of 72 white blood cells are counted on the two sides of the hemocytometer, for a total of 10 square mm

Calculation

$$\frac{72 \times 20 = 1440}{10 \times 0.1} = \frac{1440}{1} = 1440\, cells\, /\, \mu L$$

9. The hemocytometer is then disinfected by using bleach or a commercial disinfectant. It is important to soak the instrument for at least 5 min before rinsing the slide. Rinsing is accomplished by using deionized or distilled water or with 70% alcohol, and then thoroughly drying the slide with lens paper to prevent fibers and residue from accumulating on the slide

Special considerations apply to the examination of miscellaneous types of body fluids other than the major fluids of cerebrospinal fluid, semen, and other commonly encountered fluids. After determining whether the fluid is a transudate, or an exudate, based chiefly upon the specific gravity and the level of protein present, the samples are normally compared with a blood sample from the patient for comparison and correlation. As a general rule, exudates contain more protein than a transudate, as well as more cellular materials, and are evaluated as to the cause of the effusion. Causes may relate to inflammatory condition unrelated to infection, infections of a viral or bacterial nature, and may include fungal and parasitic infections, as well as malignant processes. In other words, the presence of an effusion signals a disease process of which the etiology must be determined. Examination of fluids from the following sites with pertinent clinical information is typically employed for diagnosis.

13.4.1 Pericardial Fluid

The prefix "peri-" means around, and the word root "cardi-" refers to the heart, meaning that fluid has gathered around the heart. Since friction occurs with the constant beating of the heart which is encased in the pericardial space (sometimes called sac), 10–50 mL of fluid aids in preventing mechanical inflammation between the two membranes. This tissue fluid is an ultrafiltrate of the blood plasma. This fluid is normally clear (not turbid) and is most often a straw color. When abnormal conditions arise, the amount of fluid increases and fills the sac surrounding the heart. The pressure from the accumulated fluid impedes the pumping action of the heart and further impacts upon the body's circulation. Injuries to the heart and the pericardial membrane may cause bleeding that may result in a condition called *cardiac tamponade.* The condition may also be known as pericardial tamponade, and occurs when fluid accumulates in the pericardium, the sac in which the heart is enclosed. In addition to blunt and penetrating trauma, pericarditis or inflammation of the lining of the heart will often result in the formation of an effusion around the heart, impacting its ability to pump blood through the circulatory system.

Cardiac tamponade is caused by a large or uncontrolled pericardial effusion by the buildup of fluid inside the pericardium, a condition that may occur gradually, or may occur in acute illness. Buildup over a more gradual period of time occurs in some cancers, and more dramatically in certain infections. The changes in permeability of the membranes of the capillaries as well as the pericardium result from inflammation or infection may be accompanied by the presence of red blood cells as well as white blood cells.

13.4.2 Peritoneal Fluid

When fluid builds in the peritoneal cavity, the large cavity below the diaphragm that houses the visceral organs is impacted. This fluid as in other material functions as a lubricant and will rarely consist of more than 100 mL of straw colored, clear fluid that surround the abdominal organs. The accumulation of large amounts of peritoneal fluid resulting from an effusion of fluid reveals a condition generally known as *ascites*. Large amounts, greatly exceeding the normal amount of 100 mL, may be aspirated from the cavity to provide comfort to the patient. In congestive heart failure which may also occur from effusions of fluid around the heart, results in an increase in hydrostatic pressure in the vessels. This condition is usually accompanied with decreased plasma oncotic pressure when low levels of albumin and other proteins are present in the circulating blood. In *peritonitis*, an inflammation of the lining of the peritoneal cavity, there is an accompanying increased permeability of the capillaries in the peritoneal region. Decreased drainage of this fluid by the lymphatic system often occurs in a number of malignant diseases.

13.4.3 Pleural Fluid

Pleural fluid is found in the pleural space surrounding the lungs and heart. A minimal amount of just a few milliliters of fluid will be found in the pleural cavity from normal healthy individuals. It can be stated that there is not essentially a cavity in the chest region, as virtually the entire space is filled with the lungs and the heart, along with associated vascular structures. Any accumulations of fluid in the area will mechanically impact upon the expansion of the lungs and effusions may occur when conditions arise that cause the body to react to inflammation during a state of disease. Excess fluids may also result when the lymphatic system that normally drains fluids from the area is somehow inhibited in its ability to remove the fluids.

One of the most common fluids that may require aspiration from a body cavity is that of pleural effusions related to the lungs. A number of conditions may cause problems in the thoracic cavity, and large amounts of fluid may gather there, impacting the ability to breathe by pressing on the diaphragm and upon the lungs and heart. A medical procedure called a thoracentesis is so named because it is performed by puncturing the chest or thoracic wall by a large bore needle. The purpose of the procedure is to differentiate between a transudate and an exudate. Any bacterial infection that is present in the fluid will require a Gram stain and bacterial culture of the organisms from this fluid from the chest region. When the presence of bacteria is confirmed by stain and is cultured for bacterial growth, an antibiotic sensitivity study can be performed to determine the appropriate treatment.

Since a large number of cases of congestive heart failure where excess fluid buildup occurs in the pleural cavity is due in part by a change in the portion of plasma protein called albumin and when it falls below the normal level. Remember that albumin is the chief protein factor that provides for oncotic pressure, allowing water to flow into or out of the capillaries. Although the majority of pleural fluids lack the blood clotting factors that would lead to the formation of clots in the fluid, allowances must be made for that eventuality. So the sample is collected in a heparinized tube as a safeguard against clotting, since cell counts cannot be performed accurately on clotted specimens.

Again, it is paramount that it be determined whether pleural fluid samples are exudates or transudates. As a general baseline, fluids with a total protein value of less than 3.0 g per deciliter would be described as a transudate, while those with levels of protein above 3.0 g per deciliter would be considered as being an exudate. Differentiation as an exudate may also be determined when the total protein ratio of pleural fluid to serum protein is greater than 0.5 as pleural fluid has a protein level that is greater than one-half of that of the serum level. Other useful chemistry tests are those of lactate dehydrogenase (LD) where values exceed 200 International Units (IU) for an exudate but should be somewhat higher in serum. Similar values pertaining to pleural fluid cholesterol are also significant, where the cholesterol value in pleural fluid of greater than 60 mg per deciliter indicates that the sample is that of an exudate.

13.4.4 Amniotic Fluid

Amniotic fluid is the serous fluid in which the embryo and later the fetus is suspended within the amnion, which is the inner layer of the cavity that is in contact with the amniotic fluid. The fluid, as are the other fluids discussed in this section, is designed to protect the fetus and to allow for growth and movement. The amniotic fluid is secreted by a combination of tissues, including the membrane surrounding the cavity, the umbilical cord and the organs of the fetus that include the respiratory and renal systems along with the gastrointestinal system. Fetal urine contributes a large portion of the amniotic fluid in growing amounts during the second and third trimesters, as the fetal kidneys grow and mature in their functions. The amount of amniotic fluid at the end of a normal period of *gestation* may be up to one and one-half liters and contributes a great deal of volume and weight gain in the expectant mother.

The procedure can be safely performed by the end of the fourteenth week of the pregnancy as the normal gestation period is approximately 40 weeks for humans. But the collection of amniotic fluid is primarily done during the second and third trimesters as pregnancy is divided into three equal time periods. It is during the second trimester when most genetic and developmental tests are performed. Procedures include pre-birth treatment of *erythroblastosis fetalis* or hemolytic disease of the newborn as well as the prediction of respiratory distress in the fetus. This condition might require an early *cesarean section* (C-section) as soon as the lung maturity could support life outside the uterus of the mother.

Amniotic fluid is collected by amniocentesis, a term that literally means puncture of the amnion, and may be performed through the abdomen (transabdominally) or through the vagina. This procedure should be preceded by an *ultrasound* examination, when an amniocentesis, or aspiration of amniotic fluid, is scheduled. An ultrasound examination provides a variety of information as to gestational age and the number of fetuses present in the uterus. The procedure is used to detect major fetal abnormalities, insure fetal heart functions, the location of the placenta in the uterus, and the volume of amniotic fluid. An unintended consequence of an amniocentesis is damage to the fetus, the umbilical cord, or placenta. Infection may occur, especially when a vaginal aspiration is performed, and a ruptured membrane may induce premature labor or serious hemorrhage. A rare condition sometimes occurs where the mother is exposed to the blood of the fetus and is of a different ABO group or

Fig. 13.4 Cells stained by
the Kleihauer-Betke
process for Hemoglobin F

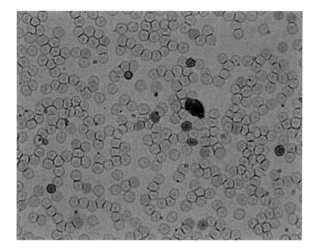

Rh type. This prompts the formation of antibodies in the mother against the blood group and type expressed by the fetus and can lead to massive blood destruction in the fetus.

The first two milliliters of fluid should be discarded since blood and maternal cells may contaminate the sample. Clear fluid is preferable and should be tested immediately to avoid deterioration of cells and chemical constituents found in the fluid. As in the collection of other body fluids, there may be a traumatic puncture which results in blood from the mother. The physical appearance of amniotic fluid is important and should be almost colorless to light straw under normal conditions. Since the first blood in the aspiration is sometimes from the patient, it is important to determine whether the blood is of maternal or fetal origin. Differentiation between fetal or maternal red blood cells is accomplished by using a test called the *Kleihauer-Bettke* stain (Fig. 13.4). Fetal stains contain a hemoglobin called *hemoglobin F* and stained maternal red cells will appear as "ghost cells." Where ghost cells are present, only the outer perimeter of the red blood cells may be observed. Fetal red blood cells will appear a refractile red color. An additional test called the hemoglobin electrophoresis can also be used to confirm the presence of fetal red cells.

Amniotic fluid as a medium for laboratory testing is growing in importance, and was traditionally used to monitor the developmental conditions provided for the growing fetus. Secretions from the intestinal system may also impart a dark and greenish color called meconium aspiration syndrome, since the fetus swallows a large amount of amniotic fluid each day (up to one-half liter). The level of the green color is described as light, moderate or heavy. *Alpha-fetoprotein* (AFP) is produced in the liver of the developing fetus and in the yolk sac. There is a minimal amount of AFP present in the amniotic fluid. But the levels are increased in spina bifida, an open neural tube defect, along with conditions of anencephaly or small brain, and in hydrocephaly, an increased level of cerebrospinal fluid causing enlargement of the skull. In cases of *Hemolytic Disease of the Newborn* (HDN), fetal lung maturity and levels of bilirubin related to destruction of red blood cells in the fetus and antibodies to the Rh factor due to passage from an Rh negative mother are monitored. *Cytogenetic* studies for prospective parents to determine if the fetus suffers from a number of genetic disorders may also be performed prior to birth of the infant. Fluids collected late in pregnancy are important in determining fetal lung development.

Another frequently-occurring and important test to determine the maturity of the fetal lungs is the determination of the *lecithin-sphingomyelin* ratio. Until about the thirty-fourth week of pregnancy, more sphingomyelin than lecithin is produced, and after this time, more lecithin than sphingomyelin is produced. Delivery before this conversion to a predominance of lecithin occurs, hyaline membrane disease of the infant may occur. The obstetrician is able from these tests to determine the best time to arrange for delivery when the medical need arises. When the lecithin to sphingomyelin (L/S) ratio is less than 2.0, the lungs of the fetus will be immature, and a ratio in the range of 2.1–3.0 is considered borderline. When the ratio reaches a level of 3.1 or greater, the fetal lungs are considered as mature and able to provide for the infant's respiratory needs.

Cell counts in amniotic fluid are of little significance when compared with the counts for other body fluids. A test that is often performed in the offices of obstetricians is that of a microscopic test called the *Fern test*. This test determines the presence of *estrogen* and *progesterone* and can be used to determine if the membranes have ruptured, but this test results in some false positive results. Mucus aspirated from the cervical region is examined microscopically after it has dried on a microscope slide. A "ferning" pattern that is likened to the shape exhibited by a palm leaf indicates the stage of the ovarian cycle and if progesterone secretion seen in large amounts in pregnancy is present (Fig. 13.5). These tests are CLIA-waived procedures and may be quite subjective in their interpretation, so are seldom performed in a licensed clinical laboratory. A substantial number of newer laboratory procedures are becoming available, based on biochemical, microbiological, and immunological methods in which amniotic fluids are used as samples.

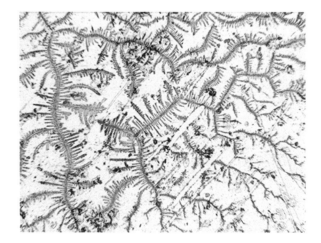

Fig. 13.5 "Ferning" pattern exhibited by drying of amniotic fluid F

13.5 Summary

Serous fluids are found in three different major cavities of the body and are formed by serous membranes that line the interior of the cavities. Cavities of the body with their special bodily fluids are formed early in the life of the human, from the beginning transformations of the zygote to specialized tissues and organs. Most of these fluids have at least some association with the liquid portion of the blood, where ultrafiltrates are formed in the cavities. These fluids are designed for protection from shock and friction, and contain constituents relative to their purposes as lubricants and nourishing liquids. In normal states, all of these fluids are clear and are colorless to light straw in color. All the major serous fluids of the body, when properly collected, stored, transported, and tested, are capable of providing valuable clinical information relative to medical conditions and the prognosis of the patient upon treatment.

The differentiation of transudates versus exudates is the first step in the testing of fluids for disease states. Fluids may form as the result of the failure to reabsorb fluids, the overproduction of fluids, and as the result of inflammation, often of a bacterial nature. A variety of tests are available to aid in the differentiation of the fluids as exudates or transudates. Generally, an exudate is more concentrated than the transudate in the amount of blood cells as well as for the levels of total proteins found in the fluids. The tests that are of clinical importance are more numerous for some body fluids than for others. Some types of tests are common among all body fluids but the normal values for specific types of fluids will vary widely. In all cases, there are specific physical properties associated with the various fluids, a chemical component that includes certain biochemical measurements, and a microscopic component for cells and infectious organisms. However, the accepted normal values for a particular component in one type of body fluid will not correlate with that of another cavity fluid.

The specimen collection procedures for the various serous fluids all require aseptic procedures, but the collection methods vary with the location of the body cavity and associated fluids. The abnormal accumulation of serous fluids is the first clue in many cases of a medical condition that may require treatment. Samples must be appropriately handled and collected based on the needs for an individual body site from which samples are being collected but valid results for diagnosis depend upon proper collection, transport and preservation of the sample. Contamination of the samples and contraction of nosocomial infection by the patient are potential hazards when procedures are conducted. Strict adherence to the proper labeling of tubes for interpretation of results, as well as prevention of deterioration of components of the fluids is mandatory.

The normal amount of fluid from each of the major body cavities will vary greatly and in some cases the amount may be too small to accurately describe the physical appearance. Increased levels of fluids may be due to either inflammatory processes or even mechanical causes that prevent normal reabsorption of fluids. Centrifugation of samples may be necessary for the recovery of sufficient numbers of cells and bacteria to conduct staining of slides for microscopic evaluation. It will be necessary to interpret the presence of blood as to whether it is the result of the collection of the fluid or is a result of a medical condition.

Special considerations are necessary for the examination of miscellaneous types of body fluids other than the major fluids of cerebrospinal fluid, semen, and other commonly encountered fluids. Major types of fluids other than blood and urine that provide valuable clinical data is from that of pericardial fluid, pleural fluid, and peritoneal fluids from the associated bodily cavities. Amniotic fluid is not always considered as serous fluids by some, but the fluid does meet the criteria established for defining serous fluids. The fluid is secreted by the inner layer of the cavity, as are the other serous fluids in which the embryo and later the fetus is suspended within the amnion, which the inner layer of the cavity that is in contact with the amniotic fluid. The fluid, as are the other fluids discussed in this section, is designed to protect the fetus and to allow for growth and movement. The amniotic fluid is excreted by a combination of tissues, including the membrane surrounding the cavity, the umbilical cord and the organs of the fetus that include the respiratory and renal systems along with the gastrointestinal system of which fetal urine is a chief contributor of amniotic fluid. The tests available for amniotic fluid are perhaps greater in number and more significant than those for other body fluids, due to conditions affecting both the mother and the unborn child.

Case #13.1
An elderly gentleman has suffered from several occurrences of respiratory infections, including pneumonia upon at least two occasions. Since his last bout with respiratory difficulties, he has had difficulty breathing, with a weak cough, and an accumulation of fluid in his lower thoracic region. This accumulation has led to a condition resembling congestive heart failure. A puncture of the thoracic wall, called a thoracentesis, is performed, and a large amount of a pleural effusion is aspirated. The fluid is referred to the laboratory for several tests.

Gross Fluid Examination:
The fluid is not of the normal consistency of body fluids, which would normally be viscous, as it is watery and somewhat cloudy.

Total protein	1.1 g/dL	Reference value = 1.0–2.0 g/dL
Cell count	WBCs = 0.421×10^9/L	Reference value $\leq 0.50 \times 10^9$/L
Blood values	Total serum protein = 7.1 g/dL	Reference range = 6.1–8.0 g/dL

Cell Differential: Predominantly lymphocytes and monocytes, few neutrophils, few RBCs.

Gram Stain: Cytofuged sample reveals no organisms; reported as a sterile culture also.

Blood cell count: 13×10^9/L.
Leukocyte differential: 71% lymphocytes and 17% neutrophils; the remainder of the cells totaled 1% eosinophils and 11% monocytes.
Reference values: WBCs 0.15×10^9/L and more than 25% neutrophils

1. In comparing the serum protein and the value of the protein of the effusion, is this an exudates or a transudate? Discuss the answer you provide.
2. What would be the significance of increased lymphocytes?
3. Why is another reason that this fluid not considered an exudate, even when the ratio of fluid to serum protein that matches that for a transudate is known?

Review Questions

1. Which of the following body fluids is not always considered as an ultrafiltrate of blood?
   a. Synovial fluid
   b. Pericardial fluid
   c. Peritoneal fluid
   d. Cerebrospinal fluid
2. A chemistry test on amniotic fluid that gives information related to neural tube deficits is:
   a. Alpha-fetoprotein
   b. Meconium
   c. Lecithin-sphingomyelin
   d. Kleihauer-Bettke
3. The "Fern test" determines the presence of:
   a. Progesterone
   b. Cervical mucus
   c. Meconium
   d. Phagocytes
4. The most obvious difference between an exudates and a transudate would be:
   a. Elevated protein in an exudate
   b. Elevated protein in a transudate
   c. Protein in transudate equal to blood
   d. None of the previous responses
5. The chief mechanism by which transudate effusions may accumulate in bodily cavities is
   a. Hydrostatic pressure
   b. Response to infectious processes
   c. Clots formation
   d. Presence of crystals
6. Which of the following would be the most accurate statement?
   a. Exudates form due to a disruption in the balance of filtration and reabsorption
   b. Transudates form due to a disruption in the balance of filtration and reabsorption
   c. Transudates are produced by inflammatory conditions involving an organ
   d. Exudates form as a result of a systemic disorder

7. Necrosis of an organ or tissue may be determined by performing:
   a. Ultrasound image
   b. Kleihauer-Bettke stain
   c. Lactate dehydrogenase
   d. Complete blood count
8. The serous fluid that could perhaps require the most extensive group of tests would be:
   a. Synovial fluid
   b. Cerebrospinal fluid
   c. Amniotic fluid
   d. Peritoneal transudate
9. A type of white blood cell found in nasal secretions during an allergic reaction is:
   a. Basophil
   b. Polymorphonuclear cell
   c. Mononuclear cell
   d. Eosinophil
10. Why is differentiation of white blood cells found in body fluids important?
   a. Differentiation provides information related to the severity of the disorder
   b. Differentiation provides information as to the type of infectious process present
   c. Differentiation is used to differentiate exudates from transudates
   d. Differentiation gives the origin of the problem as to the organ involved
11. The anticoagulant used to preserve the morphology of blood cells is:
   a. Heparin
   b. Methylene blue
   c. Glacial acetic acid
   d. EDTA
12. The type of tube used for microbiological testing of body fluids is:
   a. Sterile EDTA tube
   b. Sterile clot tube
   c. Sterile heparinized tube
   d. Any type is acceptable
13. Which of the following would not lead to an increase in the volume of the body fluid found in the affected site?
   a. The turbidity, odor, color of the fluid
   b. Decreases or increases in hydrostatic pressure
   c. Increase in capillary permeability which occurs in acute inflammatory reactions
   d. Decrease in lymphatic reabsorption, or obstructions that prevent reabsorption
14. Which of the following serous fluids would normally be crystal clear?
   a. Synovial fluid
   b. Pericardial effusions
   c. Cerebrospinal fluid
   d. Fluid from pericardial sac

15. An encapsulated yeast found in cerebrospinal fluid is often determined by:
    a. Gram stain
    b. India ink prep
    c. Acid fast stain
    d. New methylene blue dye
16. Turk's stain will:
    a. Stain red blood cells
    b. Lyse red blood cells
    c. Lyse white blood cells
    d. Provide cytopathology stains
17. Inflammation of the lining of the heart is called:
    a. Endocarditis
    b. Peritonitis
    c. Cardiac tamponade
    d. None of the previous responses
18. Oncotic pressure of the blood plasma is associated with:
    a. Glucose levels
    b. Numbers of blood cells
    c. Body fluid volume
    d. Albumin
19. Amniotic fluid, during the second and third trimesters of pregnancy, is chiefly composed of:
    a. Normal physiological saline
    b. High protein plasma
    c. Urine from the fetus
    d. Meconium
20. The test used to differentiate fetal cells from maternal cells is:
    a. Alpha-fetoprotein
    b. Lecithin-sphingomyelin
    c. Fern test
    d. Kleihauer-Bettke

Answers in Appendix C

Synovial Fluid Evaluation

14

Objectives

Describe the origin of synovial fluid

List conditions in which medical conditions may develop that are diagnosed through synovial fluid analysis

Discuss the physical properties exhibited by synovial fluid

List crystals that may be deposited in synovial fluid

Relate microscopic findings related to various medical conditions that are manifested in various diseases affecting synovial fluid

14.1 Introduction to the Testing of Synovial Fluid

Synovial fluid, sometimes known as joint fluid, is a viscous liquid that is found in all joint cavities that articulate with potential friction against each other. In addition to lubricating the synovial membranes lining the interior of joints, the fluid is found in bursae. These are sacs of fluid which serve to reduce friction between tendons and bones, as well as preventing damage to *ligaments* and *cartilaginous* tissue from friction. Synovial fluid is formed as an ultrafiltrate of the plasma across the synovial membrane. Secreted by the cells of the synovial membrane, a small amount of *mucopolysaccharide* containing *hyaluronic acid* and a small amount of protein is added. Since it is derived from plasma, synovial fluid has similar concentrations of chemicals that blood plasma does except for a high-molecular weight mucopolysaccharide that is called hyaluronate or hyaluronic acid. The presence of this chemical distinguishes synovial fluid from all other body fluids of mammals, a category that of course includes humans.

The viscosity of synovial fluid owes this unique property to the *polymerization* of hyaluronic acid, a component essential for lubrication of the joints. A general term for inflammation of the joints is arthritis or RA. This condition affects many and is related to the production of hyaluronate and its ability to polymerize, therefore reducing the viscosity of the synovial fluid present in the affected joints.

© Springer International Publishing AG, part of Springer Nature 2018
J. W. Ridley, *Fundamentals of the Study of Urine and Body Fluids*,
https://doi.org/10.1007/978-3-319-78417-5_14

Hyaluronic acid is a secretion of *synoviocytic cells* that line the joint cavities and is derived from blood plasma. Normal synovial fluid is sterile and will contain no red and few white blood cells.

A simple procedure called the *Ropes*, or *mucin clot test* has been performed for many years to determine the presence of normal synovial fluid. The test is an assay for clot formation between synovial fluid hyaluronate and acetic acid, where synovial fluid and 5% acetic acid are combined. If a solid clot in clear fluid is quickly formed, the synovial fluid is considered normal, but poor clot formation is an indicator of an inflammatory disease. In some laboratory procedures, the presence of contaminating synovial fluid may make it more difficult to dilute and perform cell counts and enumeration of crystals because of its extreme *viscosity* (stickiness).

A considerable number of immunological responses that are inflammatory processes will affect the permeability of the membranes surrounding the joint cavities, altering the amount and the quality of synovial fluid as seen in RA. Certain chemicals are implicated in the production of inflammation of the joints, as well as any traumatic injury affecting the joints. One of the most frequently encountered causes of inflammation of joints is that of bacterial infection, or the body's response to bacterial inflammation that may affect the joints of an individual. When certain chemicals, some of which are metabolic, are found in excess in the blood supply of an individual, a variety of crystal forms may form. Sometimes deposited in the joints, these may cause extreme pain requiring medical treatment for relief of pain and to prevent the formation and accumulation of crystals. A common example is gout, sometimes called gouty arthritis, where uric acid crystals are deposited from the blood into joints.

14.2   Infection Control

No specific dangers are associated with the handling of synovial fluids. But as with all body fluids, Standard Precautions mandated by governmental agencies and medical facility guidelines should be observed when transporting, handling and testing of the biological material. Equipment used for collecting the fluid should be sterile to prevent transmitting an infection to the patient, as the fluid is basically considered to be sterile. Clean and sterile containers, especially when bacterial cultures are required, should be used to avoid erroneous and confusing laboratory results from contamination of the specimen by those collecting and handling the fluid.

14.3   Routine Tests Ordered for Synovial Fluid

When joints become painful and swollen, it is necessary to determine the cause of the disorder before effective treatment for a cure or for palliative therapy can be initiated. White blood cell counts are normally the first tests that indicate the presence of infectious *synovitis* or another inflammatory condition. Microscopic

Fig. 14.1 Preparing slide of synovial fluid for Gram stain

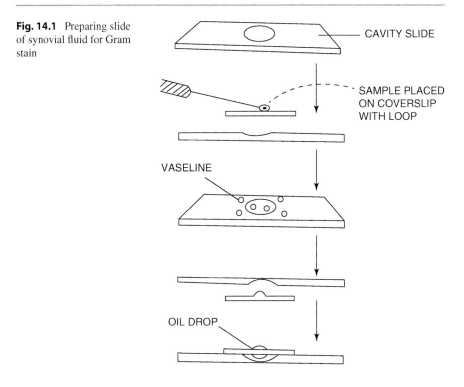

CAVITY SLIDE

SAMPLE PLACED ON COVERSLIP WITH LOOP

VASELINE

OIL DROP

examination of the morphological characteristics of any cells found and the identification of crystals that may be found is necessary to alleviate the condition. The first step for identifying the presence of bacteria that may have precipitated an acute inflammatory condition, a Gram stain is performed initially to determine the presence of and the kind of bacteria that are present, as no bacteria will be found in normal synovial fluid (Fig. 14.1). When bacterial organisms are observed following the staining of a microscopic slide containing a sample of the fluid, bacterial cultures are performed to identify the causative organism or organisms and to determine the appropriate *antimicrobial therapy*.

The differential diagnosis of joint fluids should include studies of the synovial fluid to avoid further damage to joints when the etiology of the condition is unknown. Cell counts for both red and white blood cell counts are performed unless the blood in the specimen is known to be the result of a traumatic tap. The counts for both red and white blood cells should be performed immediately as polymorphonuclear segmented neutrophils, a type of white blood cell known to be elevated in most cases of bacterial infection, will decrease rapidly after 1 h. Intact red blood cells may lyse (break down) and not be microscopically visible under certain conditions. The swelling of a joint or joints usually signals an increase in fluid (edema) that accumulates around the inflammatory site for protection and for the addition of white blood cells necessary to combat an infection (Fig. 14.2). Other responses to diseases related to synovial productions are presented in Table 14.3.

Fig. 14.2 Edema in the
extremities related to fluid
accumulation

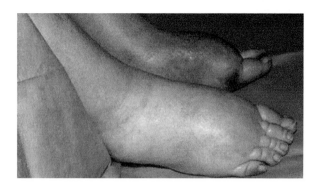

Some non-inflammatory conditions called degenerative diseases in which the cartilage and supportive tissues of the joints almost completely disintegrate will not produce the findings of those seen in acute inflammatory disorders of the joints. The degenerative types of diseases are for the most part chronic as a long-standing condition with no available cure. Those of an inflammatory nature are known as acute conditions that may be improved if not cured. In each of these disorders, the glucose and protein will be within normal ranges, even with tissue damage of the joint. The white blood cell count will be normal for synovial fluid.

14.3.1 Specimen Collection for Synovial Fluid

The prefix, arthro-, indicates a jointed appendage of the body, and the suffix, -itis, is ascribed to any of more than 100 types of joint inflammation. *Arthritides* is the plural of arthritis, a term used when an individual suffers from more than one of the approximately 100 types of arthritis.

Arthritic pain from joints of the body results in many visits to medical offices for alleviation of pain. The large joints of the body are most often involved, where bones meet and articulate against each other and provide the most prevalent sites from which synovial fluid is collected for analysis. The knee, shoulder, wrist, hip, and ankle provide most of the inflammatory processes that require medical intervention.

Normal amounts of fluid available from the various body sites largely vary with the size of the joint. The ranges may be from 0.1 to 2.0 mL and may be symptomatic of disease in more than one site or for more than one type of arthritis. Since there is minimal fluid from most anatomic sites containing synovial fluid, a "*dry tap*" where no fluid is aspirated is common, unless the synovial fluid is accompanied by an effusion. An effusion occurs when there is increased production of fluid resulting from trauma. Effusions also occur when blood accumulates in a joint following surgery or from a disease where the ability of the blood to coagulate is impacted, as in *hemophilia* or *anticoagulation therapy*, causing an increase in fluid volume.

Fig. 14.3 Aspiration of
fluid from a synovial joint

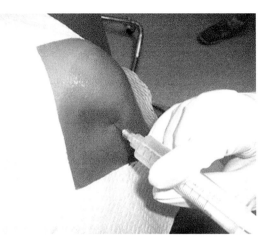

When an effusion has occurred, there may be as much as 20 mL or more of fluid
that can be aspirated for testing. During some procedures a small amount of fluid
will be found in the needle used for the puncture of the joint, even when no fluid is
found in the syringe attached to the needle. It is possible to perform some of the
tests from this small amount, such as a Gram stain for bacteria, and a culture of the
fluid for determining the species of bacteria if any is present.

The fluid is collected using a sterile needle and syringe by a process called
arthrocentesis (Fig. 14.3), which literally means "puncture of the joint." Again, the
practice of Standard Precautions is to be followed to prevent transfer of infectious
organisms during the collection of fluid. In a manner akin to that of collecting and
transporting cerebrospinal fluid, the fluid is divided into three tubes if the volume is
sufficient. A sterile tube is used for microbiological tests, and if possible, a 5 or
more mL sample is placed in this tube.

For the determination of the presence of blood cells and crystals, 5 mL of an
anticoagulant to prevent clotting and clumping of any cells in the fluid is placed into
a tube containing *sodium heparin,* the anticoagulant most commonly used for this
procedure. The heparin solution prevents clotting by interfering with the coagulation factors that may be present in the fluid. The cell count can then be more easily
performed and serves to preserve the cellular morphology of both white and red
blood cells that may be present in the fluid.

Other anticoagulants such as oxalates and powdered EDTA, as well as *lithium
heparin,* are sometimes used but may result in crystallization of the additives. When
this phenomenon occurs, it could potentially give confusing information that may
be interpreted as the presence of crystals that are contributing to an inflammatory
process. The aspirate from only small volumes of synovial fluid in the anticoagulants could artificially increase the potential for crystal formation, since the concentration of additives would be greater in the relatively smaller volume of sample than
is normally collected. Chemical and immunological tests require a red-topped tube
in which clotting can take place, if possible. Normal synovial fluid will not clot, but

the effusion of blood with its coagulation factors may cause a clot to occur. After centrifugation of the sample, the clear portion of fluid in which the clot occurs may be used for chemistry tests, such as for glucose.

14.3.2 Physical Appearance of Synovial Fluid

Synovial fluid under normal circumstances is clear and quite viscous (sticky) and the level of viscosity can be readily determined at the time of collection. When the fluid can be allowed to drip from the end of the needle, it will appear as a thin string that may be from 2 to 3 inches in length. If the string does not persist until it is more than 1 in. in length, the viscosity is less than normal, and most likely contains significantly low levels of hyaluronic acid. Some bacteria as well as certain chemicals formed by the body during inflammation, *acute phase reactants*, will produce certain enzymes that can break down hyaluronic acid. Therefore, if the viscosity is less than normal or is totally absent, it may be assumed that an inflammatory process is in effect.

Certain infectious diseases as well as inflammation induced by the presence of crystals may cause fibrin clots that form due to the components of blood that are present in the synovial fluid. There is some controversy over the use of anticoagulated samples for crystal identification by some authorities, so it would be advisable to have both an anticoagulated and a plain tube available for comparison when observing for crystals. Another precaution to be observed is the study of fluid that has been taken from a joint where steroids or another drug that is typically injected into the joints may have occurred.

• Infectious disease

Fluids resulting from an infectious process will generally be cloudy and may be turbid when elevated levels of white blood cells are present. Large amounts of bacteria may also cause the fluid to be milky or cloudy. The fluid may also exhibit a yellow or green color due to chemical components from an effusion of blood. The viscosity of the fluid will be decreased due to the previously mentioned production of enzymes and acute phase reactants that occur following an acute infection. Organisms that are common causes of infectious arthritis are those of the various species of *streptococcal* and *staphylococcal* bacteria. A well-known sexually-transmitted disease (STD) called *Neisseria gonorrhea* is also sometimes implicated in complicated cases preceded by untreated infectious diseases of the joints. Several bacterial species of the genus *Haemophilus* along with a considerable number of fungi and anaerobic bacteria are also capable of causing infectious arthritis.

There is a considerable number of less commonly encountered bacterial infections leading to infectious arthritis. Tuberculosis, a disease caused by a microorganism called *mycobacterium*, is a serious and consistently found organism in inflammatory processes of the body. There is a distinct correlation between the age of onset and the type of organism isolated from the samples of fluid. Other bacteria that may also be implicated in some infectious diseases of the synovial joints include *Chlamydia trachomatis*, a common sexually-transmitted disease. In addition to those previously named, the genera *Salmonella, Yersinia, Shigella*, and *Campylobacter* are other genera of bacterial organisms that chiefly affect the gastrointestinal system but may be implicated in symptoms related to infectious joint disease.

Most infectious diseases of the synovial joints are bacterial in nature. But increasing evidence has led to the determination that a considerable number of viruses also contribute to arthritis and *arthralgia* (painful synovial joints). *Parvovirus* infection is another somewhat common affliction that affects mostly young children and is manifested by a rash and anemia but seldom leads to chronic rheumatoid arthritis. The condition is by determining the presence of the organism through tests for DNA found in early cases demonstrating synovitis, which is a term referring to inflammation of the synovial membranes. Systemic lupus erythematosus (SLE) and parvovirus infection are quite similar and in some cases patients with SLE may also exhibit parvovirus antibodies.

The *Epstein-Barr virus* (EBV) chiefly known for producing most of the cases of infectious mononucleosis has been found to be a complicating agent for some of those with rheumatoid arthritis, aggravating the condition. *Cytomegalovirus, Herpes simplex* virus, and the *Varicella zoster* virus may also be present in the synovial fluids of patients with patients suffering from chicken pox. Even patients with HIV infections may have an increased frequency of joint symptoms. But antiviral therapy for HIV-infected individuals has led to improvement of pain associated with the musculoskeletal system of these persons.

- Non-inflammatory origin

Non-inflammatory conditions will usually yield a synovial fluid that is clear and normally viscous, since few white blood cells are present in these types of conditions. If a phase microscope is used, there may be fragments of cartilage and fibrils of *collagen*, a connective tissue, even when the specimen appears to be normal fluid. Degenerative conditions such as *osteoarthritis*, or when arthritis is caused by a traumatic injury, are examples of non-inflammatory conditions where synovial fluid may accumulate and can be collected. In those who are considered middle-aged or older, the non-inflammatory types of arthritis are found in large segments of the population.

- Inflammatory disease

Inflammatory types of disease will usually provide a synovial fluid specimen that is accompanied by an effusion that is caused by several diseases resulting from an immunological disorder. Well known contributors to this type of disorder are those of lupus erythematosus and *rheumatoid arthritis*. The synovial fluid from those with these disorders is usually of low viscosity and is accompanied by a cloudy and yellow appearance. The leukocyte count is usually only moderately elevated and fibrin clots may be found in the fluid.

• Crystal influenced disease

The most common disease where the synovial fluid provides clinical evidence of disease is that of *gouty arthritis*. True gout is known as *urate gout*, where uric acid crystals are found in the synovial fluid, and *pseudogout* may reveal *pyrophosphate* crystals in the synovial fluid. The fluid may be yellow and turbid and will often contain an elevated numerical level of white blood cells. Urate gout will cause acute bouts of the disease periodically and is genetically induced in conditions where high levels of uric acid are found in the blood. The crystal implicated in this type of gout is called *monosodium urate* or MSU.

Pseudogout frequently but not always reveals the presence of calcium pyrophosphate dihydrate in the fluid of those suffering from this condition. Crystal identification is accomplished by observing the morphology of these crystals microscopically using polarized light for the best results. Besides uric acid and calcium pyrophosphate crystals, cholesterol crystals and crystals of apatite, a major material of cartilage, may be observed.

Techniques for analyzing the chemical composition of crystals found in body fluids may include testing for certain chemical constituents, but this is rarely necessary. Microscopic analysis most frequently enables the identification of crystals of synovial fluid, of which there are a limited number, along with the patient's medical history, including current therapy. Some crystals are said to be of the cubic system are said to be isotropic, since these have consistent configurations in all directions with parallel sides. The use of polarized light utilizes a property called the refractive index. Crystals that are not included in the cubic system are said to be *anisotropic*, having two (*birefringent*) or even three refractive indices.

• Hemorrhagic fluid

Hemorrhagic fluid will contain elevated levels of red blood cells and may result from injury to the joint or to nearby bones, such as a fracture or a tumor of the bone. Effusions of blood will increase the volume of the fluid and may be a result of genetic diseases that prolong or prevent the normal clotting of blood. Persons receiving anticoagulant therapy to combat clots or to prevent certain strokes and cardiac events may also have bloody synovial fluid due to bleeding due to the treatment.

14.4   Laboratory Analysis of Synovial Fluid

Routine laboratory studies of synovial fluid include the physical properties of the fluid, microbiological studies, white blood cells count and differential, crystal identification using appropriate microscopy, and basic chemistry procedures. Normal findings are found in Table 14.1. White blood cells called mononuclear cells include lymphocytes, monocytes, *macrophages*, and synovial tissue cells are the primary cells that will be seen in normal synovial fluid. Neutrophils should account for less than 25% of the differential count. Thinly-smeared Wright stained slides are used

Table 14.1 Normal constituents of synovial fluid

Laboratory finding	Normal range of values
White blood cells count	Less than 150/mL
WBC differential neutrophils (segmented)	<25%
Lymphocytes	<75%
Monocytes	<70%
Glucose (blood level less synovial fluid level)	<10 mg/dL[a]
Protein	<10 mg/dL

[a]Blood and CSF should be roughly equivalent in absence of disease

for white blood cell differential counts and are examined microscopically to determine the percentages of the various types of white blood cells. Elevations of certain cells may indicate the presence of an infectious process by bacteria. Microscopic findings are best performed when a complete history including current diseases and medications that may have been administered is conducted.

Cellular differentiation and morphology of white blood cells and in some cases, red blood cells along with crystals that may be present comprise the most commonly performed laboratory observations of the synovial fluid sample. It is well understood that a variety of conditions may contribute to disorders of the articular joints where synovial fluid is the body fluid of choice for the diagnosis of a specific disease process that is occurring. It will be remembered from a previous section of this chapter that a disease revealed by the examination of synovial fluid may be either inflammatory or non-inflammatory and may be either hemorrhagic or crystal-induced. Overlap of symptoms, signs, and clinical data from laboratory procedures may present a challenge when attempting to achieve a definitive diagnosis. Patients are usually spurred to seek medical attention due to pain or loss of range of motion of sometimes one or even several joints. The normal ranges (Table 14.1) for cell counts and common chemistry tests routinely performed on synovial fluid follows.

14.5 Routine Laboratory Tests Performed on Synovial Fluid

In addition to microscopic cell counts and WBC differentiation, other laboratory, other tests for diagnosis of synovial joint disorders may be necessary. The presence of white blood cells in synovial fluid is more diagnostic than those of red blood cells, since bleeding may have occurred from a traumatic injury as well as having occurred from the puncture itself. It is important to prevent distortion and damage to the cells that may be present in the fluid, so smears for staining and microscopic examination must be prepared within 1 h of collection using the process called arthrocentesis, a term presented earlier. The smears will be stained using a fixative which will preserve the morphology of the cells. When a sample is extremely viscous and resists spreading onto a microscope slide, it may be necessary to add a substance called hyaluronidase, which is an enzyme that leads to the breakdown of

Table 14.2 Routine chemical tests for synovial fluid

Laboratory analysis	Interpretation of laboratory test results
Glucose	Glucose is most often slightly lower than that found in blood plasma. But in cases of joint infection and other types of inflammation, the glucose levels may be significantly lower than glucose values found in the blood due to the presence of bacteria, which may utilize available glucose
Protein	Protein levels will be increased when bacterial infections are present, and perhaps reduced in cases of viral infection
Lactate dehydrogenase	Levels of LD will be increased in those suffering from rheumatoid arthritis, infectious arthritis, or gout
Uric acid	Uric acid levels in both the blood plasma and synovial fluid are normally increased with a type of arthritis called gout

hyaluronic acid found in the synovial fluid. This substance is also commonly known as the *spreading factor.*

In addition to the determination of numbers of cells and any bacterial agents that may be present, it may also be necessary to perform chemical examinations on synovial fluid. Since synovial fluid is an ultrafiltrate of blood plasma plus hyaluronic acid, synovial fluid contains proteins that may be electrophoretically and immunologically identical to plasma proteins but should normally be found in lower levels than those of blood plasma. Routine chemical tests that may be performed on synovial fluid samples showing clinical signs of infection (Table 14.2) should include the following:

14.5.1 Crystal Analysis of Synovial Fluid

Unlike the importance of the enumeration of blood cells, the numbers of crystals will be less important as the numbers may not reflect the severity of the condition. The specific microscopic identification of crystals is important in the treatment of and prevention of future episodes of crystal-induced arthritides. As previously described, a considerable variety of crystals may be seen in synovial fluid and are identified chiefly by their respective morphological characteristics. The mechanism by which crystals are deposited in the synovial joints is not clearly understood but individual characteristics, including family genetics, the aging process and degenerative changes of the joints are all implicated.

Careful and accurate microscopic observation of crystals is the chief techniques for identifying crystals. If possible, a *phase contrast microscope* should be used to identify crystals (Table 14.3). Other examples of exogenous crystals and artifacts are those of powder from gloves worn by the practitioner performing the arthrocentesis. These granules may be introduced into the synovial cavity when the puncture site is contaminated by the powder when samples are collected, or during the administration of steroids into the cavity as therapy for reducing inflammation. Some individuals may live with deposited crystals for years before signs and symptoms appear. Sometimes, underlying diseases such as hypothyroidism,

Table 14.3 Crystals commonly found in synovial fluid

Crystal(s)	Medical condition	Description
Calcium Pyrophosphate Dihydrate (CCPD)	Pseudogout (pyrophosphate) gout; also called CPPD or deposition disease; also seen in those with degenerative arthritis	Rhomboid parallelogram in which adjacent sides are of unequal lengths and angles are not 90° (oblique)
Cholesterol crystals	Patients with long-standing arthritis; rarely seen	Flat, clear, rhombic, but with one corner neatly "punched out"
Hydroxyapatite	Apatitic gout	Crystal deposits, extremely small and barely visible with brightfield microscopy; will not show polarization (other crystals do)
Lipid crystals	Acute arthritic conditions	Maltese cross design seen with use of polarized light
Monosodium urate (MSU)	Predominantly found in acute urate gout	Structures are needle-shaped and may be found intracellularly and/ or extracellularly; sometimes confused with crystalline steroid medication
Miscellaneous crystals and artifacts	May accompany a variety of medical conditions affecting the joints	Calcium oxalate, collagen fibrils, metallic fragments arising from prosthetic joints, corticosteroids
Calcium oxalate, collagen fibrils, metallic fragments from prosthetic joints, corticosteroids	Calcium oxalate, collagen fibrils, metallic fragments from prosthetic joints, corticosteroids	Calcium oxalate, collagen fibrils, metallic fragments from prosthetic joints, corticosteroids

hyperparathyroidism and hemochromatosis are present, leading to the deposit of *calcium pyrophosphate dihydrate* crystals. The *parathyroid glands* produce parathormone (PTH) that leads to hypercalcemia described as increased levels of calcium in the blood. This may explain the presence of calcium pyrophosphate dihydrate crystals in the synovial fluid of those suffering from hyperparathryroidism, since the fluid is an ultrafiltrate of the blood plasma.

The procedure for identifying the crystals presented in Table 14.3 are among the most common crystals found in synovial fluid. In many cases these crystals are of very little clinical interest unless pain, inflammation and perhaps swelling occur.

Procedure 14.1: Crystal Identification

1. A drop of unclotted synovial fluid is placed on a glass slide, and is covered by a cover glass. Clotted specimens must be treated chemically to provide a specimen that is spread thinly enough on the slide to allow a thorough microscopic evaluation
2. It may be necessary to seal the cover glass to prevent evaporation. Clear nail polish may be used to accomplish this. A wait of 10–15 min will be

necessary for complete drying of the polish, to prevent the microscope objective from contacting the polish. A phase contrast microscope is most advantageous in determining the presence of and identification of crystals

3. Following the settling of the cells and the cover glass, place the slide on the stage of a microscope. A phase contrast microscope is best suited for this purpose, as a widely used method that reveals differences in that shows differences in the refractive index. The refractive index utilizes the different velocities of light to distinctly show the various morphological characteristics of crystals by providing significant differences in contrast

4. When a brightfield microscope is used, the crystals should be viewed at a reduced light level, and if possible, should be further evaluated by phase contrast microscopy. For the method of reducing the light level, the iris diaphragm is in a closed position and the condenser is lowered only slightly to increase the contrast of the target crystal. Do not lower the level of the light source to enable a reduction of the light level passing through the specimen

5. Insure thorough cleaning of the slides and cover glasses using alcohol before drying them by using lens paper to avoid fibrous particles that may appear as artifacts upon subsequent use. It should be noted that artifacts ordinarily have blurred and indistinct edges whereas crystals should have distinct and well-defined edges

14.5.2 Synovial Fluid Cell Count

In preparation for a synovial fluid cell count, patients suspected of having a bacterial infection of the synovial membranes and those with crystal-induced synovitis should have a microscopic count, and bacterial infections must be ruled out as the cause of the illness. An increase in white cells will indicate the need for Gram stain and bacterial culture and antibiotic sensitivity as appropriate. Repeat aspiration and analysis of synovial fluid may be necessary to monitor the response of septic arthritis to treatment in the diagnosis of conditions such as gout, where the initial aspirate does not reveal microscopic crystals. Any joint, bursa, or tendon swelling must be evaluated as to an inflammatory or non-inflammatory condition.

When the body fluid that requires a blood cell count is blood, dilute acetic acid is used as the diluting fluid. But for synovial fluid, acetic acid will cause clotting due to the mucin content of the fluid. If necessary due to an elevated count, an isotonic solution of saline (salt solution) is used with a small amount of *methylene blue* to enhance the structures of the cells. Undiluted synovial fluid, or if necessary, suitably diluted fluid, will be mounted in the hemocytometer as is the procedure for cerebrospinal fluid. Both red and white blood cells may be counted simultaneously but might be difficult for the inexperienced microscopist.

When the cell count is below 200/µL, and fewer that 25% of the cells are polymorphonuclear (segmented neutrophils), and no red cells are observed, the count is considered normal. Monocytes, lymphocytes and macrophages are normally seen in small numbers in the absence of a disease process. A low white cell count with mostly mononuclear cells may indicate a non-inflammatory condition, but an elevated white blood cell count indicates inflammation. When the percentage of polymorphonuclear cells that are observed is extremely high, the condition will be predominantly an infectious one, and most likely will be of a bacterial nature.

Procedure 14.2: White Blood Cell Count, Synovial Fluid

1. When the sample does not require a dilution due to an elevated count, a Pasteur pipette rinsed with normal saline/methylene blue stain may be used to accentuate nuclear morphology
2. After mixing the synovial fluid sample carefully by twirling and inverting the tube containing the specimen, carefully tilt the tube containing the fluid sample if necessary and place the tip of the pipette into the solution. Tilting the pipette enables sample to flow by capillary action into the pipette. Allow the pipette to fill at least half its length, then place a gloved finger over the large end of the pipette to prevent the sample from spilling from the open end
3. Insure complete mixing of the sample by holding the partially-filled pipette in a horizontal position and carefully tilting and turning the pipette to achieve consistent distribution of the cellular components of the fluid
4. Carefully deliver a small amount of synovial fluid under the cover glass on both sides of the hemocytometer slide. If a V-shaped depression is present, this step is much simpler
5. Prepare a petri dish with humidity to prevent evaporation by placing a slightly damp piece of filter paper in the bottom of the dish, before placing the hemocytometer on the paper. Allow several minutes for the slide to equilibrate to the correct level
6. Use the low-power objective (10×) to quickly scan both gridded sides of the hemocytometer to determine the presence of any white blood cells and to insure consistency of the solution. If clumps of cells are observed, the procedure must be repeated, insuring that no inconsistently heavy areas of concentration are present. Each major square of the slide should have a roughly equal distribution of white cells on both sides of the slide
7. While still using the 10× objective, count the white blood cells using a manual hand-held "clicker" or manual counter in the four corner squares and the larger center square on each of the two sides of the slide. The four corner squares and the entire center square are the most closely gridded areas are to be counted
8. Using the 40× objective, the WBCs can be tentatively classified as either mononuclear or polymorphonuclear, but a stained smear will be necessary for accurate differentiation of the cells

9. When the numbers of white cells for each of the 10 squares on the 2 sides of the chamber exceed 200, fewer squares should be counted. The number of cells counted is multiplied by the dilution factor to adjust for the numbers that would have been counted in the 10 squares. For example, if 3 squares are counted on one side of the chamber and 2 are counted on the other, the numbers are then added and then multiplied by 2, for a total of 10

10. For calculating the number of white blood cells per volume of synovial fluid, 10 large squares on the two sides of the hemocytometer are counted. The calculation of the count is achieved by multiplying the count obtained by the dilution. The volume factor is obtained by performing the following function

11. Upon completion of the procedure, the hemocytometer should be disinfected by using a 10% solution of bleach or a commercial disinfectant by soaking the instrument in the solution for at least 5 min. The slide should then be rinsed with deionized or distilled water or with 70% alcohol and then dried using lens paper

Note: Calculations of the result from the raw count requires the following steps

---

Box 14.1 Manual White Blood Cell Count Calculation

Volume factor = 1 μL (10 mm^2 × 0.1 mm) = 1

Total cells counted × dilution factor (if applicable) × volume factor = cells per μL (mm^3)

When 10 squares are counted, a volume of one microliter (1 μL) is counted. Assuming 210 cells were counted, the results would be calculated as follows:

Calculation

210 (number of WBCs counted in 10 large squares) × volume factor = 210/μL

14.6   Summary

Synovial fluid is found in all joint cavities that lubricate joints that contact each other and cushion the movement of wo bones against each other. The fluid is designed to reduce friction that could damage the cartilage and synovial membranes that come in contact. Synovial fluid is formed as an ultrafiltrate of the plasma and contains hyaluronic acid and a small amount of protein. Hyaluronic acid differentiates synovial fluid from all other body fluids of mammals. The acid also contributes to the viscosity of the synovial fluid.

Normal synovial fluid is sterile and will contain no red and few white blood cells. The Ropes, or mucin clot test, has been performed for many years to determine the presence of normal synovial fluid. Treatment of synovial fluid with acetic acid, where synovial fluid and 5% acetic acid are combined, will normally cause the rapid formation of a solid clot in clear fluid. Poor clot formation is an indicator of an inflammatory disease. For some laboratory procedures, the presence of contaminating synovial fluid may make it more difficult to dilute and perform cell counts and enumeration of crystals because of its extreme viscosity.

A considerable number of immunological responses affect the permeability of the membranes surrounding the joint cavities and will alter the amount and quality of synovial fluid. Certain chemicals as well as trauma to joints will produce inflammation of the joints, along with infections including bacteria, viruses, fungi and other infectious agents. Since body fluids provide an effective medium capable of harboring many biohazardous materials, Standard Precautions should be observed when handling the fluids.

Inflammatory conditions require microscopic evaluation of the fluid for the presence of cells and crystals are the most common tests performed on synovial fluid. When an elevated number of polymorphonuclear white blood cells are present, a Gram stain for identification of the morphology of bacteria, and a white cell count are necessary. The presence of red blood cells may be attributed to a traumatic injury as well as the damage called by the arthrocentesis.

Non-inflammatory conditions are called degenerative diseases and occur where cartilage and supportive tissues of the joints literally disintegrate for several reasons. Non-inflammatory diseases will differ in the findings of those seen in acute inflammatory disorders of the joints. The degenerative types are for the most part chronic or long-standing, with no available cure. But inflammatory disorders are known as acute conditions that may at least be alleviated. In non-inflammatory conditions, the white blood cell count will be normal for synovial fluid but elevated in inflammatory disease.

Specimens are collected by a process called arthrocentesis where a sterile needle is used to aspirate from 0.1 to 2.0 mL of synovial fluid. Where there is an effusion of blood the volume of available fluid will be greatly increased, causing swelling. Minimal fluid is found in most anatomic sites for synovial fluid, so a "dry tap" where no fluid is aspirated is common. Even when small amounts of fluid are available, tests that are possible for small amounts such as the Gram stain should be accomplished. A sterile tube is used for microbiological tests and for blood cell counts and identification of crystals. The specimen is placed into a tube containing sodium heparin, an anticoagulant to prevent clotting that would interfere with cell counts.

Synovial fluid should be clear and quite viscous (sticky) for normal individuals. Some infectious diseases as well as inflammation induced by the presence of crystals may cause fibrin clots to form since some of the components of blood that are present in the synovial fluid. Samples from patients with an infectious process will generally be cloudy and may be turbid when elevated levels of white blood cells are present. Large amounts of bacteria may also cause the fluid to be milky or cloudy.

Effusions of blood may lead to development of a yellow or green color. Viscosity will be decreased when enzymes and acute phase reactants occur during acute infection. In addition to infectious, inflammatory processes are those with a non-inflammatory origin. Synovial fluid will be clear and normally viscous, and in some of these conditions, few white blood cells are present but may yield fragments of cartilage and fibrils of collagen, a connective tissue.

Crystal influenced diseases include the common condition of gout, where monosodium urate (uric acid) crystals are found and in pseudogout, where calcium pyrophosphate crystals prevail. Crystal identification is made by observing the morphology of these crystals microscopically using polarized light for the best results. Besides uric acid and calcium pyrophosphate crystals, cholesterol crystals and crystals of apatite, a major material of cartilage, may be viewed.

Routine laboratory studies of synovial fluid include the physical properties of the fluid, microbiological studies, white blood cells count and differential, crystal identification using appropriate microscopy, and basic chemistry procedures. Cellular differentiation and morphology of white blood cells and in some cases, red blood cells along with crystals that may be present comprise the most commonly performed laboratory observations of the synovial fluid sample. Glucose values are most often slightly lower than that found in the blood plasma. But in cases of joint infection and inflammation, the glucose levels may be significantly lower than those found in the blood levels due to bacterial utilization. Protein levels will be increased when bacterial infections are present.

Case #14.1

A middle-aged man has had a previous bout of similar symptoms and now suffers from a swollen great toe of the right foot. During the next episode a year later, the knee becomes swollen and red, with excruciating pain and an inability to walk. His blood chemistry tests reveal a high uric acid level. Synovial fluid is aspirated from the knee and is sent to the laboratory for evaluation. The physician must decide if there is an association between the presence of an elevated uric acid level in the blood and the presence of an infection of the joint of the knee. The physician notes that instead of a viscous and clear solution, the fluid is watery and somewhat cloudy. The cloudy condition could be attributed both to the complications of infection or to the crystals that produce similar symptoms and signs, so further fluid analysis is warranted. The fluid is sent to the laboratory for microbiological studies including a Gram stain and culture, cell counts and leukocyte differentiation, and microscopic examination for crystals.

Gross Fluid Examination

The fluid is watery and not viscous, as the lubricating fluid of the knee joint would ordinarily be. In addition, it is considerably cloudy.

Microscopic Examination

Gram Stain: Cytofuged sample reveals no organisms and is reported as a sterile culture after a 48-h incubation.

White blood cell count: $0.12 \times 10^9/L$.

Reference values:

WBCs $0.15 \times 10^9/L$ and more than 25% neutrophils.

Total leukocytes: $4.00\text{--}11.0 \times 10\ ^9/L$.

Neutrophils: $2.5\text{--}7.5 \times 10\ ^9/L$.

Lymphocytes: $1.5\text{--}3.5 \times 10\ ^9/L$.

Monocytes: $0.2\text{--}0.8 \times 10\ ^9/L$.

Eosinophils: $0.04\text{--}0.4 \times 10\ ^9/L$.

Leukocyte differential: 71% lymphocytes and 17% neutrophils; the remainder of the cells include 1% eosinophils and 11% monocytes.

Crystal Identification: Needle-shaped crystals of a yellowish hue, morphologically suggestive of monosodium urate (MSU) crystals seen in urate gout

1. What is the name for this accumulation of fluid in a major joint?
2. How are acute infectious processes causing bacterial arthritis ruled out?
3. To what can the turbidity of the sample be attributed?
4. What is the condition most likely diagnosed?

Review Questions

1. Synovial fluid is collect by a procedure called:
   a. Lumbar puncture
   b. Phlebotomy
   c. Arthrocentesis
   d. Arteriocentesis
2. When red blood cells are found in synovial fluid, they are usually the result of:
   a. Traumatic injury
   b. Acute infection
   c. Traumatic joint fluid tap
   d. a & c
3. An effusion into the synovial cavity will:
   a. Have no effect
   b. Increase volume of fluid
   c. Decrease volume of fluid
   d. Indicate bacterial infection
4. Crystals are best observed by:
   a. Utilizing macroscopic methods
   b. Using a brightfield microscope
   c. Employing phase contrast technique
   d. Chemistry tests for properties
5. Synovial fluid will normally have:
   a. Many white blood cells
   b. Many red blood cells
   c. No red blood cells
   d. High glucose level

6. Needle-like crystals that are yellow and are characteristic of acute gouty arthritis are:
   a. Corticosteroid
   b. Leucine
   c. Monosodium urate
   d. Hydroxyapatite
7. The viscosity of synovial fluid is due to:
   a. Hyaluronic acid
   b. Protein in the fluid
   c. Bacterial infection
   d. Cartilage debris

Answers Found in Appendix C

Fecal Analysis

15

Objectives

Describe the importance of fecal examinations as compared with the importance of other body fluids

List at least two qualitative and two quantitative laboratory procedures that are performed on fecal specimens

Discuss the meaning of the term "malabsorption" as it relates to the gastrointestinal system

Explain how the inability to digest or absorb certain dietary nutrients may be manifested in the feces

Name the departments of the clinical laboratory where various procedures on fecal samples are normally performed

Provide the reason for observing Standard Precautions when handling fecal samples

Discuss the reasons for not performing quantitative red and white blood cell counts on feces

List the five basic colors found in fecal samples and reasons leading to a variety of colors found in fecal samples

List the four sugars (reducing substances) that are determined by the use of the Clinitest tablets

Discuss the need for performing an occult blood determination on a grossly bloody fecal sample

15.1 Introduction to the Testing of Fecal (Stool) Samples

In the minds of most laboratory personnel, analysis of fecal specimens fits into the category of a "necessary evil" and few enjoy such tasks. However, as the end product of metabolism in the human body, feces do provide valuable diagnostic

© Springer International Publishing AG, part of Springer Nature 2018
J. W. Ridley, *Fundamentals of the Study of Urine and Body Fluids*,
https://doi.org/10.1007/978-3-319-78417-5_15

information. Fecal samples normally contain extreme numbers of bacterial organisms and materials from the diet that may be difficult to rule out as the cause for a disorder involving the gastrointestinal tract. Studies of stool samples, while not considered strictly as a body fluid, nevertheless have similarities to fluids derived from cavities of the body. Fecal samples are often tested for fats, reducing substances that are sugars other than glucose, blood cells, and the presence of both normal and pathological bacteria. It is known that there are thousands of species of bacteria in the human gut, some of which have not been named to date. Many of the examinations performed on stool samples fall into the province of microbiology, where bacteriological and parasitological procedures are performed, but a number of tests performed on fecal samples may not even be performed in the microbiology department of a clinical laboratory.

Routine fecal examination includes macroscopic, microscopic, and chemical analyses for the early detection of gastrointestinal bleeding and liver and related biliary duct disorders, along with malabsorption syndromes. Of equal diagnostic value is the detection and identification of pathogenic bacteria and parasites. These microbial procedures are beyond the realm of this text and are best covered in a microbiology/parasitology department for the culture and isolation of bacteria to determine pathogenicity. Also, identification of parasitic organisms will not be discussed in this text. This chapter will involve studies of the secretion of digestive juices and the absorption and reabsorption of certain constituents of the gastrointestinal system and will be addressed as pertinent to body fluids analysis.

The majority of these tests may or may not be performed in the microbiology department, depending upon the complexity of the departmental organization. Most often, fecal studies are considered more applicable to the analysis of body fluids. The physiology of the gastrointestinal system includes various common activities similar to those organs associated with body cavities where the gastric organs play a role in fluid balance and reabsorption in the large intestine. As a way to determine diseases associated with the gastrointestinal (GI) system and the impact of diseases of other parts of the body on the GI system, diagnostic procedures are similar to those for other body fluids.

The normal fecal specimen with bacteria, cellulose and other undigested foodstuffs, bile pigments, gastrointestinal secretions, cells from the intestinal walls, electrolytes, and water sometimes obfuscate the medical technologist's efforts to examine a specimen extensively. Many species of bacteria make up the normal flora of the intestines that contribute to the digestive process as well as the body's recognition of certain organisms as being normal. Recent approaches to normal flora reveal that perhaps the body's development of an effective immune system is based on normal gut flora, thus the drive toward using probiotics for a healthy existence. The strong odor associated with feces may be attributed in great part to the metabolic actions of bacteria as they break down materials in the gut and give off metabolic byproducts as the result of their life cycle.

15.2   Infection Control

No specific dangers are associated with the handling of fecal samples, although organisms found normally in stool samples are capable of contaminating hands and foodstuffs, resulting in an infection of organisms broadly called *coliforms*. Decades ago, it was recognized that polio, or poliomyelitis that resulted in lifelong paralysis, was an intestinal virus excreted in feces. Therefore, washing of the hands became a passion at that time. Although polio is rarely diagnosed today, lack of effective handwashing is still a way to unwittingly become infected by a host of organisms. Today, fecal contaminants may give rise to diseases such as salmonellosis and cholera among many others. So as with the body fluids, Standard Precautions should be observed when transporting, handling, testing and disposing of the biological material. Equipment used to collect the fluid need only to be clean and should be placed in a carrying container impervious to liquids and with a tight lid to avoid leakage of watery samples.

15.3   Routine Tests Ordered for Stool Samples

Routine fecal screening tests include macroscopic observation of the color and consistency; microscopic examination for white blood cells, muscle fibers, and fecal fat. Often problems with digestion will leave large portions of undigested food materials that are readily visible macroscopically. Qualitative chemical tests for blood, microscopic examinations for the presence of white and red blood cells, and quantitative tests for digestive enzymes are routinely performed for chemical components related to digestion. Again, it is possible to discover parasites in the course of analyzing a fecal specimen. The specimen should then be referred to the lab section performing microbiological and/or parasitological procedures.

15.3.1 Specimen Collection for Stool Samples

Stool samples are collected in clean containers as stated earlier and are not required to be sterile as would most body fluids, since fecal specimens contain many strains of normally occurring organisms. It is necessary to provide clear directions to the patient or caretaker when collecting a stool sample. Clean, dry, sealable and leak-proof containers are available from laboratory supply firms to ensure proper collection and safe transport and handling by the patient and the medical staff. Patients should be made aware that samples should not be contaminated with water or with urine. Contamination by strong cleaners used in bathrooms may also adversely affect a lab's ability to recover pathogenic organisms from the sample. In addition, some tests require certain dietary regimens prior to collection, and when barium sulfate or enemas have been introduced into the bowel for radiological purposes, these specimens may provide invalid results.

15.3.2 Physical Appearance of Stool Samples

The feces of humans is of course the waste products remaining following digestion of nutrients from food, but a large percentage of the bulk of the stool is due to normal bacterial content of the sample. A stool sample's appearance is largely due to the presence of disease as well as the diet of the individual and the health status of the patient. A normal stool is light to moderately brown in color when a normal diet is established and is semisolid with a mucus coating to ease the passage of the material from the body. Normal color is imparted to stools by a combination of *bilirubin* and bile, both of which are derived from red blood cells. Small pieces of harder, less moist feces may be observed in dehydrated patients, since most of the water contained in the stool would have been absorbed by the large intestine. There are several terms in general use that are associated with various types of stool, based on the appearance or consistency of the samples.

When a patient is constipated, the samples may appear as separate hard lumps called syllabi that are hard to pass and generally reflect a condition where little moisture is contained in them. Less severe cases of constipation will reveal sausage-like stools that are lumpy in appearance. The most "normal" stools will appear as link sausages with cracks on the surface or will appear smooth and soft. Conditions of diarrhea will most often be visible as soft blobs with clear cut edges that are easily passed. In the most extreme cases, the stools will be almost all liquid, and might somewhat resemble rice water, with visible mucus. Color variations of feces are significant in humans, depending upon diet and health. Some general coloration of feces is associated with certain medical conditions, such as an infestation by the parasite *Giardia lamblia*. A characteristic yellow coloring of feces may be attributed to a common parasitic infection by an organism called *Giardia lamblia* (Fig. 15.1). *G. lamblia* is now also known variously as *G. intestinalis* or *G. duodenalis*. *Giardiasis* is frequently associated with a severe and easily transmitted type of diarrhea.

A range of colors may be present due to hemolysis. The stage of the illness that ranges from long-standing conditions such as that of melena, the excretion of dark or black stools from fecal blood to bright red blood. Bleeding of the lower gastrointestinal tract results in bright red blood often covering the exterior of the feces. Those of the upper GI tract have gone through digestion and combination with foods and the color may be darker or mahogany colored. The darker colors are related to oxidation of heme originating in hemoglobin of red cells combined with fecal matter. Other colors are described in this section relative to materials causing coloration.

15.3.2.1   Yellow

Jaundice is a condition where the stool and the color of the skin may show an obvious yellow hue. A certain category of conditions may cause yellowing of the skin, but a commonly occurring condition is that of Gilbert's Syndrome, a medical disorder that affects up to 3% of the population. The yellowing of the stool is due to a condition called hyperbilirubinemia, where an elevated level of bilirubin is present

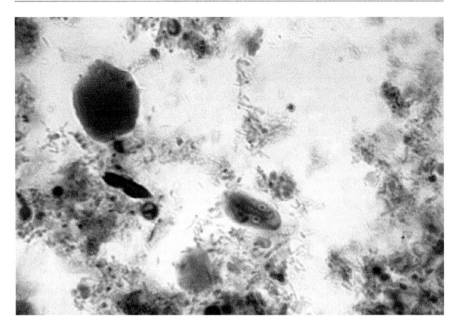

Fig. 15.1 Image of stained *G. lamblia (intestinalis)* parasite

in the blood. Hyperbilirubinemia is also associated with changes in urine color as well as of the stool, and is traced to a number of conditions related to the destruction of red blood cells, liver disease, and obstruction of the bile duct (Table 15.1).

15.3.2.2   Black

Feces appearing as a black-colored specimen may be due to the presence of red blood cells that have been lysed (destroyed) in the process of digestion that requires a period of time to occur. The term used for black stools is that of *melena* and is usually due to active in the upper area of the digestive tract, including peptic ulcers which may cause heavy bleeding. Black stools may also be seen after consuming foods that contain a substantial proportion of animal blood, and may be initially misleading, but are harmless. This black color that may be attributed to the presence of blood is caused by oxidation of the iron found in the hemoglobin of animals.

Certain prescription medications are also known to cause discolorations of the stool, including some purchased over the counter (OTC). Those requiring a prescription may be due to a bismuth preparation (Pepto-Bismol) as well as the taking of iron supplements. A number of persons may be misled by "iron poor blood" advertisements and the result is black stools, but only a very small fraction of persons in the developed countries suffer from this malady. Some foods, including vegetables and fruits such as the common beet and blueberries, along with black licorice are also capable of imparting a black color to the stool sample. The occult (guiac) reaction for blood will be positive for true bleeding, and not from dietary interfering substances.

Table 15.1 Interpretation of jaundice affecting stool and urine color

Origin of bilirubin	Clinical condition	Free, unconjugated bilirubin (bilirubinemia)	Conjugated bilirubin (bilirubinuria)	Urobilinogen (conversion of bilirubin)	Color imparted to feces
Obstruction	Cancer of bile duct; stones of gall bladder	0.1–1.5 mg/dL (normal)	Increased	Decreased or absent	White, chalky appearance
RBC hemolysis	PCH (paroxysmal cold hemoglobinuria), HDN (hemolytic disease of the newborn), ABO incompatibilities	>1.5 mg/dL	None	Increased	Dark brown
Hepatic (liver)	All types of hepatitis (infectious and chemical)	Increased	Increased	Varies from increased to absence	Normal light brown or pale

15.3.2.3 Red

The passage of fresh, bright red blood in the stools, where the cells have not remained in the intestine for a sufficient period of to be destroyed, is called *hematochezia*. This type bleeding may be form any part of the digestive tract and is quickly passed before color change occurs. Alcoholism is also a common contributor to the passing of red blood cells in the stool.

15.3.2.4 Blue

Dye treatment with Prussian blue, which will stain any iron pigments a dark blue color, may occur for treatment for poisoning by radiation and certain metals. If large amounts of sugary desserts and blue colored drinks are consumed, a stool specimen may also appear blue in color.

15.3.2.5 Whitish or Silver

A pewter grey or a tarnished silver color, sometimes described as being an aluminum color, may result from obstruction of the *common bile duct*, where little or no bilirubin is able to enter the intestine before being converted to urobilinogen by bacterial action.

15.4 Laboratory Analysis of Stool Samples

Routine laboratory studies of stool specimens include physical properties of the sample, as described by color and consistency. The quantitative number of white and red blood cells, or of white cell differentiation, although significant in other body fluids, are not of medical importance for stool specimens. Stained microbiological specimens are inconclusive, unlike in the other body fluids, except in an absence of white cells or where extremely high numbers of white blood cells exist, which would indicate a non-specific condition. There are literally thousands of species of bacteria inhabiting the human gut, and in the absence of specific bacterial morphology, it would be impossible to predict with any modicum of accuracy the presence of pathogens from a stained smear of fecal material.

15.5 Routine Laboratory Tests Performed on Stool Samples

Screening tests are often performed to determine if more specific tests are required for the diagnosis of a specific disease condition. Negative screening tests may rule out certain conditions, where absence of signs and symptoms require no further testing of the patient.

15.5.1 Occult Blood

The test for blood in the stool sample, which is often not visible macroscopically, is by far the most frequently performed fecal analysis. The tests for blood detect components of blood, and the chemical reaction used may indicate presence as "occult" or hidden in many cases. When the test for blood yields a positive result in a chemical screening test, the results must be confirmed. As discussed earlier, bleeding in the *upper gastrointestinal tract* may produce a black, tarry stool due to the length of time for the blood to traverse the length of the intestines. Bleeding may occur anywhere along the gastrointestinal system, and if it occurs in the *lower gastrointestinal tract* and is quickly excreted, results may be an overtly bloody stool.

It is necessary to test samples that are overtly bloody for occult blood also, as bleeding may occur in several areas of the digestive tract. However, because any bleeding in excess of 2 mL/150 g of stool is considered pathologically significant, and since no visible signs of bleeding may be present even with the presence of this amount of blood, chemical detection of "occult" blood is necessary. Originally used primarily to test suspected cases of gastrointestinal disease, the test for occult blood has become widely used as a mass screening procedure for the early detection of colorectal cancer. Positive test results may be followed by a colonoscopic exam if symptoms warrant. In testing for occult blood, the least sensitive reagent, *guiac*, is preferred for routine testing. This train of thought is contrary to most chemical testing procedures where a high level of sensitivity is preferred. Dietary considerations are important, as a number of food products will yield a positive result, in the absence of blood components.

The guiac reaction features the *pseudoperoxidase* activity of hemoglobin reacting with hydrogen peroxide to oxidize a colorless compound to a visible coloration. However, since pseudoperoxidase activity, the key to this reaction, is found in animal hemoglobin, and in the metabolism of certain bacteria of the intestines, as well

Fig. 15.2 Positive result
for occult blood screening
procedure

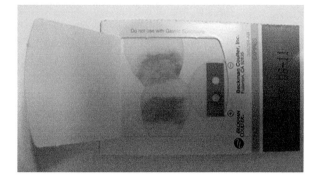

as certain vegetables, false positive results might occur. Positive results require further testing for confirming a definitive diagnosis for the presence of blood. Therefore, random samples from people with no dietary restrictions may produce fast positive reactions when tested with a reagent of great sensitivity to certain products in foods that could react with components other than blood.

The procedure is quite simple, requiring the collection of three fecal samples, one after the other, to determine bleeding at different levels of the colon. The feces sample is applied to thick paper designed for quick testing. After applying the fecal sample, one to two drops of hydrogen peroxide is applied to the reverse side of the paper from the fecal sample. Hydrogen peroxide is observed for a rapid blue color change within a few seconds (Fig. 15.2). Heme, a component of the hemoglobin molecule, catalyzes the reaction, and with no quick color change, the test is negative. Certain components of vegetables may provide a false positive result, but will occur at a slower rate than that found if heme is present.

15.5.2 White Blood Cells

Microscopic examination of the feces to determine the presence of white blood cells is performed as a preliminary procedure in determining the cause of diarrhea. When polymorphonuclear cells (neutrophils) are seen in the feces in large numbers, indications of disease affecting the intestinal wall, such as *ulcerative colitis* and infection with invasive bacterial pathogens such as *Clostridium difficile* should be suspected. Bacteria that cause diarrhea by producing of toxins rather than by invading and inflaming the walls of the intestines, viral infections, and intestinal parasites often reveal do not yield neutrophils in the feces. For this reason, presence or absence of white blood cells (neutrophils) in the feces can provide the physician with diagnostic sufficient information to initiate treatment prior to further testing for a bacterial pathogen. Only three or four neutrophils per high-power field may indicate of some sort of invasion affecting the intestines.

Specimens examined as wet preparations that are stained with methylene blue or dried smears may be stained with Gram stain or Wright's stains, enabling the differentiation of white blood cells.

15.5.3 Qualitative and Quantitative Fecal Fats

Steatorrhea refers is a condition where excess fecal fat is found in the stool specimen, and may be the result of pancreatic or intestinal disorders. Causes of this condition is often elusive, and may require a great deal of diagnostic effort to determine the cause (Table 15.2). A malabsorptive syndrome is possible when a macroscopic examination reveals a pale, frothy and malodorous sample. Decreased fat absorption is a significant finding due to a variety of several differing medical conditions. A portion of these disorders include both acute and *chronic pancreatitis*, cancer of the pancreas, *cystic fibrosis*, *cholelithiasis*, and *celiac disease*. Other serous conditions include biliary cancer obstructing the common bile duct as well as *Crohn's Disease* and *Whipple's Disease*, all of which are characterized by abnormal fat absorption in the gastrointestinal system. The presence of reduced fat absorption in the feces fat is not definitive in providing a specific diagnosis of any of these conditions where decreased fat absorption occurs. The procedure is often used to monitor a patient's prognosis while undergoing treatment for malabsorption disorders. In general there is a correlation between the qualitative and quantitative fecal fat procedures but the quantitative procedure is required to determine unstained *phospholipids* and cholesteryl esters.

Four types of lipids are typically found in feces. These four lipids found in the microscopic examination of feces are called: neutral fats, which are triglycerides, cholesterol, fatty acid salts found in soaps, and fatty acids. Presence of these lipids

Table 15.2 Evaluative causes for steatorrhea

Maldigestion	Decreased levels of pancreatic enzymes
	Pancreatic malignancy
	Cystic fibrosis
	Pancreatitis
	Zollinger-Ellison syndrome
	Resection of the ileus of the intestine
	Decreased bile
	Bile duct obstruction (stones)
	Cirrhosis including bile duct
	Severe hepatitis
Malabsorption	Damage to mucosal lining of intestines
	Tropical disease of unknown origin called *sprue*
	Celiac disease where small intestine is hypersensitive to gluten
	Obstructions in lymphatic system
	Lymphoma
	Whipple's disease

can be seen microscopically when they are stained with the dyes called *Sudan III* or IV, or with Oil Red O. Sudan III is the most routinely used stain in the clinical laboratory. Neutral fats are easily stained by Sudan III and are readily visualized as large orange to red droplets, often found near the edge of cover slip (Fig. 15.3). Note that soaps do not stain directly with Sudan dyes.

When qualitative fat studies are performed, two slides should be prepared. The first slide is for the presence of neutral fats, using a suspension of stool examined by microscope for fat droplets which stain orange or red, depending on which dye is used. When *steatorrhea* suspected, and more than 60 droplets per high-power field are seen, the result is confirmed. The second prepared slide is mixed with acetic acid, then heated, releasing fatty acids through hydrolysis of soaps and neutral fats. The number and size of the droplets found on this slide are significant and may range in size from very small up to 75 μ or more. Smaller droplets are roughly the size of a red blood cell, so care must be exercised to differentiate the presence of blood cells. When drops are small, there may be as many as 100 droplets per field, but with larger drops, much fewer droplets are seen. The number of fat droplets is increased with severity of the malabsorptive disorder, and in normal specimens fewer than ten droplets of fat per high power field (HPF) will be seen.

Quantitative levels of the excretion of fat are reported in grams per day, and in the absence of disease, fewer than 6 g per day of fecal fat is excreted. When preparing the patient for a quantitative fat excretion measurement, a diet of 100 g of fat is administered per day for 6 days, followed by collection of stool samples over a period of 3 days normally. A number of fat determinations are necessary to determine the fat content of the 72-h stool sample. These quantitative tests are important in determining the cause of any malabsorptive condition. An additional test, *phospholipase A₂* has been developed to more accurately assess acute attacks of pancreatitis. Another test, *fecal elastase*, is important in testing children with cystic fibrosis for pancreatic insufficiency.

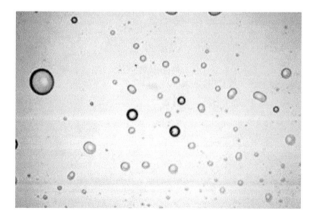

Fig. 15.3 Presence of fat bodies when stained with Sudan red

15.5.4 Muscle Fibers

Microscopic examination of feces my provide evidence of the presence of undigested striated muscle fibers, and may be helpful in diagnosing and monitoring patients with pancreatic insufficiency, particularly for patients with cystic fibrosis. Increased amounts of striated fibers can also be present in biliary obstruction and *gastrocolic fistulas*. Large numbers of meat fibers called creatorrhea (abnormal excretion of muscle fibers) often indicates a condition of impaired digestion of sluggish peristalsis and rapid evacuation of the bowel. Staining a bit of fecal metal in suspension, using a staining solution of eosin in alcohol for identification of meat fibers.

15.5.5 Trypsin

Trypsin, a *proteolytic enzyme*, is formed in the small intestine, and functions in the digestion of protein. Absence of this protein-digesting enzyme results in abdominal discomfort and malabsorption. The presence of the enzyme is screened for by placing a small amount of stool emulsified in water on a piece of x-ray paper. In the presence of trypsin, the gelatin on the x-ray paper will be digested, leaving a clear area on the film. But fecal *chymotrypsin* determinations are considered more reliable in the assessment of pancreatic function than is the absence of trypsin.

15.5.6 Carbohydrates

A positive test for reducing substances in stool samples indicates that certain sugars or carbohydrates are not being digested in the intestine. The commonly used Clinitest by Bayer Corporation, Elkhart, IN, enables differentiation of glucose from other sugars that include *lactose*, fructose, *galactose*, and pentoses. Specific tests for glucose are available to distinguish between glucose and the other reducing substances. Carbohydrate malabsorption or intolerance can also be analyzed by serum tests, but an increased concentration of carbohydrates can be determined by performing a copper reduction test on the fecal specimen. Infants will often show symptoms of intolerance to certain sugars during infancy. It is a commonly practiced action to test the feces of infants to determine the inability to metabolize a number of sugars other than glucose, particularly for that of lactose, found primarily in milk. Lactose intolerance is on the rise, it appears, among both infants and adults. An enzyme that splits lactose into glucose and galactose is called lactase, and is located on the surface of the cells lining the small intestine. Lactose intolerance is caused by reduced levels or by inactivity of lactase, preventing the lactose molecule from being split.

15.5.7 Stool Sample Cell Evaluation

Quantitative cell counts, either white or red blood cells, are not specifically indicative of the presence of or severity of a pathological condition. These procedures are not routinely performed and therefore a procedure will not be provided for cell counts in stool samples. The presence of large amounts of red or white blood cells, copious mucus, parasites, and undigested foods are the most indicative of an infectious disease or one of a malabsorptive disorder.

15.6   Summary

Some have an aversion to fecal samples, but with repetitive procedures and experience, the problem may grow less distasteful. Fecal specimens are normally tested in the microbiology laboratory for the presence of bacterial pathogens or parasites, but the growing repertoire of analytical procedures requires more specialized equipment than is found in a routine microbiology department. Several procedures are performed on feces in the chemistry department of a laboratory and some immunological or immunochemical tests are performed in specialized serological areas of the clinical laboratory.

Standard Precautions should be observed to avoid contaminating work areas and equipment that will be handled by others and should be observed in the handling of fecal samples. Both qualitative and quantitative tests are available for testing stool samples, and the handling, transport, storage and testing of samples should be accompanied by precautions to avoid becoming ill from pathogens that may be present in the sample. Certain laws and practices are required to prevent transmission of disease when specimens are sent by mail or by transport companies. Some specimens may require transport to a reference laboratory when procedures are not performed in the laboratory in which the tests are requested. In this case, specimens must be maintained in appropriate containers (Fig. 15.4) with an outside container that is impervious to liquids, with interior absorbent padding to protect handlers of the package.

The set of steps for evaluating a fecal sample is quite similar to that for the other true body fluids. Initially a physical examination is performed, which includes the color, consistency, and odor of the sample, as a macroscopic analysis for any visible abnormalities. Sometimes the sample is liquid or has strands of mucus and gross blood that is obvious as abnormal findings. Occult blood is also tested, even when the sample contains obvious blood, as one of the first chemical tests performed on the sample. Further chemical tests are performed for the presence of fats, which can be both qualitative as a stained specimen for the presence of fat bodies, and a quantitative test for total fats in a timed sample.

A microscopic exam is also performed, with an estimate of the numbers of red and white blood cells. The presence of intestinal parasites and/or their eggs may be seen on this examination. Problems with digestion and absorption of certain foods and the presence of pancreatic dysfunction will also provide clinical findings that lead to a diagnosis. For those individuals with absorptive disorders, particularly for infants who may lack certain enzymes for the digestion of sugars, a test for reducing

Fig. 15.4 Package for
transporting lab samples

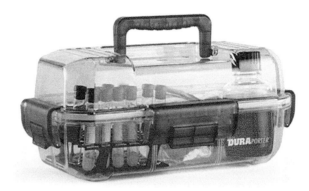

substances is performed independently of the test for glucose, the most common sugar the body uses in its metabolism.

Internet Resources
http://books.google.com/books?id=SmKGfd7DsxgC&pg=PA46&lpg=PA46&dq=f ecal+fat+bodies&source

Review Questions

1. A Gram stain of the feces is not normally important for the finding of bacteria because:
   a. Feces is usually sterile
   b. A Gram stain is for viruses only
   c. Thousands of species of bacteria are found in normal stool samples
   d. A Gram stain is for the identification of white blood cells only
2. The presence of abnormal amounts of fats in the stool is indicative of:
   a. Pancreatic disorder
   b. Diet high in fats
   c. Bacterial infection
   d. Viral infection
3. The odor given off by fecal samples is caused by:
   a. Food breakdown
   b. Viral contamination
   c. Bacterial contamination
   d. Bacterial metabolism
4. Which of the following would not be considered an abnormal condition for feces?
   a. Massive numbers of bacteria
   b. Large numbers of white blood cells
   c. Muscle fibers
   d. More than ten fat bodies/HPF

5. A large proportion of the bulk of a stool sample is accounted for by:
   a. Blood products
   b. Unmetabolized sugars
   c. Bacteria
   d. Intestinal parasites
6. The normal brown color of feces is attributed to:
   a. Mucus
   b. Undigested foods
   c. Bile
   d. Digestive cells
7. The term used for stools that are black in color is:
   a. Hematochezia
   b. Melena
   c. Jaundice
   d. Urobilinogen
8. Black, tarry stools is a sign of:
   a. Bleeding from the upper gastrointestinal tract
   b. Acute and current bleeding
   c. Foods containing blood
   d. High bilirubin levels in the blood
9. A whitish or silver color in the fecal sample is often due to:
   a. Obstructed bile duct
   b. Ingestion of bismuth
   c. Eating food from aluminum pots
   d. Increased urobilinogen in stool
10. The guiac reaction for occult blood may yield a false positive when:
    a. Peptic ulcers are bleeding
    b. The common bile duct is obstructed
    c. Large amounts of meat are eaten
    d. The patient is anemic
11. A condition called "ulcerative colitis" may result from:
    a. Active bleeding from the intestines
    b. Liver disease causing release of bilirubin
    c. Infection by *Clostridium difficile*
    d. Increase in numbers of white blood cells in stool
12. Decreased fat absorption is due to a variety of medical conditions. Which of the following would not be a cause for decreased fat absorption?
    a. Chronic pancreatitis
    b. Cystic fibrosis
    c. Acute pancreatitis
    d. Gastrocolic fistulas

13. A condition where the bile duct may be obstructed is called:
    a. Choleliathiasis
    b. Biliary cancer
    c. Celiac disease
    d. All of the previous responses
14. Sudan III is used to:
    a. Dye lipids
    b. Dye white blood cells
    c. Dye undigested muscle fibers
    d. Dye bacteria

Answers Found in Appendix C

Miscellaneous Laboratory Analyses/Gastric Fluid

16

Objectives

Provide some reasons why the study of gastric fluids differs from the other "major" fluids

Discuss the chief purpose for maintaining an acid environment in the stomach

Name an organism that can survive high acidity in the stomach

List two functions of the acid secreted in the stomach

Explain how one of the secretions of the stomach may be related to pernicious anemia

Discuss the reason for the patient to fast before undergoing a gastric analysis, and how failure to remain in a fasting state during the procedure may lead to erroneous results

16.1 Introduction to the Testing of Gastric Fluid

In addition to the "major" body fluids that were discussed in previous sections, there are several tests that are performed on a basis best described as not being "routine," but that are tested with some regularity in most medical facilities. One of these is that of studies of the bone marrow and are conducted when diseases related to the blood-making capabilities of the body require such examinations. The study of bone marrow is best reserved for a hematology course, as the sequence from juvenile cells to mature cells in their various proportions to each other is essential to a thorough understanding by the student or the laboratory professional. Since gastric juices may reveal and lead to diagnosis of a number of medical conditions, it is important to discuss this important type of lab examination along with those of other better-known body fluids.

The study of gastric contents includes several tests for a complete gastric analysis. *Gastric fluid analysis* is a medical procedure used to examine the secretions and other liquids normally found in the stomach. By means of a tube passed

© Springer International Publishing AG, part of Springer Nature 2018
J. W. Ridley, *Fundamentals of the Study of Urine and Body Fluids*,
https://doi.org/10.1007/978-3-319-78417-5_16

through the nose and through the esophagus to the stomach, gastric fluid is aspirated. The most common reason for this test is to assess for the presence of blood in the upper gastrointestinal (GI) tract. Gastric fluid is sometimes may also feasibly be tested for the presence of tuberculosis organisms when obtaining a sputum specimen is not possible. Fluid analysis testing chiefly involves analyzing the acidity of the stomach, a vital part of digestion. Aspiration by nasogastric tube also bypasses the normal bacteria found in the mouth and helps to prevent this bacteria from entering the stomach, as most normal flora (bacteria) cannot survive a high acid content.

A major organism, *Helicobacter pylori* (*H. pylori*) is an organism with an unusual shape that is culpable in the formation of peptic ulcers (Fig. 16.1). In the past, it was thought that excess acidity of the stomach was the cause of most peptic ulcers, but *H. pylori* is implicated now in the majority of peptic ulcers, chronic gastritis and stomach cancers. This bacterium found in the stomach may be diagnosed in some cases by a breath test performed by testing the breath before and after drinking a solution that reacts to *H. pylori* by release of carbon dioxide. This organism is often present in large numbers and may be easily visualized microscopically from a simple methylene blue preparation. Certain food-borne illnesses may also be caused by bacteria that are able to reach the stomach when contaminated food is ingested, causing "food poisoning." Gastric fluids are not an ultrafiltrate of blood as are many of the other major fluids but is the product of cellular secretion from specialized cells found in the gastric mucosa, the fluids of which are chiefly involved with digestion.

Due to the development of non-laboratory procedures for the evaluation of gastric functions, these tests are often more precise, less time consuming, and less uncomfortable for the patient. Routine examination of *gastric contents* in the clinical laboratory, although diminishing in numbers, has not been completely eliminated from the menu of tests offered by many clinical laboratories. Of major interest in the laboratory analysis of gastric secretion is the measurement of *gastric acidity* and is considered useful in the diagnosis and treatment of peptic ulcers, *pernicious anemia, Zollinger-Ellison syndrome*, and for monitoring surgical procedures.

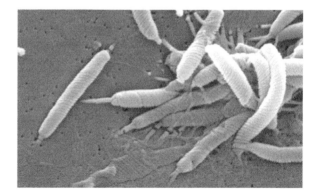

Fig. 16.1 Microscopic depiction of *H. pylori* colonizing intestine

Additional procedures now in use for the detection of these disorders include direct examination of lesions by endoscopy, improved radiologic techniques, and pH-sensitive electrodes that will transmit *pH* readings when passed into the stomach. Measurement of serum gastrin levels, cytologic examination of gastric contents for malignant cells, and immunologic testing of serum for the presence of *anti-intrinsic factor* and *antiparietal cell antibodies* seen in pernicious anemia are types of testing offered. The sophistication of these procedures has in some instances reduced the diagnostic role of actual gastric acidity titration to a secondary concern. However, gastric analysis is still used in difficult diagnostic cases and for confirming results obtained by other methods.

16.2   Infection Control

Although gastric fluids, due to the highly acid environment of the stomach, is essentially free of bacteria, it is advisable to handle gastric contents carefully. In cases of a bleeding peptic ulcer, fresh blood may contain *bloodborne pathogens*. Gastric fluids have not been known as a means for transmitting of infectious disease to others including TB or HIV-1 even when blood is present, but gastric contents should still be collected, transported and handled with reasonable care.

16.3   Routine Laboratory Tests for Gastric Fluid Studies

For a number of years it was believed that gastric acidity existed in two phases, and that acid with a pH of <3.5 represented "free" acid as hydrochloric acid, and the remainder of the acid was "combined" or was an organic acid where the two acids were measured separately. Currently the measurement of overall H$^+$ concentration is the recommended procedure. The major test performed on gastric fluids includes the titration of the acidity of the contents of the stomach using sodium hydroxide with phenolphthalein as an indicator. A number of hormones related to digestion are also found in the gastric fluids but are not normally tested for as a quantitative procedure. The wall of the stomach is lined with millions of glands called gastric glands, which secrete up to 800 mL of gastric juice during a meal. Several kinds of cells found in the gastric glands include parietal, chief and mucus secreting cells, as well as hormone secreting cells called *endocrine cells*, which secrete *pepsin, rennin,* and *gastrin*, and perhaps others.

Additional routine evaluations of gastric specimens include physical appearance, pH and volume. Normal gastric fluid contains mucus and is pale gray. In a fasting state, food particles should not be present as this would indicate an incomplete digestive process. The presence of large amounts of bile producing a yellowish to greenish color and the appearance of blood in the sample should be reported. When the contents called the basal samples (hourly collections) are collected, a gastric stimulation test is performed. A drug called *Pentagastrin* or one that is similar and that stimulates gastric acid stimulation is administered subcutaneously and after

15 min, four more specimens are collected at 15-min intervals for a period of 1 h. These post-stimulation samples are again titrated for their acidity and the results of the four samples are averaged. The *maximal acid output* (MAO) is obtained from these averages. The *peak acid output* (PAO) is determined by averaging the results of the two highest values.

16.3.1 Specimen Collection of Gastric Fluid

Ordinarily the patient from whom a sample from the stomach will be obtained should be fasting overnight before collection. A tube is inserted through a patient's nose and into the stomach. After a few minutes allowed to adjust from any discomfort of having a tube pushed into his or her nose, the patient is assisted to a sitting position (Fig. 16.2). Specimens are aspirated through the tube with the use of a syringe every 15 min for usually a 90-min period. The first two samples are observed for the presence of blood and volume but are then discarded to avoid results that might be impacted by the stress experienced by the patient.

No beverages are to be drunk during the procedure, and no saliva should be swallowed by the patient but is expectorated to avoid dilution of the fluids in the stomach. The four remaining samples, collected over a period of an hour, are used for determining the entire basal acid output by the parietal cells of the stomach that secrete *hydrogen chloride* (HCl) and intrinsic factor. Alcohol and medicines such as antacids and others such as *adrenergic blockers* and *adrenocorticosteroids* should be avoided for up to 3 days before the test is performed.

16.3.2 Physical Appearance of Gastric Fluid

For the normal gastric juice, the appearance is of a pale gray and translucent material that is slightly viscous. Mucus will most likely be evident in the samples from the majority of individuals. A faintly pungent odor is detectable and after a 12 h fast, there should be no food products visible. However, if food particles are present, a

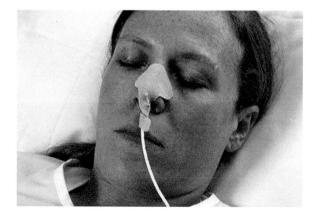

Fig. 16.2 Patient inserted with a nasogastric tube

pyloric obstruction may be present. Large amounts of bile will impart a yellow to greenish appearance in a patient with a healthy digestive system. The liquid secreted by the glands in the lining of the stomach is the focus of a gastric analysis and without bleeding or infection, the gastric fluids will be unremarkable. With the advent of more sophisticated testing procedures, the determination of gastric acid and intrinsic factor are performed and confirmed for both digestive purposes where anemia might occur from a lack of intrinsic factor. With the increasing rate of bypass surgery, there are conditions with the decreased cell mass of the stomach's lining that require administration of vitamin B_{12} and other adjunctive therapeutic medical support.

16.3.3 Gastric Fluid Cell Count

Unlike other body fluid studies, cell counts are not indicated for this type of sample. The presence of intact red blood cells might indicate current heavy bleeding. Cells from the stomach suspected as being malignant cells should be analyzed by surgical biopsy for evaluation.

16.4 Summary

Gastric fluid is a physiological liquid that results from the secretion of hydrochloric acid by the parietal cells in the stomach. These cells are also responsible for the production of intrinsic factor necessary for the intestinal absorption of *vitamin B_{12}*. Specimen collection involves the aspiration of gastric contents that are collected by nasal or oral intubation of the patient. Following the initial aspirations, Pentagastrin or a similar medication is administered subcutaneously. Another set of collections is initiated over an hour's time period, at 15 min intervals, is collected and the resulting values are averaged and examined for abnormalities.

The basic test performed on gastric fluids is that of the basal gastric acidity and was originally the only one. Properly preparing the patient for the procedure in order to produce meaningful results is essential. Improper instructions to the patient as to the protocol required to obtain a meaningful sample may result in erroneous results. Patients must be informed of personal responsibility for complying with requirements mandatory for obtaining meaningful laboratory values.

Again, the previous steps provided refers to the basal, or fasting, specimen, the initial collection steps in a gastric analysis. The basal specimen is a 1-h collection, usually consisting of four 15-min specimens, after discarding the first two samples. Although the 90-min test is most preferable, any other time frame may be used, including a single 1-h collection. Several test variations are available, but all utilize the same principle, which is to introduce a gastric stimulant to the patient following the basal collection. The volume, pH, titratable acidity and acid output of the initial samples constituting the basal specimen are determined before proceeding to the second step, that of stimulating the secretion of acid, and testing of the resulting secretions.

Therefore, following the basal portion of the procedure, a post-stimulation gastric acidity is performed and results from this process are compared with results obtained from the basal samples. The inability to produce gastric acidity cannot be determined solely from the analysis of the basal gastric secretion, so additional tests must be performed, again with proper preparation and stimulating the patient to induce heavy secretions of fluid. Specimens collection is continued and are tested for possible increased volume and acid content. Commonly used stimulants include Pentagastrin, histamine, and *Histalog*.

Review Questions

1. What is the major reason that gastric juices are not considered a "major" body fluid?
   a. Not an ultrafiltrate of blood
   b. Does not possess significant cells
   c. Not often performed
   d. All of the previous responses
2. The organism, *Helicobacter pylori*, is implicated in:
   a. Lack of adequate digestion
   b. Food poisoning of certain types
   c. Anemia from low intrinsic factor
   d. High acidity
   e. Peptic ulcers
3. A condition that is rarely found when examining gastric fluids is:
   a. Presence of malignant cells
   b. Extremely low acidity
   c. Lack of white blood cells
   d. Large amounts of mucus
4. Why would the gastric juices prevent the presence of many pathogens in the stomach?
   a. Low acidity inhibits bacterial growth
   b. Most bacteria in the stomach is normal flora
   c. No blood cells are found in gastric content
   d. None of the above
5. Which of the following would not be a hormone found in gastric juices?
   a. Pepsin
   b. Rennin
   c. Vitamin B_{12}
   d. Gastrin
6. Gastric glands may secrete up to mL during a meal.
   a. Up to 80 mL
   b. More than a liter
   c. Generally none is secreted
   d. 800 mL

7. Gastric fluid is generally collected by:
   a. Subcutaneous aspiration
   b. Vomiting
   c. Nasal tube aspiration
   d. Blood samples

Answers Found in Appendix C

Microscope Use and Care

17

Objective(s)
Discuss the history of the microscope
Identify the basic parts of the microscope
Understand the use of the coarse and fine adjustments
Clean the oculars, objectives and stage of the microscope
Describe the basic types of microscopes used in the clinical laboratory
Demonstrate proper transporting of and storage of the microscope

17.1 History of the Evolution of the Microscope

Antoni van Leeuwenhoek is most often accorded the title of the father of the microscope that led to the development of today's complex instrument called a microscope although others have been credited with breaking ground for its improved versions. The development of the modern microscope actually began in the 1200s, AD, with the development of a crude microscope that is a forerunner of those in use today. The earliest version of the *magnifying glass* that was called the first "microscope" included the magnifying glass used to concentrate the sun's rays onto a flammable surface and was called a *"burning glass,"* a characteristic based on its ability to start a fire when the sun's rays were sharply focused on kindling material such as paper and dry, rich wood or dried leaves.

Improving upon the magnifying glass, the *glass lens* was thought to have been discovered by *Roger Bacon* in 1268. Bacon recorded in his observations during that time that a person who examined written letters or any other minute objects through a crystal or glass of some other transparent substance, and it were shaped like a portion of a glass sphere or bass, with the convex side toward the eye, he would see the objects with greater clarity and they will appear larger to him. So in addition, such an instrument would aid those with visual difficulties to see an individual written character of a narrative through magnification.

© Springer International Publishing AG, part of Springer Nature 2018
J. W. Ridley, *Fundamentals of the Study of Urine and Body Fluids*,
https://doi.org/10.1007/978-3-319-78417-5_17

It has been alleged that Bacon accidentally broke a *crystal sphere* and used the shards of glass to make observations not visible earlier, giving rise to continuing observations. With some of the glass pieces *convex* and others *concave*, the images he was using for observation were clearer and larger. The *glass lens* that was devised due to his observations were miraculously used to improve the vision of those with defective human eyes. Lenses were apparently used to develop eyeglasses shortly after Bacon's observations, aiding improvement in the visual acuity of some over the next several decades. In 1299, a letter from a resident of Florence stated that as old age weighted him down, he found great difficulty in reading or writing unless using modified glass lenses called spectacles.

One of the five senses such as that of eyesight is necessary for observing clinical signs and to examine clinical specimens in order to detect conditions of disease as laboratorians do. Although *macroscopic* vision as seen by the naked eye is useful to an extent for many purposes in the practice of medicine, the amount of detail, even of blemishes and potential tumors of the skin, require *magnification*. Medical practitioners insisted on further manipulations of the primitive lenses developed earlier, and these efforts led to the development beyond that of spectacles and magnifying glasses to the instruments we know today as the telescope and the microscope. Several hundred years had elapsed after the earlier discoveries of the miracles of glass in certain shapes before a means was found of arranging glass lenses on a framework which amplified extremely small objects heretofore not visible with the naked eye. These led to the discovery of a microscopic life that caused or contributed to infectious diseases, which opened the way to even further experimentation and observations. Manipulations of these lenses caused small objects and organisms to appear larger, and distant objects, such as heavenly bodies, appear closer. The earliest simple microscope was merely a tube with a plate for the object at one end and a lens at the other end that gave a magnification less than ten times the actual size. Today's modern microscope called a compound microscope commonly possesses a 10-power ocular, which multiplies the power of each of normally four objectives by a factor of 10, allowing for visualization of extremely small objects.

Several related developments in the seventeenth century led to a number of useful theories regarding the anatomy of organs of the body. *Marcello Malpighi* confirmed *William Harvey's* blood circulation theories and documented his discoveries of the microscopic morphology of the liver, kidneys, bone, nerve tracts, and the inner layer of the epidermis which still bears Malpighi's name. *Robert Hooke* was another major contributor to the field of microscopy, demonstrating the anatomy of plant cells and the presence of other objects, both animate and inanimate.

Hooke was an inveterate mechanical tinkerer and also developed and modified a simple compound microscope called the Jansen microscope into a more modern version. After the compound microscope, the next major development was in lenses. Half a century later, following the invention of the compound microscope, Robert Hooke and Antoni van Leeuwenhoek together found that lenses with short focal lengths would provide for better magnification, using double convex lenses which we see today in modern microscopes. This development led to better resolution and magnification power. Advances based on these developments enabled *Robert Koch* to discover bacteria such as those that caused tuberculosis and *cholera*, medical scourges at the time. But although others contributed directly to the development of the microscope, Antoni van Leeuwenhoek is generally considered the father of modern microscopy.

17.2   Basic Types of Microscopes Used in a Clinical Laboratory

The basic microscope used in the laboratory today is that of the light microscope, also known as the compound *bright-field microscope* (Fig. 17.1). The term "compound" indicates that two sources of magnification are used in conjunction with each other, as discovered by the earlier pioneers, amplifying the degree of magnification. Another type that is in wide use for certain applications in the clinical laboratory is that of the *phase-contrast microscope*. This microscope provides for ease

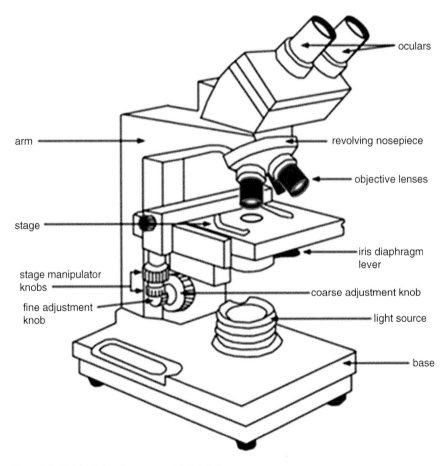

Fig. 17.1 Bright field microscope with labeled parts

of viewing unstained and transparent specimens that are difficult to visualize on unstained slides of specimens. In the procedures where the phase-contrast microscope is used, the background appears black and the specimen is brightly lighted, the opposite of the view obtained when using a bright-field microscope where the background is clear and bright.

Two other types of microscopes may be employed in the clinical laboratory but are less common than the two previously described microscopes. The *epifluorescent microscope* is used to visualize objects that have been coated with antibodies against the object, such as human cells or even microbiological organisms. The objects are stained with a fluorescent dye and enables identification of certain areas within a cell or on the surface of the cell or organism. The electron microscope is seldom used in the general clinical laboratory but is found in many research laboratories. Electronic waves enable an indirect visualization of extremely small particles such as viruses, and other objects too small to be seen with the bright-field microscope. Due to the expense incurred in the purchase of these instruments and the amount of time required for specimen preparation, the electron microscope is found generally in teaching hospitals and research laboratories.

17.3   Parts Included in the Bright-Field Microscope

Regardless of the brand and type of construction of the basic microscopes used in the medical laboratory, the following mechanical elements are common to all of the bright-field, epifluorescence and phase contrast microscopes. Descriptions of the construction of electron microscopes are beyond the scope of this section.

17.3.1 Microscope Arm

The arm is the part of the microscope that provides for structure in the connection and the arranging of the functional parts of the microscope and attaches the area where the *oculars* or *eyepieces* are located to the base, which provides stability to the microscope while it is being used.

17.3.2 Mechanical Stage

The stage is located between the objectives and the light source that is located in the base of the microscope.

17.3.3 Eyepieces or Oculars

The eyepieces generally consist of lenses within tubes that are adjusted to allow for the individual differences in the eyes of the users of the microscope. This process is called the interpupillary adjustment, which allows the oculars to correspond with the distance between the pupils of the eyes. After the interpupillary distance is established, the second adjustment of the oculars is that of the dioptic positioning. This adjustment allows for refractive differences in the eyes of the microscopist. The eyepieces almost exclusively have a magnifying power of 10×, a number that amplifies the power of each objective as the ocular and the objective operate jointly in the process of magnification. A *monocular microscope* has only one eyepiece but is seldom used in a clinical laboratory. The *binocular microscope* with two eyepieces is most commonly found in the clinical laboratory, and usually includes a device for adjustments to allow for differing distance between the eyes for individuals as well as for differing focal lengths when the eyes have different refractive errors in an individual.

17.3.4 Nosepiece and Objectives

The underside of the upper horizontal portion of the arm attaches to a circular, revolving nosepiece where usually at least three objectives are mounted by screw-type attachments into the nosepiece. The nosepiece revolves, enabling ease in changing the objectives to different powers of magnification. Objectives are commonly of low power (10×), high-power (40×) and *oil immersion* (100×). Some microscopes contain four objectives where the fourth objective is of an intermediate strength in a range between the three common objectives as presented. Each of these objectives are multiplied by the 10-power ocular to achieve a magnification factor of each objective multiplied by the power of 10, i.e., the 40× objective, when multiplied by the strength of the ocular, will achieve a multiplication of 400 times the object's actual size. The degree of magnification while retaining a clear image is limited, and this is called the resolving power, which is greatly affected by the quality of the objective lenses, where the better *resolving power* of a microscope dictates the price of the instrument.

17.3.5 Light Source and Relationship of the Condenser and Iris Diaphragm

Using the proper light is essential to the optimal use of the microscope. The microscope light source is found in the base of the microscope and is accompanied by the condenser and the iris diaphragm. The condenser focuses the light from the light source by moving the condenser in an up and down direction until the desire amount of light is achieved. Generally, the lowering of the condenser is necessary for viewing transparent or unstained objects, and raising of the condenser is required for darker stained specimens such as blood smears. The iris diaphragm controls the amount of light that strikes the objective by operator adjustments, enabling a desirable image for examination. The light path extends from the oculars through the body tube, through a prism, to the objectives (Fig. 17.2). The light source extends

Fig. 17.2 Illumination
path in the compound
microscope

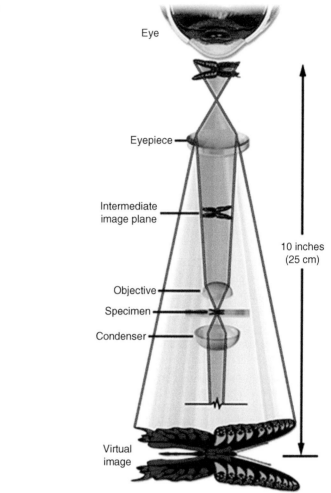

illumination upward from the base of the microscope, through the condenser and
through the specimen.

17.3.6 Procedure for Aligning Illumination Source

Proper alignment of the light source is necessary for good resolution, as poor alignment causes poor resolution and may even depict artifacts that are not included in
the target object. An uneven lighted field of vision results from improper alignment.
The diaphragm, sometimes referred to as the field diaphragm, is located under the
stage and should be properly aligned in order to obtain the best lighting required to
obtain proper contrast for the visualization of certain objects and parts of objects,
such as the granular appearance of cells.

When alignment is not performed by a service company, the technician or technologist may find it necessary to perform the task. Microscopes using must be routinely checked for correct alignment. For best results, the experienced microscopist may find it necessary to make adjustments before each use of the microscope for instruments employing Köhler illumination. Alignment of the light source is accomplished by manually aligning and focusing the illumination to determine whether the correct optical components are in focus with respect to the light source image planes and the specimen image planes. Alignment of optical components on the specimen image plane is basically performed by first loading a test specimen on the stage. For this adjustment, the specimen is placed directly below the low power objective before the light source is turned on and the specimen is brought into sharp focus by moving either the objective or the specimen.

The field diaphragm is then partially closed and the edges of the diaphragm are brought into focus by adjusting the condenser in an up or downward position. The focus can be adjusted by raising or lowering the condenser lenses and diaphragm. At this time the edges of the diaphragm and the specimen should appear in focus and should be centered in the field of vision. The field diaphragm image is centered using he condenser adjustment knobs. Finally, the field diaphragm is reopened to just outside the field of view. The iris diaphragm of the condenser is then adjusted to the desired level of contrast, and it may be necessary to also adjust the light intensity by use of the rheostat located on the base of the microscope. The lowest intensity of light necessary for achieving an acceptable image is advantageous for the life of the bulb as well as eliminating eye strain.

17.3.7 Coarse and Fine Adjustment

The coarse and fine adjustment knobs are most often found as one attachment to the arm of the microscope, and just above the base of the instrument. The inner of smaller knob is the fine adjustment and the larger knob that surround the fine adjustment is manipulated to more quickly move the objective(s) closer to the viewing field. The *coarse adjustment* should not be used when using the higher power objectives, as the objective may strike the object being viewed, unless the microscope is engineered to eliminate this risk. The distance between the objective and the object being examined is called the *working distance*. The distance between the slide and the high-power objective is quite small. Even though modern microscopes are said to be parfocal, meaning the nosepiece can be rotated through several different objectives, slight misplacement of the slide may result in damage to the objective, resulting in considerable expense. Therefore, only the fine adjustment should be manipulated when the high-power oil objective is being used to prevent possible damage to the objective and perhaps the slide.

Microscopes are operated as finely tuned instruments and must be maintained and handled carefully for optimum operation. A microscope that is not properly adjusted and maintained results in possible errors of identification as well as eyestrain and fatigue following prolonged use of the microscope. It is sometimes necessary to seek professional help in certain instances. Most facilities enter into an agreement where a commercial company sends trained specialists that adjust and replace parts that may be necessary for continued good operation. Good quality microscopes are expensive but will last for many years when properly cared for.

17.4   Use and Care of the Microscope

- The microscope should be carried with two hands, with one hand under the base to support the entire microscope. Care should be taken to prevent the oculars from falling to the floor or a hard surface, resulting in damage to them. The microscope is always placed carefully on a surface to avoid vibration and jarring.
- When not in use, the microscope should be kept covered to eliminate dust and environmental hazards from damaging the instrument. The cover is removed before attaching the electrical cord to the outlet and turning on the illuminating light. The microscope should be stored with the low-power objective I position, and the nosepiece in its lowest position. The open aperture of the stage should be centered so the stage does not extend to the side or forward, allowing collisions storage cabinets.
- Using stabilizing clamps attached to the stage, place the slide on the stage.
- Initially, the stage should be in the most elevated position.
- The *scanning objective* is used to locate the object and to focus the image using the coarse adjustment knob.
- Finalize the focusing process, using the fine adjustment knob to bring the object into clear focus and in the center of the field of view.
- Bring the low power objective (40×) into place.
- Focus on the object using minor adjustments with the inner fine adjustment knob.
- Again, the stage is moved to center the object in field of view and adjust light level as desired.
- Rotating the nosepiece, bring the high power objective into place.
- Again, using only the fine adjustment knob, focus on the object, and again adjust the light level as necessary while centering the object.
- When it is necessary to use the oil objective, after focusing on the target object using the high-power objective, rotate the nosepiece until the objectives are free of the slide. Place a drop of immersion oil on the slide where the light source appears through the aperture in the stage.
- Rotate the nosepiece until the oil immersion objective (100×) is immersed into the oil drop. Again, using the fine adjustment knob, focus on the target object.
- Care of lenses require routine cleaning with lens paper both before and after use. Paper other than lens paper is capable of inscribing scratches on the lenses. Objectives should be carefully cleaned and dried. NEVER leave oil on the objectives as the sealant may be affected by oil and cause seepage into the interior of the objective, which results in considerable cost for replacement objectives.

Safety Point

When body fluids, as a wet mount, or unfixed tissue specimens are examined, they are capable of producing disease. The microscope should be regularly cleaned with a disinfectant when sued in a biohazardous area. Disconnect the electrical cord from the microscope before any disassembly or when illuminator bulbs are being replaced.

17.5 Preparation for Storage when Finished with Using the Microscope

- Remove the slide from the stage
- Using absorbent wipes, remove an oil or debris from the stage
- Rotate the nosepiece until the lowest scanning objective is in place
- Return the stage to its highest elevated position
- Turn off the illuminating light source
- Secure the electrical cord by rolling it up if the microscope is to be stored in cabinet
- Wipe off the oculars with lens paper and replace cover
- Storage for later use requires use of a cabinet for protection of the instrument

17.6 Precautions to Be Observed

- NEVER use the coarse adjustment knob when on HIGH power
- Never leave the oil immersion objective in oil. Remove excess oil with lens paper
- When the target object is lost from view, begin the initial process of using the microscope again

17.7 Summary

Microscopes are designed to enable the user to visualized very small cells and organisms too small to be seen with the naked eye, and that are applicable to disease states. Blood cells, tissue cells, parasites and urine sediment are all elements that require the practice of microscopy. The use of the microscope requires skill and practice in order to optimize the practice of microscopy necessary to provide for good identification and evaluation of a number of body fluids.

There are three basic types of microscopes used in the clinical laboratory. The light microscope, the phase contrast microscope, and the electron microscope are used for varying functions, but the light microscope is the type most commonly used in the medical laboratory. A less commonly employed microscope is that of the epifluorescence microscope, which enables visualization of objectives that have been stained by fluorescent dyes. These dyes are often combined with antibodies which attach to certain areas of a particular cell or organism. The term "compound" microscope refers to one that possesses two oculars, and the monocular scope is seldom seen in the laboratory.

The basic parts of a microscope a number of sections of the microscope, and are all similar in their design and function. The oculars are designed and are adjustable to adapt to the shape and setting of the eyes. The microscope arm holds the oculars and is attached to the base of the microscope by a barrel or tube. The oculars and the objectives are magnifying glasses that operate in conjunction with each other. They operate by multiplying the power of the magnification of the oculars (usually ×10), and the objectives range from 10× up to 100× for most microscopes. The objectives are attached to a revolving nosepiece that enable ease of movement from low power to high power as needed. The 100× objective is used in conjunction with immersion oil to reduce the incident light that may interfere with obtaining sharp images of cells and their internal structures.

Adjustments with fine and coarse focusing knobs and skillful manipulation of the iris diaphragm, and the condenser enable the experienced microscopist to quickly obtain an acceptable view of the target image. The stage is designed with an orifice to enable light to pass through the sample on the stage, and usually has clamps to stabilize the slide being observed. Phase contrast microscopes enable the viewing of unstained cells, which are transparent, and for platelet counts and unstained urinary sediment which are best observed by this type of microscope.

Microscopes are expensive investments that require careful use and routine maintenance in order to optimize their use. Objectives must be carefully cleaned with lens paper before and after use, and care must be taken to avoid immersing the objectives that are not oil-immersible, to prevent damage to the surface of the lens inside of the objective. Lens cleaner is available and must be of a good quality in order to best care for the microscope. And finally, transport of the microscope where the entire instrument is supported to prevent dropping of the oculars and objectives, or even the entire microscope (Fig. 17.3). When the objectives, light

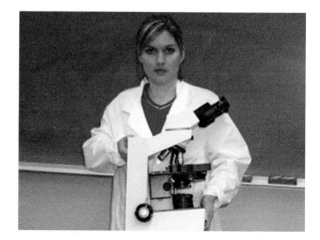

Fig. 17.3 Proper transport of the microscope to avoid damage by dropping

source and oculars are improperly aligned, the results produced by the instrument leaves a great deal to be desired, and may require professional adjustment to correct the defect.

Review Questions

1. Describe the proper cleaning procedures used for the objectives.
2. List the major types of microscopes and the uses for each of them.
3. What are the powers of the three most common objectives, and in conjunction with the ocular lenses, what is the magnification for each?
4. When is it advantageous to use a phase contrast microscope?
5. Name the major components of the bright-field microscope.

Answers Found in Appendix C

Appendix A: Reference Ranges for Urine Chemistry Values

The following values are provided for common chemistry tests performed in a clinical laboratory, but thousands of tests are possible, chiefly by reference laboratories, and all but the most common procedures are beyond the scope of this textbook. Slight differences will be noted for the clinical findings for the constituents and analytes determined in the testing of urine and other body fluids. Differences will be found in various publications based on sources of information used by the author, as well as the method used in the various procedures, and for population groups from differing geographic locations based on cultural practices and diet as well as the individual laboratory performing the diagnostic test. Most differences between ranges presented in publications and by the clinical facilities will be insignificant, and extreme values will indicate a disease state regardless of the values that are published (Table A.1).

© Springer International Publishing AG, part of Springer Nature 2018
J. W. Ridley, *Fundamentals of the Study of Urine and Body Fluids*,
https://doi.org/10.1007/978-3-319-78417-5

Table A.1 Normal urinalysis chemistry values

Analyte	Normal range	Clinical data	Note
Protein	Less than 15 mg/dL	Elevated pH may result in false positive result	Strenuous exercise may reveal transient proteinuria
Microalbumin	Random sample: 0–45 mcg/mL	Elevated in some diabetics	Not detected by routine "dipstick" methodology; requires specific test strip
Blood	Less than 0.010 mg/dL; 3 RBCs/µL	Positive hemoglobin or intact RBCs found in urological and nephrological conditions along with bleeding disorders	Trace reaction varies among individuals; menstruation may result in positive reaction
Leukocyte esterase	Negative results	Result of small or greater indicates increase in leukocytes (10/µL)	Elevated glucose and some antibiotics may cause reduced test results
Nitrite	Negative results	False negative results from short bladder incubation of urine	Pink spots or edges on test strip should not be reported as "positive"
Glucose	Less than 30 mg/dL	Specific for glucose; aids in differentiating between glucose and other reducing substances	Ketone bodies may reduce sensitivity of test
Ketone	Negative results	Correlates with carbohydrate or lipid metabolism in diabetics	Starvation, stress, pregnancy and frequent strenuous exercise may yield trace results
pH	From 4.6to8.0	Bacterial growth leads to alkaline results	Artificially altering pH may be used in treating urinary calculi
Specific gravity	1.001–1.035	Strip differ from other methods as it measures dissolved ions rather than concentration	Highly alkaline urine and increased protein levels may cause higher results
Bilirubin	0.02 mg/dL (not detectable)	Specific for bilirubin; aids in detection of liver diseases	Atypical colors may indicate bile pigments; interfere with results
Urobilinogen	>1.0 mg/dL	Increased in hemolytic and hepatic disease	Differentiates between biliary and liver diseases

Appendix B: Example, Material Safety Data Sheet

Not to Be Used as Actual MSDS*

- The following example is merely provided to show the governmental regulations that must be provided for reference when one is exposed and to be sued for training of those who will handle the product. The complexity of the requirements to be provided by the manufacturer related to research before a product is released for consumption is staggering. Copies of MSDS's are required for all medical treatment facilities and for commercial businesses who must maintain a current MSDS for each product they use.

Material Safety Data Sheet (Sample)

Simple All-Purpose Cleaner Scrubbing Pad

Version No. 1322509 Date of Issue: February 2010 *ANSI-Z400.1-2003 Format*

Product Name: Simple All-Purpose Cleaner Scrubbing Pad

Additional Name: Concentrated Cleaner Pads

Manufacturer's Product Code Numbers: *Please Refer to Manufacturer's Catalog*

Company: Moonshine Endeavors, Inc.
　　　　　1490 Atlantic Boulevard
　　　　　O'possum Haven, VA 20649 USA

Telephone: 888-202-3666; Fax: 212-429-1508

Emergency Phone: Chem-Tel 24-Hour Emergency Service: 866-405-8024

Use of Product: An all purpose cleaner with scrubbing pad for manual scrubbing purposes (on water-safe surfaces).

Section 2: Hazards Identification

Emergency Overview: CAUTION. Mild eye irritant.

Simple All-Purpose Cleaner is a dark green liquid with a mint odor (includes green cellulose scrubbing pad).

HMIS Rating:

Health = 1 = slight

© Springer International Publishing AG, part of Springer Nature 2018
J. W. Ridley, *Fundamentals of the Study of Urine and Body Fluids*,
https://doi.org/10.1007/978-3-319-78417-5

Fire = 0

Reactivity, and Special = 0 = minimal

Eye Contact: Mild Eye and Mucous Membrane Irritant.

Skin Contact: No adverse effects expected in typical use conditions. Prolonged exposure may cause skin dryness. Use of gloves and skin moisturizer after washing may be indicated.

Ingestion: May cause stomach or intestinal upset if swallowed (due to detersive properties.)

Inhalation: No adverse effects expected in normal conditions. Ventilation should be present when using Simple All-Purpose Cleaner over a prolonged period of time.

Carcinogens: No ingredients are listed by IARC,OSHA, or NTP as a suspected carcinogen.

Medical Conditions: No medical conditions known to be aggravated by exposure to Simple All-Purpose Cleaner.

UN Number: Not Required

Dangerous Goods Class: Non-hazardous

Section 3: Composition/Information on Ingredients

Ingredients: The only ingredient of Simple All-Purpose Cleaner with established exposure limits is undiluted 2-bis-theranol. Based upon chemical analysis, Simple All-Purpose Cleaner contains no known EPA priority pollutants, heavy metals or chemicals listed under federal and state lists for toxic organic and inorganic materials. All components of Simple All-Purpose Cleaner are listed on the TSCA Chemical Substance Inventory. This product does not contain any ingredients covered by the provisions of 29 CFR 1910.1200.

Section 4: First Aid Measures

Eye Contact: Reddening may develop. Immediately remove contact lenses if applicable and rinse the eye with large quantities of cool water. Seek medical attention if irritation persists.

Skin Contact: Minimal effects, if any; rinse skin with water, rinse shoes and launder clothing before reuse. Reversible reddening may be eliminated by thoroughly rinsing area and get medical attention if reaction persists.

Swallowing: Essentially non-toxic. Several glasses of water will dilute material but do not induce vomiting.

Inhalation: Non-toxic. Exposure to concentrate may cause mild irritation of nasal passages or throat; remove to fresh air. Get medical attention if irritation persists.

Section 5: Fire Fighting Measures

Simple All-Purpose Cleaner is stable, not flammable, and will not burn. No special procedures required.

Flash Point/Auto-Ignition: Not flammable. Extinguishing Media: Not flammable/non-explosive.

Flammability Limits: Not flammable. Special Fire Fighting Procedures: None required.

Section 6: Accidental Release Measures

Personal Precautions: Avoid contact with eyes. Do not rub eyes with hands during cleanup. No special precautions for dermal contact are needed. Wash hands thoroughly after cleaning up spill or leak.

Method for cleaning up: Recover usable material by convenient method, residual may be removed by wipe or wet mop. If necessary, unrecoverable material may be washed to drain with large quantities of water.

Section 7: Handling and Storage

Special Precautions: No special precautions are required. **This product is non-hazardous for storage and transport according to the U.S.**

Department of Transportation Regulations. Simple All-Purpose Cleaner requires no special labeling or placarding to meet U.S. Department of Transportation requirements.

UN Number: Not Required

Dangerous Goods Class: Non-hazardous

Section 8: Exposure Controls/Personal Protection

Exposure Limits: The Simple All-Purpose Cleaner formulation presents no health hazards to the user when used according to label directions for its intended purposes. Mild skin and eye irritation is possible (please see Eye contact and Skin contact in section IV.) No special precautionary measures required under normal use conditions.

Ventilation: No special ventilation, precautions or respiratory protection is required during normal use. Large scale use indoors should provide an increased rate of air exchange.

Human Health Effects or Risks From Exposure: Adverse effects on human health are not expected from Simple Green®, based on 20 years of use of Simple All-Purpose Cleaner without reported adverse health incidence in diverse population groups, including extensive use by inmates of U.S. Federal prisons in cleaning operations.

Eye protection: Simple All-Purpose Cleaner is a mild eye irritant; mucous membranes may become irritated by concentrate. Eye protection not generally required. Wash hands after using wipes.

Skin protection: Simple All-Purpose Cleaner is not likely to irritate the skin in the majority of users. Repeated daily application to the skin without rinsing, or continuous contact on the skin may lead to temporary, but most often a reversible irritation. Rinse completely from skin after contact.

General hygiene conditions: There are no known hazards associated with this material when used as recommended. The following general hygiene considerations are recognized as common good industrial hygiene practices:

– Avoid breathing vapor or mist.
– Avoid contact with eyes.
– Wash thoroughly after handling and before eating, drinking, or smoking.

Appearance & Odor: Cleaner is a dark green liquid, pad is a fibrous green matrix; exhibit a cinnamaldehyde odor.

Specific Gravity: 1.010 ± 0.010
Vapor Pressure: 18 mmHg @ 20 °C; 23.5 mmHg @ 26 °C
Vapor Density: 1.3 (air = 1)
Evaporation: >1 (butyl acetate = 1)
Water Solubility: 100%
Density: 8.5 lbs/gallon
Boiling Point: 100.6 °C (212 °F)
pH: 9.5 ± 0.3
Ash Content: At 600 °F: 1.86% by weight
Nutrient Content: None
Freezing Point: Approx −9 °C (16 °F)
Phosphorus: 0.3% by formula
Nitrogen: <1.0% by weight
Sulfur: 0.6% by weight (barium chloride precipitation)
If product freezes, it will reconstitute without loss of efficacy when brought back to room temperature and stirred.
VOC Composite Partial Pressure: 0.006 mmHg @ 20 °C
Volatile Organic Compounds (VOCs): Cleaner meets CARB & BAAQMD regulations.
CARB Method 310 3.8%
SCAQMD Method 313 2.8%
Section 10: Stability and Reactivity
Stability: Stable
Materials to Avoid: None known
Hazardous Decomposition Products: None observed
Toxicology information is based on chemical profile of ingredients and extrapolation of data from similar formulas.
Acute Toxicity: Oral LD50 (rat) >5 g/kg body weight*
Eye Irritation: Moderate/Mild reversible eye irritation may occur based on relevant laboratory studies. This potential is reduced by immediate rinsing of eyes in case of eye contact.
Dermal Irritation: Mild, reversible skin irritation may occur based on relevant laboratory studies. A 6-h exposure to human skin under a patch did not produce irritation
Repeat Exposure Via Skin Contact: Based on relevant laboratory studies, no toxic effects are expected to be associated with daily skin exposures (with up to 2 g/kg/day tested for 13 weeks on rabbits). Skin irritation may, however, occur with repeated exposures.
Reproductive Effects Assessment: Based on relevant laboratory studies (CD-1 mouse 18-week fertility assessment continuous breeding), no adverse effects on reproduction, fertility, or health of offspring are expected.
Material Safety Data Sheet: **Simple All-Purpose Cleaner All-Purpose Cleaner Simple All-Purpose Cleaner Scrubbing Pad**
Section 12: Ecological Information

Hazard to wild animals & aquatic organisms: Low, based on toxicological profile.

Biodegradability: Readily biodegradable based on biodegradation profile, PRO/FT CBT-AC 014-7 "Ready Biodegradability: Closed Bottle Test" OECD, and OECD 302B laboratory tests

Environmental Toxicity Information: It is important not to allow the runoff from cleaning into closed systems such as decorative ponds. Always protect closed systems with tarps or dikes if necessary.

Section 13: Disposal Considerations

Dispose of materials and containers in accordance with all applicable local, state and federal laws. This product is non-hazardous for transport according to the U.S. Department of Transportation Services UN Number: Not required Dangerous Goods Class: Non-hazardous

Section 15: Regulatory Information

*Reportable components:

All components are listed on: EINECS and TSCA Inventory

No components listed under: Clean Air Act Section 112

TSCA /TRI SARA Title III

Reporting: This product contains 2-pentoxyethetheranol which is subject to the reporting requirements of Section 313, Title III of Superfund Amendments and Reauthorization Act of 1986 as Category N230—Certain Glycol Ethers.

RCRA Status: Not a hazardous waste. **CERCLA Status:** No components listed

CA PROP. 65 Status: No components listed

Section 16: Other Information

PREPARER:

Questions about the information found on this MSDS should be directed to:

SUNSHINE MAKERS, INC.—TECHNICAL DEPARTMENT

15922 Pacific Coast Hwy. Huntington Harbour, CA 92649

Phone: 800/228-0709 [8am–5pm Pacific time, Mon-Fri] *Fax:* 562/592-3830 *Email:* infoweb@simplegreen.com

CAGE CODE 1Z575

GSA/FSS - CONTRACT NO. GS-07F-0065J

Scrubbing Pad GSA/BPA—CONTRACT NO. GS-07F-BSIMP

National Stock Numbers & Industrial Part Numbers: Retail Numbers:

Simple Green Part Number NSN Size Part Number Size

13012 7930-01-342-5315 24 oz spray (12/case) 13002 16 oz Trigger (12/case)

Scrubbing Pad 10224 7930-01-346-9148 Each (24/case) ****International Part Numbers May Differ.**

Disclaimer The information provided with this MSDS is furnished in good faith and without warranty of any kind. Personnel handling this material must make independent determinations of the suitability and completeness of information from all sources to assure proper use and disposal of this material and the safety and health of employees and customers. Sunshine Makers, Inc. assumes no additional liability or responsibility resulting from the use of, or reliance on this information.

Appendix C: Summary Question Answers

Review Questions, Chapter One

1. Name the three types of examinations performed during the evaluation of body fluids.
   Physical or macroscopic, chemical and microscopic
2. Discuss uses of a urine analysis for the evaluation of a patient
   Metabolic diseases, infectious conditions of the urinary tract, toxicology, therapeutic drugs, drugs of abuse, physiological processes of kidneys
3. What are the visible characteristics examined for with the macroscopic examination of urine and other body fluids?
   Clarity, color, volume
4. Why is a urine such a valuable and effective means of discovering a number of diseases?
   Urine is easily obtained and yields a variety of clues as to certain medical conditions. Many metabolic and infectious diseases cause changes in the appearance, chemical and microscopic findings.
5. In what way is urine similar to body fluids other than whole blood?
   Urine and other body fluids are ultrafiltrates of the blood and contain various, and usually lower, levels of certain chemicals when compared with levels of these chemicals in blood

Review Questions, Chapter Two

1. What is the importance of quality assurance?
2. Quality assessment would be best described as:
3. What is meant by quality control? Describe key elements of a quality control program.
4. When a new procedure is adopted, what would be an initial responsibility of the clinical staff of the laboratory?
5. The primary goal of an effective quality assurance program is:

© Springer International Publishing AG, part of Springer Nature 2018
J. W. Ridley, *Fundamentals of the Study of Urine and Body Fluids*,
https://doi.org/10.1007/978-3-319-78417-5

Review Questions, Chapter Three

1. Name three specimen types that are NOT included in the list of samples that are significant sources of infection in medical laboratory employees.
   Urine, sweat, tears
2. The two bloodborne pathogens which require training as mandated by the federal are:
   HIV and HBV
3. The most common disinfectant used for cleaning work surfaces in the laboratory is:
   Sodium hypochlorite (Chlorox)
4. The agency that requires a medical facility to provide adequate protective equipment which includes gloves is:
   Occupational Safety and Health Administration
5. When washing the hands, which of the following activities is not a requirement?
   e. Hands should be washed with the fingers pointed in an upward position
6. Centrifuging of a specimen is likely to create:
   An aerosol
7. Which of the following legislative regulations led to the standards required of ALL medical laboratories?
   c. Clinical Laboratory Improvement Amendments of 1988
8. Name the three categories of laboratory tests that were established by CLIA '88.
   Waived, moderate and highly complex tests

Review Questions, Chapter Four

1. Blood flow though a nephron of the kidney follows which of the following paths?
   b. Afferent arteriole, peritubular glomerular capillaries, efferent arteriole
2. The electrolyte affected by rennin-angiotensin-aldosterone hormone is:
   d. Sodium
3. The daily volume of urine excreted depends would be affected by:
   d. All of the above
4. Why is an adequate flow of blood, or perfusion, important to the kidneys?
   The kidneys need oxygenated blood for maintaining cellular functions, and the kidneys must have a significant flow of blood in order to filter toxins from the plasma.
5. Which of the following would not be a function of the renal system?
   c. Blood, formed in the bone marrow, is stimulated by a kidney hormone called EPO
6. The hormone most responsible for the regulation of sodium in the blood is:
   c. Aldosterone
7. The test used to determine the concentrating ability of the kidneys is:
   c. Osmolality

8. The three ways for determining the specific gravity of a urine sample includes all except:
   c. Weighing a given urine sample

Review Questions, Chapter Five

1. How are body fluids other than urine and blood formed?
   d. a & b
2. Elements found in the examination of urine that has no clinical significance is:
   b. Artifacts
3. Body fluids include all of the following except:
   e. All of the above are body fluids
4. Intracellular fluid is contained:
   c. Inside cell walls
5. *Most* of the fluids in the body are derived from:
   c. Foods and water
6. Organs and tissues that play a major role in water balance include all except:
   e. All of the above organs are involved
7. The term commonly used for the body fluid compartments of the human body are:
   b. Intra- and extracellular fluids
8. The concentration of greatly influence the volume of body fluids found in various areas of the body?
   b. Concentration of electrolytes
9. The term "osmolality" is best related to:
   a. Concentration of dissolved materials
10. The term "phagocytosis" refers to:
    d. Eating of the body's cells
11. The disease called gout is based on the presence of:
    d. Presence of monosodium urate crystals

Review Questions, Chapter Six

1. Why is it necessary to calculate the protein from a 24-h urine specimen rather than merely documenting a semi-quantitative level found in a random urine sample?
   The volume of urine varies during a 24-h period, affecting the amount of protein that may be present at one given time. A quantitative result will more accurately determine the extent of the loss of protein in the urine.
2. What is critical to remember when using a preservative for a urine sample when a bacterial culture will be performed?
   The preservative used in this type of sample should only affect the pH of the sample which would not destroy the bacteria. The preservative chosen should

retard the growth of any bacteria present, preventing them from growing rapidly, to include any small levels of skin contaminants that may be present in the sample.

3. List the special requirements necessary when collecting a specimen for drug analysis, and give the reasons for these requirements when collecting, storing and transporting of the samples.

   Drug screenings when not handled properly may affect the potential employment or retention of an employee, as well as result in the incarceration of an individual if the specimens are not properly identified. A significant amount of information is required even when a random sample is collected, and a specific protocol must be followed to safeguard the identity and validity of the sample. The sample should be protected and monitored throughout the collection, storage and transport of the sample to the testing site, a process called Chain-of-Custody.

Review Questions, Chapter Seven

1. The most common disorders of the urinary system are based on:
   a. Bacterial infection
2. The basic organs included in the urinary system include all of the following except:
   c. Uterus
3. The kidney is responsible for a number of important functions. They normally include all of the following except:
   d. Formation of crystals
4. The chief functional unit of the kidney is:
   a. Nephrons
5. The blood flow to the kidneys includes approximately what percentage of the total volume of the blood that nourishes the body?
   b. 33 %
6. The flow of blood within the kidney is controlled by the functions of a complex hormone system that includes all except:
   a. Antidiuretic hormone
7. The glomerular flow rate of water containing low-molecular-weight substances that flow through the glomeruli of the kidneys per minute is:
   c. 120 mL/minute
8. The correct pH (acidity or alkalinity) of the blood of the human body is maintained by:
   d. b & c
9. Which of the following would greatly affect the specific gravity of the urine?
   d. All of the previous responses
10. Which of the following statements is true regarding the value of using osmolality rather than osmolarity for the measurement of non-dissociable substance?
    c. Osmolality is not affected by changes in temperature, atmospheric pressure

11. What is the physical or colligative property used to measure the concentration of solutes in the urine, serum or plasma?
    b. Freezing point depression
12. The stimulation of ADH is *most* effectively triggered by:
    a. Changes in NaCl concentration
13. Which of the following is/are components of Liddle's Syndrome?
    a. Extreme hypertension
14. A disease caused by a malfunction of ADH is that of:
    b. Diabetes insipidus
15. The simplest and most easily treated urinary tract infection (UTI) is called:
    a. Cystitis
16. Acute pyelonephritis will produce a positive nitrite reaction due to:
    a. Presence of certain bacteria
17. The kidney condition referred to as the sterile inflammatory process is:
    d. Glomerulonephritis
18. Rheumatic fever is precipitated by:
    b. Poststreptococcal infections
19. Blood tests that may be elevated during the acute stages but will return to normal along with the urinalysis results are:
    b. Blood urea nitrogen, creatinine
20. The disease characterized by progressive kidney failure but is accompanied by lung disease is called:
    b. Goodpasture's syndrome
21. A condition that is characterized by massive proteinuria and associated edema is that of:
    a. Nephrotic syndrome
22. Acute renal failure is often characterized by:
    c. Anuria or oliguria
23. A group of disorders called "amino acid disorders" usually refer to:
    d. All of the above
24. Various states within the US require tests at birth to detect hereditary metabolic disorders. The one required by all states is that of:
    c. Phenylketonuria
25. Fanconi's Syndrome is best described as an X-linked disease that is:
    d. All of the above
26. Metabolic acidosis may progress to an acute medical condition due to:
    d. All of the above
27. A precursor to the neurotransmitter serotonin is:
    b. Tryptophan
28. Porphyrins are the intermediate compounds in the production of:
    d. Heme

Review Questions, Chapter Eight

1. Arguably, the most important constituent in urine that may cause the majority of interferences with accurate results, is that of:
   d. Ascorbic acid
2. Measurement of the specific gravity of the urine is important in:
   d. All of the above
3. Which of the following could affect the evaluation for protein in a urine sample?
   b. Alkaline pH
4. Which of the following may be most important in assessing kidney damage?
   d. Protein
5. The presence of nitrites in a urine sample is indicative of:
   c. Certain bacteria
6. The test pad on the dipstick for measuring blood would be negative in the presence of:
   d. Hemosiderin
7. Light chain immunoglobulins in the urine would be indicative of:
   c. Multiple myeloma
8. Glycosuria, or glucose in the urine in abnormal amounts, would be present in:
   d. Diabetes mellitus
9. The finding of glucose in the urine would not be affected by:
   d. All of the above
10. The confirmatory test for bilirubin in the urine is:
    c. Ictotest
11. Which of the following is not one of the three ketone bodies?
    b. Prednisone
12. Precipitation tests are used to test for:
    d. Proteins
13. A test for urobilinogen would indicate:
    f. a & c
14. Tests for bilirubin in the urine would include evaluation for:
    c. Liver disease

Review Questions, Chapter Nine

1. In the examination of urine sediment, which of the following would be the most prominent indicator of *early* renal disease?
   c. White blood cells
2. Which of the following statements would not be true regarding findings in urinary sediment?
   b. Bacteria is always found microscopically in cases of cystitis
3. Those suffering from the nephritic syndrome will always exhibit:
   d. Elevated blood albumin

4. The most predictive of the severity of renal disease would be the presence of:
   c. Waxy casts
5. For confirming the presence of fat globules in the urine, which of the following would be included in completing the microscopic examination?
   c. Staining with a Sudan stain
6. Renal epithelial cells originate from the:
   d. Collecting ducts
7. Urinary casts are formed in:
   a. The distal convoluted tubule and collecting ducts of nephrons

Review Questions, Chapter Ten

1. Where would tests that are not routinely performed in the routine hospital laboratory be sent for further evaluation?
   d. To a reference lab
2. One of the contraindications of using a urine preservative is:
   a. Some analytes may be destroyed
3. Urine screening tests except for microscopy can legally be performed by:
   d. All of the previous responses
4. A urine sample is comprised primarily of:
   d. Water
5. The most important component of the following list in the evaluation of urine is:
   a. Chemical constituents
6. Which of the following would not require a confirmatory test when a positive result was obtained by dipstick chemistry?
   b. Leukocyte esterase
7. Urinary sediment would be used to determine the presence of:
   d. Yeasts
8. Which of the following findings would not be particularly important in diagnosing an illness related to the urinary tract?
   d. All of the above would
9. High levels of metabolism of fats for energy would give a positive result of:
   d. Ketones
10. Musty odors of the urine may sometimes be attributed to:
    b. Phenylketonuria
11. The clarity of urine is referred to as:
    a. Turbidity
12. The specific gravity of urine using the refractometer compares the sample with:
    b. Air
13. Urobilinogen is formed directly from:
    c. Bilirubin
14. The chemistry test performed on urine that is most sensitive to sunlight is:
    d. Bilirubin

15. The chemistry test performed on urine that is most sensitive to high alkalinity is:
    b. Protein
16. A species of bacteria that is able to convert nitrates to nitrites is:
    c. *Escherichia coli*
17. The best type of specimen for a complete urinalysis is:
    a. Fresh
18. Most test results provided by urinary dipstick are:
    b. Semi-quantitative
19. The purpose of centrifuging a urine sample is to:
    b. Concentrate the sample results
20. The Clinitest is used to:
    c. Detect reducing sugars

Review Questions, Chapter Eleven

1. The most common condition for which a lumbar puncture is performed is for the diagnosis of:
   d. Meningitis
2. The centrifuged supernatant from cerebrospinal fluid is pink to yellowish. The most likely cause is:
   c. Subarachnoid hemorrhage
3. As a result of a traumatic spinal tap, which of the following patterns would be observed from a sequential collection of CSF?
   a. More red color in tube #1
4. When polymorphonuclear cells are increased in a CSF sample, the likely cause is:
   b. Bacterial meningitis
5. Viral meningitis is usually diagnosed by:
   d. a & b
6. Excess cerebrospinal fluid is retained in the ventricles of the brain in which of the following?
   b. Hydrocephalus
7. Under normal conditions, glucose and protein levels in the CSF would be:
   c. Lower than that found in blood
8. Which of the following is used to prevent infection of the CNS during a lumbar puncture?
   c. Povidone-iodine
9. The most commonly diagnosed demyelinating disease of the CNS is:
   b. Multiple sclerosis
10. Intracranial pressure is monitored during a lumbar puncture. When the pressure drops significantly following aspiration of a small amount of CSF, the likely reason is:
    e. a & c

11. The origin of blood found in CSF can be determined by:
    b. Test for D-Dimer Fibrin
12. Cytocentrifugation is chiefly used for:
    a. WBC cellular differentiation
13. When doing a *preliminary* differentiation of leukocytes while using a hemocy-tometer, which of the following would be used to enable an estimate of the types of cells present?
    a. WBC cellular differentiation
14. Which of the following would be elevated following hypoxia with an impact on the brain?
    d. Lactate
15. A decreased CSF protein might result from:
    b. Tears of the lining of the brain
16. An increased CSF protein might result from:
    e. a & c
17. A decreased CSF glucose may be the result of which of the following:
    a. Delay in testing
18. An increased CSF glucose may be the result of which of the following:
    c. Diabetic coma

Review Questions, Chapter Twelve

1. What is the most common test performed to determine causes of infertility in a couple?
   d. Complete sperm count
2. Which of the following is most cost effective in determining causes of infertility?
   c. Complete sperm count
3. Which of the following would not be a factor in determining sperm motility?
   c. Vasectomy
4. Which of the following is the best way for collecting sperm samples?
   c. Masturbation
5. The most important component to be considered in determining a male's fertility status is:
   c. Sperm count
6. The semen should be collected on which of the following schedules to detect a man's fertility status based on a semen analysis:
   d. All of the above
7. Sperm counts are performed based on the following units of measurement:
   d. Count per milliliter (mL)
8. Sperm cells that are for the most part aligned head to tail is exhibiting which of the following?
   a. Immunological response
9. Semen should liquefy within:
   c. Within thirty minutes

10. A more dilute semen sample would most likely show:
    b. Decreased count per unit

Review Questions, Chapter Thirteen

 1. Which of the following body fluids is not always considered as an ultrafiltrate of blood?
    d. Cerebrospinal fluid
 2. A chemistry test on amniotic fluid that gives information related to neural tube deficits is:
    a. Alpha-fetoprotein
 3. The "Fern test" determines the presence of:
    a. Progesterone
 4. The most obvious difference between an exudates and a transudate would be:
    a. Elevated protein in an exudates
 5. The chief mechanism by which transudate effusions may accumulate in bodily cavities is
    a. Hydrostatic pressure
 6. Which of the following would be the most accurate statement?
    b. Transudates form due to a disruption in the balance of filtration and reabsorption
 7. Necrosis of an organ or tissue may be determined by performing:
    c. Lactate dehydrogenase
 8. The serous fluid that could perhaps require the most extensive group of tests would be:
    c. Amniotic fluid
 9. A type of white blood cell found in nasal secretions during an allergic reaction is:
    d. Eosinophil
10. Why is differentiation of white blood cells found in body fluids important?
    b. Differentiation provides information as to the type of infectious process present
11. The anticoagulant used to preserve the morphology of blood cells is:
    d. EDTA
12. The type of tube used for microbiological testing of body fluids is:
    c. Sterile heparinized tube
13. Which of the following would not lead to an increase in the volume of the body fluid?
    a. The turbidity, odor, color of the fluid
14. Which of the following serous fluids would normally be crystal clear?
    c. Cerebrospinal fluid
15. An encapsulated yeast found in cerebrospinal fluid is often determined by:
    b. India ink prep
16. Turk's stain will:
    b. Lyse red blood cells

17. Inflammation of the lining of the heart is called:
    a. Endocarditis
18. Oncotic pressure of the blood plasma is associated with:
    d. Albumin
19. Amniotic fluid, during the second and third trimesters of pregnancy, is chiefly composed of:
    c. Urine from the fetus
20. The test used to differentiate fetal cells from maternal cells is:
    c. Urine from the fetus

Review Questions, Chapter Fourteen

1. Synovial fluid is collect by a procedure called:
   c. Arthrocentesis
2. When red blood cells are found in synovial fluid, they are usually the result of:
   d. a & c
3. An effusion into the synovial cavity will:
   b. Increase volume of fluid
4. Crystals are best observed by:
   c. Employing phase contrast techniques
5. Synovial fluid will normally have:
   c. No red blood cells
6. Needle-like crystals that are yellow and are characteristic of acute gouty arthritis are:
   c. Monosodium urate
7. The viscosity of synovial fluid is due to:
   a. Hyaluronic acid

Review Questions, Chapter Fifteen

1. A Gram stain of the feces is not normally important for the finding of bacteria because:
   c. Thousands of species of bacteria are found in stool samples
2. The presence of abnormal amounts of fats in the stool is indicative of:
   a. Pancreatic disorder
3. The odor given off by fecal samples is caused by:
   d. Bacterial metabolism
4. Which of the following would not be considered an abnormal condition for feces?
   a. Massive numbers of bacteria
5. A large proportion of the bulk of a stool sample is accounted for by:
   c. Bacteria
6. The normal brown color of feces is attributed to:
   c. Bacteria

7. The term used for stools that are black in color is:
   b. Melena
8. Black, tarry stools is a sign of:
   a. Bleeding from the upper gastrointestinal tract
9. A whitish or silver color in the fecal sample is often due to:
   a. Obstructed bile duct
10. The guaiac reaction for occult blood may yield a false positive when:
    c. Large amounts of meat are eaten
11. A condition called "ulcerative colitis" may result from:
    c. Infection by *Clostridium difficile*
12. Decreased fat absorption is due to a variety of medical conditions. Which of the following would not be a cause for decreased fat absorption?
    d. Gastrocolic fistulas
13. A condition where the bile duct may be obstructed is called:
    d. All of the previous responses
14. Sudan III is used to:
    a. Dye lipids

Review Questions, Chapter Sixteen

1. What is the major reason that gastric juices are not considered a "major" body fluid?
   d. All of the previous responses
2. The organism, *Helicobacter pylori*, is implicated in:
   e. Peptic ulcers
3. A condition that is rarely found when examining gastric fluids is:
   a. Presence of malignant cells
4. Why would the gastric juices prevent the presence of many pathogens in the stomach?
   a. Low acidity inhibits bacterial growth
5. Which of the following would not be a hormone found in gastric juices?
   c. Vitamin B_{12}
6. Gastric glands may secrete up to mL during a meal.
   d. 800 mL
7. Gastric fluid is generally collected by:
   c. Nasal tube aspiration

Review Questions, Chapter Seventeen

1. Describe the proper cleaning procedures used for the objectives.
   Objectives should be carefully cleaned and dried using only lens paper. NEVER leave oil on the objectives as the sealant around the lens of the objective may be

affected by oil and cause seepage into the interior of the objective, which results in considerable cost for replacement objectives.

2. List the major types of microscopes and the uses for each of them.
Bright-field microscope—for general microscopy
Phase contrast—for use when viewing transparent and unstained specimens
Epifluorescent microscope—when viewing cells or organisms coated with antibodies that are coated with a fluorescent dye
Electron microscope—research and teaching purposes where extremely small objects are to be visualized

3. What are the powers of the three most common objectives, and in conjunction with the oculars, what is the magnification for each?

10 power	100 times actual size
40 power	400 times actual size
100 power	1000 times actual size

4. When is it advantageous to use a phase contrast microscope?
When transparent and unstained objects are to be studied

5. Name the major components of the bright-field microscope.
Arm
Oculars
Objectives
Base
Stage
Condenser
Iris diaphragm
Light source
Fine and coarse adjustments

Appendix D: Case Study Answers

Case Study 5.1

1. What type of stain did the laboratory technologist most likely use for this test?
   Prussian blue dye
2. What are the cells called that contained the granules?
   Siderophages
3. What would be the likely condition from which the accident victim is suffering?
   A cerebral hemorrhage has occurred, with leaking of fresh blood into the sub-arachnoid space of the skull

Case Study 6.1

1. What other test(s) would he perform?
   A 2-h glucose tolerance
2. If the blood glucose values are elevated, what condition would he most likely consider?
   Type II diabetes
3. What would be the best way to approach treatment for this patient?
   Prescribing a special diet and regular exercise

Case Study 6.2

1. Should the laboratory technologist accept this sample?
   No, the sample should be in a bag with a tamper proof seal to prevent exchange of the sample during transportation; a donor consent form is required
2. Would the sample results stand up in a court of law?
   No, it has been improperly transported and does is not accompanied by a signed donor consent form

© Springer International Publishing AG, part of Springer Nature 2018
J. W. Ridley, *Fundamentals of the Study of Urine and Body Fluids*,
https://doi.org/10.1007/978-3-319-78417-5

Case Study 7.1

1. What are the abnormal values?
   Leukocyte esterase, protein, leukocytes
2. What is a reason for a negative nitrite result when bacteria were seen microscopically?
   The bacteria may not be a species capable of reducing nitrate to nitrite
3. What is the probable diagnosis for this patient?
   Acute glomerulonephritis

Case Study 7.2

1. What are the abnormal values found in this report?
   Leukocyte esterase, protein, erythrocytes. leukocytes
2. What is a reason for a negative nitrite result when bacteria were seen microscopically?
   The bacteria may not be a species capable of reducing nitrate to nitrite
3. What would likely be seen upon Gram staining the urine sediment?
   In addition to the blood and epithelial cells, bacteria should be seen
4. Can *S. saprophyticus* be the causative agent for a urinary infection
   Yes, in somewhat rare cases
5. What is the most probable diagnosis for this patient's condition.
   Acute glomerulonephritis

Case Study 7.3

1. What are the abnormal values found in this report?
   High specific gravity, positive ketones, high level of glucose
2. What is the reason for yeast cells being found?
   Commonly found in urine of persons with glycosuria
3. Why is the specific gravity elevated?
   High levels of glucose will increase the specific gravity as a dissolved constituent
4. What is the probable diagnosis for the young man's condition?
   Diabetes mellitus

Case Study 7.4

1. What are the abnormal values found in this report?
   Color, character, protein, blood, microscopic erythrocytes
2. What is the clinical significance of the patient's medical history?

He has suffered from several throat infections, although he did not seek medical attention for most of them.

3. What is the probable diagnosis for the condition from which the patient is suffering?

The facial edema and the presence of protein and red blood cells in the urine, accompanied by dysmorphic erythrocytes, suggest a post-streptococcal autoimmune condition. In some instances, this condition leads to a chronic condition called rheumatic fever.

Case Study 7.5

1. What are the abnormal values found in this report?

Pale color and frothy, high levels of protein, fatty bodies and casts

2. What could contribute to the white froth of the sample?

Fatty bodies and protein

3. What could contribute to the general and the facial edema?

Albumin, which contributes greatly to oncotic pressure, moving tissue fluids into the blood vessels, is low due to the extreme loss of protein, of which albumin is a component.

4. Explain the presence of oval fatty bodies.

Severe glomerular damage is attributable to the presence of fat bodies in the urine.

5. What would be the most likely diagnosis for this patient?

Nephrotic syndrome

Case Study 7.6

1. What are the abnormal values found in this report?

Hazy character and blood

2. What could contribute to the blood in the sample?

Fresh red cells indicate current bleeding

3. What could contribute to the general nausea?

Extreme pain

4. What would be the most likely diagnosis for this patient?

Urinary calculi (kidney stones)

Case Study 7.7

1. What other characteristics of this disease might be observed?

Anemia, diarrhea, delirium

2. What dietary material is deficient in those suffering from this condition?

Tryptophan-poor diet of salt pork, cane syrup and cornmeal

3. What will be the likely diagnosis of this man's condition?
Pellagra

Case Study 8.1

1. What are the abnormal values found in this report?
Color, high levels of bilirubin
2. If the urine were shaken, what would the laboratory technician expect to see?
Yellow bubbles in the urine
3. Explain the differences between high levels of urobilinogen and of bilirubin.
High levels of bilirubin are related to liver disease or to hemolytic conditions of the red blood cells. Bilirubin passes through the bile duct and into the intestine, where bacterial action converts the bilirubin to urobilinogen.
4. What is the probable diagnosis for the condition from which this woman is suffering?
Since the urobilinogen is normal but the bilirubin level is high, the bilirubin is being prevented from reaching the intestine. This is most likely due to an obstruction of the bile duct by gall bladder "stones."

Case Study 8.2

1. What are the abnormal values found in this report?
4+ amorphous crystals and slight turbidity
2. What could contribute to the turbidity of the sample?
Sediment that has accumulated due to dissolved materials in the urine
3. Explain the presence of the amorphous crystals.
During refrigeration, amorphous phosphates formed, due to the alkaline urine sample. The technician did not allow the urine sample to warm to ambient temperature which may have caused the amorphous sediment to dissolve.
4. What would be the most likely diagnosis for this patient?
No medical abnormality is traced to the urine values

Case Study 9.1

1. What are the abnormal values found in this report?
Dark with cloudy character, Positive Leukocyte esterase but negative leukocytes for microscopic evaluation, Positive reaction for blood, but rare RBC for microscopic evaluation
2. What could contribute to the turbidity of the sample?
The technologist noted that the sample felt cool to the touch; perhaps sample was refrigerated before transport to the laboratory

3. Explain the presence of the amorphous crystals.
   Alkaline pH and refrigeration would result in amorphous phosphate crystals
4. What would be the most likely reason for the disparity in the chemical analysis and the microscopic findings? Please explain fully.
   The sample may have been delayed in its transport to the laboratory, and was refrigerated, leading to the formation of amorphous phosphates, due to an alkaline pH
   The chemical presence of protein, leukocyte esterase, and blood indicate that both erythrocytes and leukocytes were initially present in the sample; the presence of protein may have indicated the presence of casts

Case Study 10.1

1. What are the abnormal values found in this report?
   Color, high levels of bilirubin
2. If the urine were shaken, what would the laboratory technician expect to see?
   Yellow bubbles in the urine
3. Explain the differences between high levels of urobilinogen and of bilirubin.
   High levels of bilirubin are related to liver disease or to hemolytic conditions of the red blood cells. Bilirubin passes through the bile duct and into the intestine, where bacterial action converts the bilirubin to urobilinogen.
4. What is the probable diagnosis for the condition from which this woman is suffering?
   Since the urobilinogen is normal but the bilirubin level is high, the bilirubin is being prevented from reaching the intestine. This is most likely due to an obstruction of the bile duct by gall bladder "stones."

Case Study 11.1

1. What would be the procedure most probably performed upon this child?
   Lumbar puncture
2. What would be the significance of increased lymphocytes?
   Viral infections most often result in an increased lymphocyte count
3. Upon microscopic examination of the CSF from this patient, cells resembling lymphocytes were seen in great numbers. In addition to being white cells called lymphocytes, what is the other possibility for a causative organism?
   A yeast called *Cryptococcus neoformans*
4. What is the next step to confirm the organism suggested in the previous question?
   India ink prep
5. What would be the most likely diagnosis for this patient?
   Meningitis caused by *C. neoformans*

Case Study 12.1

1. What is/are the abnormality(ies) found in this semen evaluation, if any?
   Delayed liquefaction
2. What would be the most likely solution to the problem(s) if any are present?
   Delayed liquefaction would prevent ease of movement of the sperm cells to the cervix, as they would most likely be enmeshed in a viscous fluid from which they could not escape

Case Study 13.1

1. In comparing the serum protein and the value of the protein of the effusion, is this an exudates or a transudate?
   Since body fluids are considered a transudate when the total proteins are low, this is a transudate. The normal ratio of pleural protein in comparison to that of blood, a ratio of greater than 0.5 would be an exudate. The calculation below shows this is markedly a transudate.
   Ratio calculation: $1.1/7.1 = 0.15$
2. What would be the significance of increased lymphocytes?
   Viral infection is indicated
3. Why is another reason that this fluid not considered an exudate, even when the ratio of fluid to serum protein that matches that for a transudate is known?
   An exudate is obtained from an accumulation of plasma proteins and cells, and gives a much more concentrated sample, with higher values than those of transudates.

Case Study 14.1

1. What is the name for this accumulation of fluid in a major joint?
   Effusion related to an inflammatory exudate (may be infectious or crystal-induced)
2. How are acute infectious processes causing bacterial arthritis ruled out?
   Both Gram stain and cultures were negative
3. To what can the turbidity of the sample be attributed?
   Elevated white cell count and possible crystals
4. What is the condition most likely diagnosed?
   Urate gout, since the presence of MSU crystals are consistent with this diagnosis, and an infectious condition was ruled out since the Gram stain and bacterial cultures were negative.

Glossary

Abdominopelvic Combination term for the body cavity below the diaphragm; encompasses the gastrointestinal system and the genitourinary system

Acetoacetic acid A ketone body, CH_3COCH_2COOH, formed when fats are incompletely oxidized. It appears in urine in abnormal amounts in starvation and in untreated diabetes, primarily type 1 diabetes

Acetone It has a sweet, fruity, ethereal odor and is found in the blood and urine of diabetics, in those with other metabolic disorders, and after lengthy fasting. It is produced when fats are not properly oxidized due to inability to oxidize glucose in the blood

Acid phosphatase An enzyme that works under **acid** conditions and is made in the liver, spleen, bone marrow and the prostate gland

Acid-base disorders Acids and bases are used to used to maintain a slightly alkaline pH of the blood; interaction of hydrogen ions and bicarbonate ions are the chief components involved in this process

Acidity Refers to a preponderance of hydrogen ions leading to an acid pH

Acute glomerulonephritis In general, glomerulonephritis refers to a sterile inflammatory condition that often follows a Group A, Beta-hemolytic streptococcal infection that is characterized by edema, hematuria, and proteinuria; may include RBCs and casts of RBCs

Acute interstitial nephritis Renal dysfunction with inflammation of the renal interstitium but no glomerular or vascular abnormalities. Pyelonephritis, drug toxicity, septicemia, graft rejection, and immune disorders are related to this condition

Acute phase reactants A group of proteins are produced and activated or released in during the acute phase of a reaction to a pathogen; includes complement, fibrinogen; C-reactive protein; glycoprotein, serum amyloid A, and proteinase inhibitors

Acute tubular necrosis Failure of the kidney tubules resulting most often from cessation of blood supply to renal tubes following trauma

Addis count Quantitation of solid components in a 24-h urine specimen; has largely been replaced by more specific laboratory procedures

Adrenergic blockers Substances that prevent sympathetic nerve transmission

© Springer International Publishing AG, part of Springer Nature 2018
J. W. Ridley, *Fundamentals of the Study of Urine and Body Fluids*,
https://doi.org/10.1007/978-3-319-78417-5

Adrenocorticosteroids Hormones produced by adrenal cortex of the superior portion of the kidney; may be synthetically produced

Agglutination Physical phenomenon of clumping of complexed particles, such as antigens and antibodies or between red blood cells and coated latex particles

Aldosterone A mineralocorticoid hormone produced in the adrenal cortex; important in the facilitation of potassium exchange for sodium in distal renal tubule; results chiefly in sodium reabsorption

Aliquots Small representations of a large amount of specimen; ie., a few mLs of a 24-h urine specimen

Alkalinity State of being alkaline with a pH of greater than 7.0

Alkaptonuria Inherited condition where large amounts of homogentisic acid is found in the urine through incomplete metabolism of tyrosine and phenylalanine; results in oxidation and darkening of urine as a clinical manifestation of the disease

Alpha-fetoprotein Antigen normally present in the human fetus and in certain disease states of adults; important in diagnosing open neural conditions

Alveoli tiny air sacs located at the very ends of the bronchioles of the lungs where an exchange of oxygen and carbon dioxide occurs

Alzheimer's disease Chronic and degenerative cognitive disorder that progresses to complete disability

Ambient Surrounding conditions; term often used when referring to room temperature

Amer. Assn. of Blood Banks Professional group that accredits and governs blood banks

Amino acids Organic molecule of which proteins are constructed; contains a nitrogenous amino group (NH_2) and a carboxyl (COOH) group

Aminoaciduria Presence of excessive levels of amino acids in the urine; a low level is found in healthy individuals

Ammonia Alkaline gas resulting from breakdown of amino acids and proteins; converted to urea in liver

Amniocentesis Puncture of the fetal amniotic sac and aspiration of fluid from the sac

Amniotic fluid Fluid surrounding the developing fetus

Amorphous phosphates Shapeless and small crystals found in some alkaline urine samples

Amorphous sediment General term referring to the presence of amorphous phosphates and amorphous urates

Amorphous urates Shapeless and small crystals found in some acid urine samples

Amyloidosis Deposition of protein-containing fibril-shaped components that are deposited in tissues

Analgesics Drug that relieves pain

Analyte Material that is being tested for to determine levels of the product

Anemia Literally means "without blood" and refers to low levels of red blood cells or hemoglobin content of the red blood cells

Angiotensin Vasopressor that elevates blood pressure and is produced when kidneys release renin

Anorexia Decreased appetite or loss of appetite

Antibodies Substance produced by B-lymphocytes called plasma cells as a reaction to the presence of pathogens and incompatible substances

Antibody titer Serial dilutions to determine a semi-quantitative level of a certain antibody

Anticoagulant Substance that delays or prohibits the formation of a clot in blood

Antidiuretic hormone (ADH) Naturally occurring hormone that lessens the formation of urine: also is produced as a synthetic agent

Antigens Any substance that is capable of causing the production of antibodies in one with a normal immune system

Antimicrobial therapy Medication such as an antibiotic against bacterial microorganisms or other preparations that react specifically against fungal elements

Antinuclear Production of antibodies against the DNA of cellular nuclei

Antistreptolysin O Antibody against the exotoxin produced and used for identification of infections by Group A Beta-hemolytic streptococci

Antoni van Leeuwenhoek Person generally given credit for producing the forerunner to today's modern light microscope

Anuria Lack of urine production

Aquaporin Cell membrane that allows water to flow into and out of cells

Arachnoid mater Spider web-like lining of the central nervous system

Arachnoid villi Tufts or projections of the arachnoid membrane

Argentaffin cells Those that react with silver salts to produce black or brown color

Arteriole stenosis Narrowing of small arteries

Arthralgia Pain in synovial joints

Arthritides Inflammation of joints due to inflammation as well as of other origins

Arthrocentesis Puncture of the membrane of a synovial joint for aspirating fluid

Articular Point where two structures such as bones move against each other

Artificial insemination Mechanical injection of spermatozoa into the uterus

Ascites Accumulation of fluid causing engorgement of a body cavity; refers primarily to the peritoneal cavity

Ascorbic acid Water soluble vitamin C, a strong antioxidant

Aspartate aminotransferase Intracellular enzyme found in high concentrations in the liver, brain, and muscles; high levels indicate necrosis of tissue

Aspermatic Without production of spermatozoa

Astrocytes Neuroglial cells of the central nervous system that are important components of the blood-brain barrier

Astroglia Make up the neuroglial tissue

Atrial natriuretic hormone (ANH) Secreted by the atrial tissue of the heart and influences blood pressure, volume and circulatory output

Atrial natriuretic peptide (ANP) Peptide hormone secreted by myocytes of the cardiac atria; influence salt and water excretion

Autoimmune reaction   Medical conditions where the body does not recognize tissues of the organism and reacts against them

Bacillus subtilis   Small rod-shaped Gram-positive bacterium that produces an antibiotic similar to penicillin and is used to determine sterility

Bacteria/yeast   Bacteria and yeasts cells are not normally present in urine, unless bacterial contamination occurs

Bacteriostatic   Inhibits bacterial growth but does not kill the organisms

Bartholin's glands   Pair of small mucus glands located on each side of the wall of the vestibule of the vagina

Basophils   White blood cell that dyes a basic color; release histamine and chemicals that cause dilation of blood vessels, enhancing capillary permeability

Bayer Diagnostics Clinitek   Instrument used to optically determine color changes in chemically impregnated pad of urine dipsticks in the presence of a number of analytes

Bence-Jones protein   Proteinuria due to increased serum protein levels is excretion of Bence Jones protein by persons with multiple myeloma-this protein coagulates at temperatures between 40 and 60 °C

Berger's disease   Pathological condition of the kidneys where an immunoglobulin, IgA, causes deposits of the IgA antibody in the glomeruli

Beta-hydroxybutyric acid   Ketone body that is a derivative of butyric acid and is elevated in both blood and urine ketosis

Bicarbonate ion HCO_3^- (bicarbonate ion) is important in regulation of the pH of the blood

Biconcave   As in a red blood cell, both sides of the disc-shaped cell are thinner in the middle, creating a "central pallor"

Bilirubin   Yellow pigment that arises from red blood cell lysis

Binocular microscope   Microscope with two oculars

Biohazards   Materials of a biological origin that may harbor or transmit infectious diseases

Birefringent   Refers to the ability of some crystals or other objects to rotate or polarize light beams, becoming visible when view with polarizing filters

Blastoderm   Germinal disk containing early development stages of the embryo on the surface of the egg yolk

Blood urea nitrogen   Originates from the breakdown of amino acids for energy production, resulting in nitrogen containing urea

Blood–brain barrier (BBB)   Structures that prevent the passage of certain drugs and constituents of the blood plasma from passage into the brain

Boric acid   Preservative commonly used for inhibiting the growth of bacteria, which would destroy certain components of a body fluid

Bowman's capsule   Widened and cup-shaped end of a renal nephron where glomeruli are located

Bright-field microscope   Microscope which receives illumination from a direct light source

Burning glass   Hand-held magnifying glass

Calcitriol   A form of vitamin D that is responsible for regulating calcium metabolism

Calcium oxalate   A crystal form of calcium present in some kidney stones

Calcium pyrophosphate dehydrate   Deposition often found in gouty arthritis

Calculus (urine, body fluids)   Deposits of minerals, often called a "stone"

Campylobacter   Bacterial organism often implicated in presence of peptic ulcers

Candida albicans   Species of yeast found in moniliasis, infection of urinary tract

Candidiasis   Condition of infection with the organism *Candida albicans*

Carbohydrates   Group of chemicals comprised of C, H, and O; includes sugars, glycogen, starches, dextrins and cellulose

Carbonates   Strong alkali as a salt of carbonic acid

Carcinoid tumors   Tumor from neuroendocrine cells of intestinal tract, bile ducts pancreas, and other organs; secrete serotonin

Cardiac tamponade   Increased pressure on the heart inhibits filling with blood during diastole

Cartilaginous   Contains dense connective tissue related to cartilage

Casts   Casts only elements found in the urinary sediment that are unique to the urinary tract

Catecholamines   Amine derived from the amino acid tyrosine, and have dramatic effect on nervous and cardiac function; include epinephrine, dopamine

Catheterized specimen   Urine sample obtained by use of sterile tube inserted into the bladder via the urethra

CDCP   Centers for Disease Control and Prevention

Celiac disease   Malabsorption in the intestine resulting in diarrhea and weight loss; often results from immunological response to wheat products

Centrifuge   Instrument used to separate heavier particles from solution by rapid spinning, using centrifugal force to obtain layering of constituents

Cephalexin   Cephalosporin antibiotic that is effective against mostly Gram-positive bacteria, but against limited number of Gram-negative species

Cerebral herniation   Tearing of the brain tissue of the cerebrum

Cerebrospinal fluids   Main reason for evaluation of CSF to determine meningitis, stroke or trauma to the brain or spine

Cervix   Part of an organ resembling a neck

Cesarean section   Surgical extraction of a fetus from the uterus

Chain of infection   Tracing the transmission of an infective organism from its origin

Chain-of-custody   Documentation of the steps in the transport of a biological specimen; sometimes of a legal nature

Chlamydia trachomatis   A species of bacteria that may be the causative agent in genital infections of men and women; less frequently in other organ involvement

Chlorhexidine   Strong topical antiseptic agent

Cholelithiasis   Presence of gall bladder stones

Cholera   Causative agent, *Vibrio cholerae*, infects the small intestine, resulting in profuse water and secretory diarrhea, leading to dangerous dehydration

Chondrocytes   Cartilage cell

Chorionic villus   Vascular projections from the chorion of the fetal portion of the placenta

Choroid plexus   Comprised of cells that produce the cerebrospinal fluid (CSF) in the ventricles of the brain and in the subarachnoid space around the brain

Chronic glomerulonephritis   Variety of disorders that produce continual or permanent damage to the glomerulus. Elevated serum levels of blood urea nitrogen, creatinine, and phosphorous and decreased serum calcium levels are seen in the progression to end—stage renal disease

Chronic pancreatitis   Long-standing inflammation of the pancreas

Chymotrypsin   Digestive enzyme secreted by the pancreas

Ciliated   Possesses long hair like cilia extending from periphery of the cell

Citric acid   Weak organic acid essential is a central metabolic pathway called the citric energy cycle

CLSI   Clinical and Laboratory Standards Institute

CLIA   Clinical Laboratory Improvement Amendments

Clinitest   Tablet test for presence of reducing substances in urine and feces

Clostridium difficile   Bacterial organism causing necrosis of intestine when colonized

Coagulate   Congeal or form a gel-like material

Coarse adjustment   Microscopic adjustment that is used prior to finely focusing the image

Coelom   Tube-like opening

Coitus interruptus   Halting act of copulation to collect semen sample

Coliforms   General term for types of bacteria found in the intestines

Collagen   Strong, fibrous protein found in connective tissues

CAP   College of American Pathologists

Colligative properties   Any property that depends on the number of solute particles in a solution, but not the identity of the particles, but how they physically interact

Colonoscopic exam   Endoscopic examination of the lower gastrointestinal system

Color   Refers to the hue imparted to body fluids by the constituents contained in the biological sample

Color-blind   Genetic inability to differentiate between certain colors; affects males most frequently

Common bile duct   Tube-like passage that is formed by the union of the common duct from the liver, the cystic duct from the gall bladder, and the pancreatic duct

Complement   Group of proteins that directly destroy organisms and cells following opsonization, or coating of the cell or organism

Computerized tomography   Commonly known as the CAT scan; tomes or leaf-like radiographs are integrated by computerized programs to produce detailed imagery of an organ or parts of the entire body

Concave   Having a depressed or hollow surface

Condenser   Substage lens of the microscope that condenses light for illumination of a target object

Congestive heart failure   Accumulation of fluids in the pericardium that impacts upon the function of the heart

Contaminants   Organisms or chemical materials that affect the sterility of materials or proper reactions by chemicals

Convex   Curved evenly and outwardly from a surface

Coproporphyrins   Precursor to heme that is found in feces and urine

Cortex   Renal cortex is the outer layer of the kidney and is made up of the glomeruli of the nephrons and the proximal convoluted tubules

Cortisol   Glucorticoid hormone of the adrenal gland cortex

Cowper's gland   Bulbourethral glands of the male reproductive system

Creatinine   Waste product derived from the metabolism of phosphocreatine

Creatinine clearance   Procedure designed to determine the glomerular flow rate (GFR)

Creatine kinase   Enzyme that catalyzes transfer of phosphate between creatine and phosphocreatine

Crohn's disease   Inflammatory disease of the bowel where patches of deep-seated inflammation occurs in the gastrointestinal system, ranging from the oral cavity to the anus

Cryptococcus neoformans   A pathogenic species of yeast like fungus that may cause meningitis

Crystals   Crystalline formation of chemicals into stone-like configurations

Cushing's syndrome   Group of symptoms and signs caused by excessive exposure to glucocorticoid hormones

Cystic fibrosis   Chronic genetic disease that affects multiple body systems; causes chronic obstructive pulmonary disease with frequent lung infections, as well as other severe manifestations

Cystinuria   Hereditary condition with excretion of large amounts of cystine, lysine, arginine, and ornithine in the urine; recurrent urinary calculi usually accompany the disease

Cystitis   Bladder inflammation due to urinary tract infection

Cytocentrifugation   Process where special cytofuge is used to slowly rotate and accomplish a thin area of cellular distribution which is then stained for microscopic examination

Cytogenetic   Related to study of chromosomes as to structure and function

Cytological   Examinations based on cellular presence and morphology

Cytomegalovirus   Specific herpes-virus organism capable of causing viral damage to developing fetus

Cytometry   Counting of and measuring of cells

D-dimer fibrin   A fibrin degradation product (FDP) is a small protein fragment found in the blood following formation of a blood clot is degraded by fibrinolysis (destruction of fibrin clot)

Deciliter   One tenth of a liter, or 100 mL (mL)

Decontamination   Procedure in which a contaminant or an undesirable element has been introduced to a specimen is remedied; cleaning of work surfaces with an effective antiseptic solution to prevent transmission of infectious organisms

Dehydration   Removal of water from the body or from a chemical preparation

Deionized water   Process where all charged particles (ions) have been removed from the water, to be used as a solvent

Demyelinating   Removal or destruction of the myelin sheath surrounding nerve tissue

Denature   To deprive a chemical of its natural character or physical properties, rendering it harmless or unable to react chemically

DOT   Department of Transportation

Diabetes insipidus   Refers to a condition in which the kidneys are unable to conserve water due to lack of effective antidiuretic hormone (ADH)

Diabetes mellitus   Group of metabolic diseases characterized by high blood sugar (glucose) levels, that result from defects in insulin levels or defects

Diabetic nephropathy   Diabetic nephropathy leading to reduced glomerular filtration is a common occurrence in persons with diabetes mellitus can first be predicted by detection of microalbuminuria

Diapedesis   Refers to the passage of blood cells through intact vessel walls, moving from the vascular system to surrounding tissues

Diaphragm   Chief muscle involved in inspiration of air into lungs; thin, dome-shaped sheet of muscle that inserts into the lower ribs

Diluent   Refers to a diluting agent for preparation of medications and reagents for laboratory procedures

Distal convoluted tubule   Tubules of the nephron that are located the greatest distance from the glomerulus where reabsorption of sodium and elimination of hydrogen ions occurs

Diuretics   Medication designed to increase the rate of urination

Diurnal   Functions that occur over a 24-h period

Dry tap   A dry tap occurs when the puncture of a body site for aspirating fluid results in no yield of sample

Ductules   Small or minute ducts

Dura mater   The dura mater is the outermost of the three layers of the meninges, membranes that surround the brain and spinal cord

Dysmorphia   Refers to misshapen structures, such as red blood cells that are not of a normal biconcave and disc-like shape

Eczema-like rash   May appear as a ringworm-like rash of circular, itchy, scaling patches and is related to a variety of medical conditions

Edema   Swelling, or enlargement and engorgement of tissues

Effusion   Refers to excess fluid that accumulates in the pleural cavities of the body

Ejaculate   The ejection of semen, that may carrying sperm, unless aspermatic, from the male reproductive tract

Electrolytes   The term "electrolyte" is any substance occurring as free ions that make a substance capable of conducting electric impulses

Electrophoresis   Laboratory procedure that provides for the separation of charged molecules on a specially prepared plate that is exposed to an electric current

End—stage renal disease   A chronic condition where kidney disease is an almost complete failure of the kidneys to fulfill their metabolic functions

Endocarditis   Inflammation of the innermost layer of heart tissue

Endocrine cells Specialized glandular secretory tissue cells that secret specific into the blood (internally) rather than on an epithelial surface

Engineered Controls Systems including hardware and software designed to protect health care employees and patients

Eosinophils Specialized white blood cells with coarse distinct granules and a bilobed nucleus that are important in immune responses during an allergic attack

Ependymal Refers to tissue cells which line the ventricles of the brain

Epididymis Part of the male reproductive system; long and narrow, tightly-coiled tube connecting the efferent ducts to the vas deferens

Epinephrine Secreted by the adrenal gland when the sympathetic nervous system is stimulated

Epithelial cells Renal epithelial cells are the most significant type as they indicate tubular necrosis

Epstein-Barr virus A herpesvirus family that is one of the most common viruses to infect humans

Erythroblastosis fetalis Hemolytic disease of the fetus and newborn as a result of blood group or type difference between mother and fetus; results in anemia and may be life-threatening

Erythrocytes Red blood cells that carry oxygen and carbon dioxide

Erythrophagia Term that indicates destruction of red blood cells by phagocytes (macrophages) that ingest cells and foreign materials

Erythropoietin (EPO) Natural hormone produced by the kidney but that is also available as a synthetic version, promotes the formation of red blood cells in the reticuloendothelial system (bone marrow)

Escherichia coli Commonly encountered Gram negative rod-shaped bacterium common in urinary tract infections

Estrogen The main sex hormone in women that is responsible for menstruation cycles and reproduction

Exposure incidents Scenario where a person comes in contact with a potentially biohazardous material

Extracellular fluid Fluid found outside the cell, and often surrounding the cells

Extrachoroidal CSF resulting from origins other than extrachoroidal formation and comes in part from ultrafiltration from cerebral capillaries

Exudates Exudates produced by conditions that directly involve membranes of the particular cavity, including infections and malignancies

Eyepieces Cylindrical projections from the optical tube of the compound microscope, usually equipped for a 10-power magnification

Fallopian tubes Two tubes that are included in the reproductive organs; responsible for transporting the egg from the ovary to the uterus

FDA Federal Drug Administration

Fecal analysis As an end-product of body metabolism, fecal exams provide diagnostic information to determine gastrointestinal bleeding, liver

Fern test Important in the detection of leakage of amniotic fluid from the amnion surrounding the fetus during pregnancy

Fertility Ability to reproduce

Fine adjustment   Adjustment knob on the microscope used for final adjustments to focus on fine details of microscopic structures

Foley catheter   Tube for insertion into bladder to potentiate urination; contains a bulb associated with the tip of the catheter that is injected with water to maintain the position of the catheter in the bladder; sometimes called an "indwelling catheter"

Formalin   Dilute formaldehyde that dessicates tissues and is used for preservation of tissue samples. Frequently seen in children and young adults following respiratory tract infections caused by certain strains of' group A streptococci

Fructose   A monosaccharide with 6 carbon atoms; found in juices and syrups and contains same simple formula as glucose

Galactose   Monosaccharide that is an isomer of glucose

Gamma globulin   Portion of total protein, the gamma portion, is a blood plasma protein which includes antibodies against infective organisms

Gastric acidity   Presence of hydrogen ions that prevent passage of bacteria to intestines and that aids in the breakdown of food to digestible states

Gastric contents   Includes ingested food, mucus, digestive enzymes

Gastric   Gastric acidity results from the secretion of hydrochloric acid by the parietal cells in the stomach. Cells also responsible for production of hormones and other products

Gastrin   Hormone of the mucosal tissue of the pyloric area of the stomach that stimulates the production of gastric acid

Gastrocolic fistulas   Opening or communication creating a passageway between the gastric epithelium and epithelium of the colon; may be malignant or benign and is sometimes a complication of a gastric ulcer or gastroenterostomy (mouth-like opening)

Gastrointestinal system   Includes all of the digestive organs from the mouth to the anus

Gelatinous   Resembling a gel

Genitourinary system   Series of organs that comprise the reproductive and excretory organs of the lower peritoabdominal cavity and associated external genitalia

Gentian violet stain   Topical gentian violet that may be used to treat some types of fungal infections of the mouth, skin and genitalia

Gestation   Period of elapsed time or required period for development of an embryo or fetus

Giardia lamblia   Parasite that causes a condition called giardiasis, contracted from contaminated food and water, and colonizes the intestines; may progress to other tissues of the body

Glomerular filtrate   Includes water, waste products, salt, glucose, and other chemicals that have been filtered out of the blood and are for the most part reabsorbed before liquid is excreted from the body

Glomerulus (p. glomeruli)   Refers to a capillary tuft involved in the initial step of filtering blood as products to eliminate in the urine; surrounded by Bowman's capsule in the nephrons of the kidney

Glucose   Basic monosaccharide used as energy sources by the body

Glucose tolerance test   Administration of a measured amount of glucose, after which blood and urine are tested periodically to determine adequate levels and functions of insulin

Glycogenesis   Term refers to the synthesis of glycogen, as glucose molecules are added to chains of glycogen for storage

Glycolysis   The metabolic pathway that converts glucose $C_6H_{12}O_6$, into pyruvate as the major energetic process in living cells

Glycoprotein   Compound that includes a carbohydrate and a glucose molecule

Glycosuria   Indicates detectable levels of glucose in the urine

Gonads   Reproductive organs that produce sperm cells in males and eggs in females

Goodpasture's syndrome   An autoimmune condition that occurs if an individual's immune system mistakenly attacks and destroys healthy body tissue

Gout   inflammatory, metabolic condition that results in high levels of uric acid that may deposit uric acid crystals in joints of the body

Gouty arthritis   Arthritic condition of the synovial joints due to uric acid deposition

Gram negative bacilli   Rod-shaped bacteria that stain a pink color when Gram stain methodology is used

Gram positive anaerobic   Organisms that stain Gram positive (purple) and grow in the absence of or reduced levels of oxygen

Gram stain   A method for staining bacteria for initial evaluation, using a four-reagent methodology

Group B streptococci   A grouping of Gram positive cocci that can be passed to an infant during delivery

Guaiac   A method used to detect the presence of occult blood in fecal samples

Haptoglobin   Binds hemoglobin iron to facilitate transfer of this molecule for recycling of iron by producing a molecular complex that is too large to be excreted by kidneys, resulting in conservation of iron

Helicobacter pylori   Bacterial organism that may colonize stomach, and is implicated in the formation of peptic ulcers

Hematochezia   The passage of bright red, bloody fecal samples usually signifies bleeding of the large intestine

Hematospermia   Presence of blood in the semen

Hematoxylin   Type of stain used for staining tissue samples for pathological examination

Hematuria   Gross or microscopic blood in the urine

Heme   Non-protein portion of a hemoglobin molecule that contains iron

Hemocytometer   Specialized slide the is marked into microscopic grids and is used for quantitation of cells and other microscopic entities

Hemoglobin   Iron-containing pigment of red blood cells that is capable of carrying oxygen throughout the body

Hemoglobin F   Fetal hemoglobin mostly occurs at the form of hemoglobin that transports oxygen around the body of the developing baby during the last 7 months of pregnancy

Hemoglobinuria Presence of hemoglobin in the urine

Hemolytic disease of the newborn Antibody-antigen incompatibility between the mother and the developing fetus may result in destruction of the baby's red blood cells when gamma globulin antibodies pass across the amniotic barrier

Hemophilia Blood coagulation disorder in which one or more clotting factors are missing, resulting in spontaneous bleeding and in minor accidents causing bruising

Haemophilus influenza Bacterial microorganism named for its occurrence in the sputum of patients with influenza, where it was first discovered; not always confined to the respiratory system

Hemorrhagic fluid Liquid sample of body fluid that contains blood

Hemosiderin Molecule concerned with iron storage; aggregate of ferritin molecules

Hemosiderin-haptoglobin Hemoglobinuria is the result of lysis of red blood cells from the urinary tract, or by intravascular hemolysis with filtering of hemoglobin through the glomeruli

Hemostasis The cessation of blood flow from a wound by the formation of a clot from factors present in the blood

Heparinized Use of heparin, an anticoagulant, to preserve blood in a liquid state

Hepatitis Generalized inflammatory condition of the liver

Hepatitis B (HBV) One of the types of hepatitis as a result of the hepatitis B virus

Herniation Abnormal protrusion of an organ or tissue through a tear; common herniations are inguinal and abdominal

Herpes simplex Herpes simplex virus organisms, of which there are several types, occurs primarily around the mouth or genital area; signs of the condition consists of painful blisters or ulcers that are found most often on the mouth, lips and gums, or genitals

Histalog Betazole hydrochloride is used in a test for measuring maximal production of gastric acidity or lack of acidity (anacidity)

Histopathologic Pathologic conditions determined by microscopic study of diseased tissues and organs

Homeostasis Refers to the body's ability to remain physiologically stable or "as is" through regulation of metabolism by controlled reactions

Homocystinuria Considered a somewhat mild inherited disorder that affects the metabolism of the amino acid methionine

Homovanillic acid A major metabolite of dopamine, a neurotransmitter, plasma levels of *homovanillic acid* are used as a peripheral measure of dopamine activity

Hormones A chemical messenger that is released by tissues or glands in one part of the body that transmits messages that affect cells in other tissues and organs

Human Immunodeficiency Virus (HIV) Retrovirus (RNA) that causes infections that may lead to Acquired Immunodeficiency Syndrome (AIDS)

Humoral immune complexes Refers to a humoral (plasma-based) immune response involving combining of antibody and antigen, forming a complex

Humors Refers to fluids and semifluids found in the organs and tissues of the body

Hyaluronate (also called hyaluronic acid) Functions chiefly in synovial joints as a tissue lubricant

Hydrocephalus Accumulation of abnormal volumes of cerebrospinal fluid, resulting in changes in increased intracranial pressure and neurological manifestations

Hydrogen chloride A strong acid composed of hydrogen and chloride molecules

Hydrogen ions Positively charged ions (H^+) that are strongly reactive in the acidification of solutions

Hydrogen peroxide A commercial bleaching product that is colorless and syrupy; decomposes readily by releasing an oxygen molecule, converting to water

Hydrolysis Reaction in which water is an active reactant in the formation of a solution such as that of a salt dissolved in water

Hydrophilic molecules The molecules that attract water molecules, such as those with polar covalent bonds

Hydrostatic pressure A position of equilibrium where fluids are not moving

5-hydroxyindoleacetic acid Compound is the main metabolite of serotonin in the human body, and is chiefly tested for in the chemical analysis of urine samples

Hydroxylase An enzyme that introduces hydrogen into a substrate

Hyperbilinuria High levels of bilirubin in the urine

Hyperbilirubinemia High levels of bilirubin in the blood

Hypercalcemia High levels of calcium ions in the blood

Hyperglycemia High levels of glucose in the blood

Hypernatremia High levels of sodium in the blood

Hypoglycemia Low levels of glucose in the blood

Hyponatremia Low levels of sodium in the blood

Hypovolemia Low levels of fluids in the blood

Hypoxia Low levels of oxygen

Iatrogenic Term applied to adverse results from a medical mistake or injury

Ictotest tablet Procedure used to determine the presence of reducing substances other than glucose in urine or feces

IgG An immune globulin that is a particular class of antibodies

Immunoassays Laboratory procedure designed to detect the presence of immunological molecules

Immunofluorescence Process for detecting antibodies that have been "tagged" with fluorescein-labeled proteins

Immunoglobulins Plasma polypeptides produced by B-lymphocyte plasma cells in response to infection by pathogens and other foreign materials

Immunohematology A study of the genetics of blood cells in which ABO groups and Rh types are expressed

Immunophenotypic Technique that employs division based on cell surface antigens and cytoplasmic antigens to differentiate conditions including lymphomas and leukemias into subgroups

India ink prep Microscopic method used to differentiate C. neoformans from lymphocytes, chiefly in cerebrospinal fluid

Indican Potassium salt present in perspiration and urine that is formed when bacteria common to the gastrointestinal system convert tryptophan to indole; also refers to a yellow glycoside as a precursor to a dye called indigo

Indirect testing   Procedures that employ identification of antibodies formed against an organism rather than detection of the organism itself

Indole   Substance present in feces, formed through bacterial decomposition of tryptophan; intestinal obstruction causes absorption of indole that is eliminated as indican

Infection/Exposure Control Committee   Interdisciplinary group often based in a medical center, that is responsible for policies designed to protect both patients and employees from contagious and toxic materials

Insulin   Hormone secreted by beta cells of the pancreas, which controls the cellular absorption of sugars, proteins and fats

Intact red blood cells   In hematuria, microscopic examination can be used to differentiate between hematuria and hemoglobinuria

Internal quality control   Employs techniques where controls developed within the facility rather than obtained from outside commercial enterprises

Interstitial   Refers to a position of occurring in spaces between cells or organs

Intracellular   Refers to components that are present inside a cell

Intracranial   Presence within the skull

Invagination   Refers to an infolding or inward growth within a space

Iodophor   Contains iodine and a chemical carrier that frees iodine in solution

Isoleucine   An essential amino acid derived from the diet

Isopropyl alcohol   "Rubbing' alcohol designed primarily as a skin disinfectant and for topical application

Isotonic   Having equal pressure between two fluids

Joint Commission   The primary accrediting agency for health care facilities

Ketoacid   Substance the increases in blood as a result of faulty metabolism of carbohydrates that may occur in diabetes mellitus

Ketoacidosis   Condition characterized by increased levels of ketone bodies; occurs primarily in patients with inadequate insulin production

Ketones   Substances containing two carbon atoms, and a carbonyl group (C=O)

Ketonuria   Presence of ketone bodies in the urine

Kidney function tests   Chemical procedures that determine the presence of waste products in the blood that are traced to malfunctions of the kidney filtration process

Kidney infarctions   Necrotic tissue that has formed in the kidney; attributed to trauma that reduces blood flow to the kidneys or other disease processes

Kleihauer-Betke   Staining procedure used to determine the presence of fetal red blood cells in the expectant mother's blood, which may occur due to exchanges of blood transplacentally

Kupffer   Term applied to phagocytes found in the liver

Lactate   Process of secreting milk

Lactate dehydrogenase   Enzyme that catalyzes lactate oxidation, and is elevated in tissues such as the blood, lungs, liver, and primarily the heart; lysis of red blood cells will result in an elevated LD

Lactoferrin   Enzyme released by neutrophils and macrophages that combine with iron in the blood

Lactose   Disaccharide sugar that hydrolyzes into glucose and galactose

Lavage   The process of "washing out" a bodily cavity

Lecithin-sphingomyelin   Test which determines the ratio of lecithin to sphingomyelin, to evaluate the maturity of fetal lungs

Leucine   An essential amino acid that must be derived from the diet

Leukemias   Group of malignancies affecting the formation of blood cells

Leukocyte esterase   Test performed on urine samples, to determine the presence of white blood cells that may be either whole cells or lysed cells

Leukocytes   White blood cells; frequent finding in the routine urinalysis is the presence of leukocytes that chiefly indicate a bacterial infection

Liddle's syndrome   Relatively rare hereditary disorder where the kidneys excrete retain too much sodium and water, resulting in high blood pressure

Ligaments   Fibrous connective tissue that binds articular bones together to limit motion and tissues that support certain organs

Light microscopes   Microscopes that utilize an artificial light to illuminate a target object

Lipids   Hydrophobic (water fearing) fat products, a group of naturally occurring molecules that include fats and fat-soluble vitamins

Lipiduria   Presence of fat bodies in the urine

Lipophages   Phagocytes that ingest fat cells

Lithium heparin   Lithium salt of heparin (lithium heparin) is used as an anticoagulant; vacuum tubes for phlebotomy usually identified by green stoppers

Loop of Henle   Structure is a long, U-shaped portion of the tubule that provides a conduit for urine within each nephron of the kidney

Lubricant   Any substance designed to reduce friction between moving parts, such as a joint

Lumbar puncture   Procedure that is also called a spinal tap; cerebrospinal fluid (CSF) surrounding the brain and spinal cord, is tested for hemorrhage, infection and other abnormalities

Lupus erythematosus   Autoimmune disease of a chronic nature; SLE may affect a single organ or multiple organs including the skin, joints, kidneys, and other organs

Lymphocytes   Type of white blood cell that is increased during viral infections

Lymphomas   Malignant growth originating from lymphocytes

Lyophilized   Also known as freeze-drying or cryodesiccation; involves a dehydration process that is primarily used to preserve a perishable material such as quality control specimens

Lyse   Destruction or breakdown of cells, tissue

Macrophages   Type of white cell known as "big eaters," and originates from large white cells called monocytes

Macroscopic   Capable of being seen by the naked eye

Malaise   General lethargy, inattentitiveness, and feelings of fatigue

Maltose   Sugar that is a disaccharide formed by two molecules of glucose

Mannitol   Mannitol is also called a sugar alcohol and is used in some foods and pharmaceuticals

Manometer   Refers to an instrument designed to measure pressure, such as atmospheric pressure

Maple syrup urine disease   An autosomal recessive metabolic disorder that is also called branched-chain ketoaciduria

Marcello Malpighi   Early user of the microscope to study anatomy and physiology of the body, particularly that of the kidney

Material safety data sheet   Informational form provided by the manufacturer, outlining product data and safety procedures associated with the use of the product

Matula   Cup-shaped container used in the Middle Ages for collection and physical observation of urine samples

Medial tubule   Collecting tube of the nephron, located between the proximal and distal portion of the tubule

Medicaid   Federal and state coordinated health insurance program for low income individuals and families

Medicare   Federal health insurance program for retired and disabled individuals who are collecting Social Security benefits

Medulla   The medulla oblongata is the lower half of the brainstem

Melanuria   Excessive levels of melanin in the urine

Melena   Term used to describe black, tarry, and foul-smelling stools

Melituria   General term for "sugar" in the urine

Meninges   Three layers of specialized epithelium inside the skull that encase and protects the central nervous system

Mesoderm   One of the three primary germ cell layers found in an early embryonic stage of development

Mesothelial   Term used for the membrane that forms the lining of several body cavities such as the parietal and abdominal regions

Metabolic acidosis   A condition called metabolic acidosis occurs when the body accumulates too much acid; often occurs when the kidneys are not removing enough acid from the blood and excreting it via the urine

Metastatic   Spread particularly of a malignancy from one organ or type of tissue to another organ or body part of another region of the body

Methemoglobin   Form of hemoglobin that cannot transport oxygen; the ferrous ion has been oxidized to a ferric ion

Methylene blue   Dark green dye that imparts to biological samples a distinctly blue color

Microalbumin   Detection of albumin utilizes a test for diagnosing kidney disorders and often conducted after a diagnosis of hypertension or diabetes

Microbial   Refers to organisms visible only microscopically

Microbiology   Study of organisms too small to be seen with the naked eye

Microhematuria   Hematuria that is visible only with the use of a microscope

Micturition   Act of urinating

Mid-stream clean catch   Refers to collection of urine samples where the initial urine stream is discarded and the mid portion of the sample is collected

Millimeter   Term used in the metric system for one one-thousandth of a meter

Mineralocorticoid   Type of steroid hormone that influences retention of or elimination of salts through the urine

Moniliasis   Another term to describe candidiasis, a yeast infection manifested in the examination of urine samples

Mononuclear cells   Generally refers to white blood cells which have an uninterrupted nuclear material, often in a concentrically circular form; monocytes and lymphocytes are mononuclear

Mononucleosis   Viral infection primarily by the Epstein-Barr virus, resulting in fever, sore throat, and swollen lymph glands of the neck; blood cell morphology often reveals abnormal forms of lymphocytes and

Monosodium urate   Monosodium urate crystals often form in a disorder of purine metabolism called gout; crystals may precipitate in the synovial joints, causing redness and swelling of the affected areas

Mucin clot test   Adding of acetic acid to normal synovial fluid, forming a clot to determine the normalcy of the sample

Mucoid   Similar to tenacious, thick mucus

Mucopolysaccharide   Gel-like, thick material found in basement cells of membranes and present in mucus secretions and synovial fluid

Mucoprotein   Polysaccharide; Tamm-Horsfall protein found in urinary casts is included

Multiple myeloma   Cancer found in the bone marrow that affects proliferation of plasma cells

Multiple sclerosis   Autoimmune disease that affects the central nervous system

Mycobacterium   Term for a yeast-like organism that is the causative organism for tuberculosis and leprosy

Myocardial   Term that refers to the muscles of the heart

Myoglobin   Myoglobin is a protein found in muscle tissue, reacts positively with the chemical test for hemoglobin on urine dipsticks

Necrosis   Death of tissue

Neisseria gonorrhea   Diplococcal form or bacteria that is sexually transmitted

Neisseria meningitidis   Bacterium that is frequently associated with meningitis

Neoplasms   Abnormal new growth, often malignant, of tissue in animals

Nephrogenic   Term associated with diabetes insipidus; a defect in the small tubules of the kidneys where water is hormonally influenced to be reabsorbed causes an individual to pass large amounts of urine

Nephrons   Functional units of the kidneys where excretion and reabsorption occurs

Nephrotic syndrome   Condition is characterized by massive proteinuria, (>3.5 g/day), edema and high levels of serum lipids, accompanied by low levels of serum or plasma albumin

Nephrotoxic agents   Toxic chemicals and drugs, primarily antibiotics, analgesics, and radiographic contrast agents cause shock and injury to the kidneys

Neubauer hemocytometer   Standardized slide with grids designed for microscopically accomplishing accurate counts of cells and other entities found in body fluids

Neutrophils Type of white blood cell that has a segmented nucleus, and is increased chiefly in bacterial infections; neutrophils are capable of becoming phagocytic

Niacin Niacin (nicotinic acid) is the B3 vitamin and is sometimes used to lower cholesterol and triglycerides

Nitrate Nitrogenous compound found in urine samples

Nitrite The reagent strip test for nitrite provides a rapid screening test for the presence of certain bacteria that reduce nitrates to nitrites

Nitrogenenous Containing nitrogen atoms

Nonrenal Indicates conditions other than those associated with the kidneys

Nosepiece and objectives Essential components of a light microscope

Nosocomial Diseases contracted during hospitalization or during a medical procedure

OSHA Occupational Safety and Health Administration

Oculars Eyepieces of a microscope

Odor A physical and noticeable property that may be detected by the olfactory senses of the receiver. Certain odors are found in infectious processes due to metabolic byproducts of microorganisms, and by materials ingested and excreted through the urine, feces, perspiration, etc

Oil immersion Use of immersion oil is necessary for certain microscopic examinations to eliminate light scatter by focusing light beam through the sample being observed

Oliguria Low output of urine over a certain time period

Oncotic pressure Refers to colloidal pressure exerted by proteins, chiefly albumin, in blood plasma that results in water moving into the blood vessels

Opaque Sufficiently turbid as to prevent visibility through the material

OPIM Other potentially infectious materials other than blood

Orthostatic Certain medical conditions are tested for by having the patient in a standing position, such as for proteinuria and blood pressure measurements

Osmolality Osmolality is more accurate reflection of concentration of dissolved

Osmolarity The clinical significance of osmolarity includes the initial evaluation of renal concentrating ability, monitoring the course of renal disease, monitoring fluid and electrolyte therapy, establishing the differential diagnosis of hypernatremia and hyponatremia and polyuria, and evaluating the secretion and renal response to ADH. Normal serum osmolarity values are between 275 and 300 mOsm

Osmoles An osmole (Osm or osmol) is a non-international standard (SI) unit of measurement that indicates the number of moles of a chemical compound that contribute to the concentration

Osmometer An instrument used for measuring osmotic strength of a solution or colloidal mixture

Osmotic Refers to pressure required to cause movement of a fluid across a semipermeable membrane

Osteoarthritis Most common form of arthritis; degenerative condition in a joint caused by cartilage loss where pain and stiffness are symptoms

Ovaries Organs of the female where ova (eggs) are produced, nurtured and released

Ovum Egg produced by the female during a menstrual cycle

Papanicolaou stain Stain used for preparing female cervical specimens for microscopic evaluation

Parathyroid glands Parathormone is secreted by the parathyroid glands to control metabolism of calcium

Parietal layer Forms the wall of the cavity; parietal cells are found as gastric glands of the stomach that secrete hydrogen chloride and the intrinsic factor

Parvovirus Serious viral infection that affects the gastrointestinal or cardiac systems of dogs; a human version also exists

Passive transfer Transfer of fluids from one are to another that does not require energy in order to occur, such as in osmosis

Pathogens Microbiological organism that contribute to a disease process

Pathological Medical condition caused by a disease process

Peak acid output Stimulated by pentagastrin, as the total acid output of the stomach by averaging the two highest consecutive collections

Penicillin One of the early antibiotics discovered

Pentagastrin Preparation used to stimulate secretions by the parietal cells of the stomach

Pentoses A sugar categorized as a monosaccharide, containing five carbon atoms

Pepsin Term for an enzyme found in the stomach that aids in the digestion of proteins by splitting them into smaller pieces called peptides

Perfusion Passage of fluids through the vessels of a specific organ or tissue to provide oxygen and nutrients

Pericardial tamponade Medical condition where compression of the heart occurs as blood or other body fluids build up between the myocardial muscles and the pericardium covering the heart

Pericardium Epithelial lining surrounding the heart

Peritoneal Refers to cavity of the abdominal and pelvic regions

Peritonitis Inflammation of the lining of the abdominopelvic region

Permeability Ability to pass into or out of one compartment through a membrane and into another compartment

Pernicious anemia Characterized by a decrease in red blood cells that occurs due to the inability of the body to properly absorb vitamin B_{12} from the gastrointestinal tract due to a lack of intrinsic factor

PPE Personal Protective Equipment (gowns, gloves, etc.)

Petri dish Flat, lidded plate containing a nutritive agar to facilitate bacterial growth for identification leading to treatment of bacterial infections

pH The acidity or alkalinity of a solution based on an excess of either H^+ (low pH) or OH^- (high pH) ions

Phagocytes White blood cells with a tendency to ingest microorganisms

Phase contrast microscope The phase microscope reveals internal structures of cells and organisms and makes it possible to study living cells

Phenylalanine   Essential amino acid used for the synthesis of proteins in the body, but must be obtained from the diet since the body cannot synthesize phenylalanine

Phenylketonuria   Somewhat rare inherited condition where a newborn lacks the ability to properly break down the amino acid called phenylalanine

Pheochromocytoma   Rare variety of adrenal gland tumor; results in excretion of excessive amounts of the hormones epinephrine and norepinephrine, resulting in abnormalities of heart rate, metabolic functions and blood pressure

Phospholipids   A class of lipids that are a primary component of cell membranes; somewhat resistant to water surrounding the cells

Phosphorous   An element found in bone and other tissues of the body

Pia mater   A somewhat delicate inner layer of the three layers of the meninges, the membranes surrounding the organs of the central nervous system

Plasma   Liquid portion of blood

Pleomorphic   Significant differences in sizes of various cells and organisms

Pleural   Refers to the thoracic cavity

Pneumoencephalography   Diagnostic radiographic procedure where some of the CSF is drained from the cranium and air or gas is injected before X-ray films are made

Podocytes   Epithelial cells of the visceral layer of a renal glomerulus; contain fingerlike radiating processes

POLs   Physician office laboratories where certain "waived tests" or those that require no personnel qualifications of those performing the procedures

Polymerization   Chemical process where small molecules called monomers are attached chemically to produce a very large chainlike molecules

Polymorphonuclear cells   White blood cells with segmented nuclei that are also called neutrophils

Polyuria   Excretion of large volumes of urine

Porphobilinogen   One type of porphyrin that normally breaks down into heme porphyrin; excessive levels may be found in the urine of those with acute or congenital porphyria

Porphyria cutanea tarda   Most common subtype of porphyria due to deficient levels of the enzyme uroporphyrinogen decarboxylase

Porphyrins   Intermediate compounds in production of heme-blockage-can be inherited or acquired

Porphyrinuria   Presence of porphyrins, precursors to hemoglobin, in the urine

Postanalytical   Handling of laboratory results following an analytical procedure

Post-prandial   Procedure performed following a meal or ingestion of a measured material such as glucose

Postrenal   Conditions of the urine following secretion from the kidneys

Poststreptococcal   Refers to conditions following a streptococcal infection that may be the result of a recurrent infection

Postural   Position of the body during a procedure

Povidone-iodine   Antiseptic used to cleanse the skin prior to certain procedures

Preanalytical   Processes performed prior to beginning the analysis of a specimen

Precipitation   Aggregation or formation of a solid or larger particles in a solution

Prerenal Event that occurs before the kidneys are involved, such as reduction of blood circulation to the kidneys

Preservatives Any material used to prevent the deterioration of a test sample

Proficiency testing Testing of commercially provided specimens to a laboratory for testing to determine the accuracy of the procedures performed in the facility

Progesterone Female hormone instrumental in the regulation of ovulation and menstruation

Prostate gland Accessory reproductive organ located directly beneath the bladder in the male; secretes to the sperm during the slightly alkaline fluid that forms part of the seminal fluid, a fluid that carries sperm

Prostatic hyperplasia Abnormally enlarged prostate gland

Prostatitis Inflammation of the prostate gland

Protein Demonstration of proteinuria in a routine analysis does not always signify renal disease but requires confirmatory testing. Major pathologic causes of proteinuria include glomerular membrane damage, disorders affecting tubular reabsorption of

Proteinuria Presence of significant levels of protein in the urine

Proteolytic enzymes Refers to enzymes that break down proteins into the smallest entities

Protozoan Refers to organisms of the microscopic one-celled parasitic protozoans

Pruritis Intense itching of the skin

Prussian blue A dye used to stain iron inclusions in cells and organisms

Pseudogout Accumulations of crystals called calcium pyrophosphate dihydrate and causes similar symptoms as that of the true gout, where uric acid crystals are the causative agent

Pseudoperoxidase A class of biological substances that includes hemoglobin and that act as does peroxidase; catalyzes a reduction-oxidation reaction between hydrogen peroxide and several other organic compounds

Pyelonephritis Acute pyelonephritis most frequent in women, often resulting from untreated cases of cystitis or lower urinary tract infection by bacteria

Pyknotic Refers to cells where nuclear chromatin in a cell is undergoing necrosis (death) or apoptosis (self-destruction)

Pyrophosphate Refers to the crystal found in cases of pseudogout

Pyruvic acid Occurs naturally in the body and is an end product of the anaerobic metabolism of starches and sugars

Pyuria Condition of leukocytes in the urine

Quality assurance Program for an institution that includes processes for insuring quality of results for all procedures performed

Quality control Determination of precision, or reproducibility, is the purpose of performing quality control procedures

Quantitative Determinations that provide a numeric value of the results of the procedure

Radiographic dye Dyes used in X-ray procedures that provide for contrast in order to obtain more clinically significant images

Red blood cells   Finding of red blood cells other than an occasional cell is abnormal

Reflux nephropathy   A medical condition caused by a variety of reasons where the kidneys are damaged by the backward flow of urine into the kidneys

Refractile   Capable of refracting light from the surface

Refractometer   Instrument that provides an accurate determination of the concentration of dissolved substances in a liquid by comparisons of refractive qualities of the substance when compared with air

Relative centrifugal force   The RCF is a constant that is independent of the type of centrifuge used; The actual equation is RCF $= 1.12R(RPM/1000)^2$ and it should be noted that the RPMs (revolutions per minute) are not equal to the RCF

Renal blood flow   Reduced circulation to kidneys will result in damage to the filtering capability of the kidneys; the kidneys receive as much as 25% of the body's blood supply continuously

Renal failure   Result of acute tubular necrosis may result from renal vasoconstriction, direct tubular damage from nephrotoxic agents

Renal function test   Used to assess health and function of the nephrons; renal functions include renal blood flow—reduced circulation to kidneys

Renal pelvis   Structure is funnel-like with an enlarged, dilated proximal part of the ureter through which urine flows from the kidney to the urinary bladder

Rennin   Rennin is also known as chymosin, and is a proteolytic enzyme synthesized by cells in the stomach

Resolving power   Ability of a microscope to produce clear and sharp images of closely placed objects

Reticuloendothelial   Components of the bone marrow and lymphoid tissues where mononuclear phagocytic system functions occur

Retroperitoneal   Cavity behind the peritoneum where the kidneys are located

Rhabdomyolysis   Breakdown of muscle fibers may damage kidneys by the release of muscle fiber products including myoglobin into the bloodstream

Rheumatic fever   Severe inflammatory disease that can develop after an repeated infections with Streptococcus bacteria from strep throat or scarlet fever; kidneys, heart, joints, skin, and brain tissues may be affected

Rheumatoid arthritis   Chronic autoimmune condition that leads to inflammation of joints and surrounding tissues, including entire organs of the body

Robert Hooke   Thought to be the first individual to study and record cells, making drawings of them, through the use of a microscope

Robert Koch   Built on the work of Louis Pasteur; primarily studied diseases of anthrax and tuberculosis

Roger Bacon   English philosopher and scientist who taught physics and applied his knowledge of geometry to optics; described spectacles fully in one of his works and perhaps provided the background for the later development of the microscope

Ropes test   Also known as the mucin clot test that reflects the polymerization of synovial fluid hyaluronate (hyaluronic acid)

Salicylates   Salicylic acid is the active property of the well-known aspirin; found naturally in some plants and possesses anti-inflammatory, analgesic, and anti-pyretic (lowers fever) properties

Salmonella   Genus of a bacterium that may cause "food poisoning"

Scleroderma   Term means "hardened skin;" disease of the connective tissues that results in damage to skin, blood vessels, muscles, and internal organs

Segmented neutrophils   Type of white blood cell that provides protective measures against invasive bacteria; also called "polymorphonuclear" cell

Semen   Most often received of miscellaneous body fluids, both for infertility studies as well as postvasectomy cases

Seminal fluids   Presence or absence of viable sperm, acid phosphatase in rape cases

Seminal vesicles   Consists of a pair of small tubular glands located near the prostate gland; secrete fluids into the ejaculatory ducts of male mammals

Serotonin   One of the neurotransmitter, thought to be a mood elevator; is involved in the transmission of nerve impulses; synthesized in the body from the amino acid tryptophan

Serous cavities   Any cavity of the body where fluids that are an ultrafiltrate of the blood is found

Serous effusion   Increase of fluids derived from the blood and as a result of inflammation or infection; also may result from some mechanical causes

Serous fluids   From cavities of body, such as pleural, pericardial, and peritoneal are ultrafiltrates of plasma

"Sharps" container   Rigid container used for disposal of needles, scalpels, broken glass and any other materials potentially capable of causing injury when handled

Shigella   Genus of bacteria that infect the digestive tract and may produce symptoms of diarrhea, cramping, vomiting, and nausea

Siderophages   Phagocytic cells containing iron pigments

Sinusoids   Irregularly shaped and sized tubular space for the passage of blood, that function as capillaries and venules in the liver, spleen, and bone marrow

Sleep apnea   Cessation of breathing, may be due to airway obstruction, during sleep

Sodium bicarbonate   Strong buffer used for reducing the acidity of chemicals as well as being important in adjusting the pH of the body; often used as an antacid for gastric "heartburn"

Sodium chloride   Known as common salt or table salt, the chemical compound NaCl is important in many bodily functions and is maintained at precise levels in the blood plasma during health

Sodium heparin   Common and stable form of anticoagulant used for preventing clotting of blood both in vivo and in blood samples where procedures require plasma as a test sample

Specific gravity   The specific gravity for urine is directly proportional to urine osmolality, the solute concentration or density of the urine when compared, depending upon methodology used, with water or air, as well as a chemical screening test to determine ion concentration

Spermatozoa   Male germ cells instrumental in fertilizing the female ova

Spermicidal   Any preparation that will render the sperm cell harmless or kills it

Sphincter   Term for muscles that serve to tighten or close an opening of a structure of the body

Squamous epithelial cells   Flattened cells that are the building blocks of epithelial tissue, which lines lumina of the body and forms large sheets that cover the entire outer surface of mucosal tissue

Standard precautions   Set of practices designed to protect the health care provider and the patient form becoming infected

Staphylococcal   Refers to the *Staphylococcal* genus of bacteria, some species of which are pathogens of the body, while other species are found as normal flora

Steatorrhea   Passing of fat bodies in the fecal sample

Streptococcal   Refers to the *Streptococcal* genus of bacteria, some species of which are pathogens of the body, while other species are found as normal flora

Streptococcus pneumoniae   A gram-positive, catalase-negative coccal form of bacteria that is an important human bacterial pathogen; commonly found in the nasopharynx (back of the nose) of healthy people and under certain conditions may colonize the respiratory system, causing serious disease

Streptococcus pyogenes   A common bacteria of the skin, the Lancefield group A, Beta-hemolytic strain is capable of causing strep throat (streptococcal pharyngitis), impetigo, and other skin and organ infections

Streptokinase   An exoenzyme of streptococcal organisms that is used to dissolve blood clots in blood vessels, causing heart attacks and strokes due to clots of the brain

Subluxation   Dislocation of two articular bone ends in a synovial cavity

Sucrose   A carbohydrate, the organic compound commonly known as table sugar, may also be identified as saccharose, and is commonly obtained for human use from sugar cane or sugar beets

Sudan III, IV   Classes of stains used in biological tests, chiefly for the microscopic detection of fat bodies in stool samples

Sulfonamides   Sulfonamides are bacteriostatic (stop growth) antimicrobials effective against both Gram-positive and Gram-negative organisms; most effective in early treatment of uncomplicated cases of cystitis

Sulfosalicylic acid   Used as a precipitating agent for proteins found in urine samples

Supernatant   Following centrifugation, where solids are precipitated, the resultant fluid is called the supernatant

Suppurative   Term describing a general production of pus (white blood cells)

Suprapubic aspiration   Use of a needle to aspirate urine from the urinary bladder

Syndrome   Group of symptoms commonly found in a particular disease

Synovial fluids   Joint fluid is viscous, formed as an ultrafiltrate of the plasma

Synovial membrane   Connective-tissue membrane lining the joint cavity and producing the synovial fluid

Synoviocytic cells   Type of cells (fibroblastic) that line joint cavities

Systemic lupus erythematosus   Also known as SLE, lupus is a chronic autoimmune disorder that may affect the skin, joints, kidneys, and other organs; sometimes organ specific or may involve multiple organs and systems

Tamm-Horsfall   Term for a glycoprotein secreted by the renal epithelium that is a component of all renal casts

Testes   Term for testicles of the male, the male sex glands are located behind the penis in the scrotum; testes produce and store sperm

Tetracycline   Broad spectrum antibiotic effective in treating certain bacterial infections such as urinary tract infections, chlamydia and skin rashes such as acne

Thorax   Region of the body housing the lungs and heart

Thrush   Oral infection by the yeast *Candida albicans*; common in infants

Thyroxine   Hormone produced by the thyroid glands

Toluene   Aromatic hydrocarbon that may be toxic to developing fetuses; commonly used as an industrial solvent in industrial plants

Toxicology   Study of toxins, their sources and effects they may have on the body

Transabdominally   Refers to a radiologic visualization across the abdominal wall or through the abdominal cavity

Transcellular   Smallest portion of extracellular fluid as a component of total body water; confined within spaces that are lined by epithelial cells

Transferrin   Transferrin is a glycoprotein that binds iron tightly but reversibly; tests for transferring are used to study iron metabolism and the causes of anemia

Transudates   Systemic disorder that disrupts the balance in regulation of fluid filtration and reabsorption, such as changes in hydrostatic pressure created by congestive heart failure or nephrotic syndrome, are transudates; transudates are effusions that form due to trauma and hydrostatic changes

Traumatic puncture/tap   Refers to a puncture of a body cavity, particularly the cerebrospinal cavity, where blood is introduced into the sample

Trichloroacetic acid   Reagent used to precipitate protein from a urine sample, as a confirmation of a positive qualitative determination made by a urine chemical dipstick

Trichomonas vaginalis   Common protozoan transmitted sexually

Triglycerides   Type of fat found in the blood and is a major source of energy

Trypsin   One of the three principal digestive chemicals of the stomach, and produced by the pancreas, trypsin is a proteolytic enzyme or proteinase that splits dietary protein into smaller segments

Trypan blue   A vital stain that is used to differentiate between live and dead tissues, by staining necrotic tissue blue

Tubulo-interstitial nephritis   Medical condition of the kidneys where spaces between the kidney tubules become inflamed

Turbidity   Clarity or lack of clarity in a fluid that is caused by suspended particles in the solution

Turk's solution   Gentian violet stain used to stain the nuclei of white cells

Two-hour post prandial   Refers to a period of time following the ingestion of a meal or a prescribed dose of glucose

Tyrosine   One of the 20 or more amino acids to synthesize proteins in the cells

Tyrosinemia   Presence of tyrosine in the blood

Tyrosyluria   Presence of tyrosine in the urine

Ulcerative colitis   A bowel disease that primarily impacts the large intestine and rectum; characterized by abdominal pain and cramping that is alleviated following a bowel movement

Ultrafiltrates   With reference to the kidneys, ultrafiltration occurs at the membrane separating the capillaries and the resulting filtrate in the renal corpuscle or Bowman's capsule in the kidneys

Ultrasound   Instruments using high-frequency sound waves, reveal images of organs and structures of the body's interior

Urate gout   Gout as a result of the deposition of uric acid crystals

Urea   A nitrogen-containing chemical compound found in urine

Urea nitrogen   A common laboratory procedure determines the kidney's ability to filter wastes from the body by measuring the level of protein breakdown in the body and its presence in the blood

Uremia   Abnormally high concentrations of nitrogenous substances in the blood as a measure of the kidney's failure to filter toxic wastes for elimination from the body

Ureters   Tubes that are paired and transport urine from the kidneys to the bladder where it is stored for excretion

Urethra   Tube that extends to the exterior of the body where urine is excreted as a waste product

Urethritis   Inflammation of the urethra

Uric acid   Term for a chemical compound that is formed when the body breaks down substances called purines

Urine sediment   Solid components such as cells and crystals from a urine sample that is centrifuged, leaving a button of sediment

Urinometer   Device with a flotation bulb used to determine the specific gravity of a solution compared with that of water

Urobilin   Bile pigment in part giving the yellowish color to urine; produced by reduction of bilirubin by intestinal bacteria and excreted by the kidneys

Urobilinogen   A bile pigment that results from the degradation of bilirubin by the intestinal bacteria

Urochrome   Thought to be the end product of hemoglobin breakdown

Uroerythrin   Term for a reddish pigment, a chromophore known to be adsorbed by the amorphous urate sediment in refrigerated samples

Urogenital system   Contains the urine excretory organs, the kidneys, ureters, bladder, and urethra, as well as the reproductive organs of the male and the female mammal

Uroporphyrins   Includes any of several porphyrins produced by oxidation of uroporphyrinogen

Uroscopy   Ancient practice of macroscopically examining a sample of urine

Valine An essential amino acid used for the construction of proteins that must be obtained through the diet in adequate quantities

Vanillylmandelic acid End-stage metabolite of the catecholamines epinephrine and norepinephrine

Varicella zoster A highly contagious viral organism, *V. zoster* is one of the eight known herpes viruses that infect humans and other vertebrates; causes chicken-pox (varicella) in children and shingles

Vasectomy Cutting of or tying off the vas deferens to prevent pregnancy of one's mate

Vasoconstriction Tightening of or lessening the potential volume of a blood vessel

Vasopressin An antidiuretic also known as ADH (anti-diuretic hormone), is released by the pituitary gland and prevents loss of water from the body

Venereal disease Any of a number of diseases caused by the sexual transmission of microorganisms

Ventricles Refers to large chambers of the lower heart and the spaces of the brain where CSF is secreted and found

Viability Capable of living, developing, or reproducing when favorable environmental conditions are met; term also used for a fetus or newborn that is capable of living outside the uterus

Viscosity "Stickiness" of a solution

Vitamin B$_{12}$ This vitamin is essential for making red blood cells and a functional nervous system

Vitreous In medicine, the term refers to the gelatinous body found in the eyeball

Waived Tests Those deemed simple enough by the Clinical Laboratory Improvement Amendments to be performed by non-laboratory Personnel; chiefly performed in physician office labs (POLs)

Wet mount Simple slide preparation where a suspension of material is mixed with a solvent, covered with a cover slip, and examined microscopically

Whipple's disease Rare medical condition of malabsorption that occurs as perhaps a result of an intestinal infection that prevents the small intestines from properly absorbing nutrients

Wright's stain Used for identifying blood cells, chiefly, and for enhancing the morphology of them; stain is a combination of acid dye (red 'eosin') and a basic dye (blue 'methylene blue') for use in staining of a blood smear

Wright's-Giemsa Combination of Wright's stain for cellular morphology, with the additional Giemsa stain developed to show distinguishing characteristics of intracellular parasites

Xanthochromic Having a yellow or yellowish color or hue

Yersinia *Yersinia pestis*, previously called *Pasteurella pestis*, is a Gram-negative rod-shaped contracted through the consumption of undercooked meat products, unpasteurized milk, and contaminated water; *Yersinia enterocolitica* is another species of this genus that is capable of causing severe illness

Zollinger-Ellison syndrome Medical condition in where increased production of the hormone gastrin occurs

Bibliography

American Diabetes Association (2013) Standards of medical care in diabetes—2013. Diabetes Care 36:S11

Bellomo R, Kellam JA, Ronco C (2012) Defining acute renal failure: physiological princples. In: Applied physiology to intensive care medicine. Springer, Berlin

Bradbury S (1968) The microscope: past and present. Pergamon Press, Oxford

Brandes SB, Johnson MH (2013) 1102 piss prophesy, uroscopy, and the symbol of the matula in paintings from the high middle ages and renaissance. J Urol 189:e451

Brunzel NA (2013) Fundamentals of urine and body fluid analysis, 3rd edn. Elsevier, Philadelphia, PA

Centers for Disease Control and Prevention (2013) CDC features: wash your hands. Centers for Medicare and Medicaid Services, Centers for Disease Control and Prevention. http://www.cdc.gov/features/handwashing/. Accessed 27 Sept 2016

Chow G, Schmidey JW (1984) Lysis of erythrocytes and leukocytes in traumatic lumbar punctures. Arch Neurol 41:1084–1085

Clinical and Laboratory Standards Institute (2004) Clinical laboratory safety: approved guideline, 2nd edn. NCCLS, Wayne, PA. NCCLS document GP17-A2. isbn:1-56238-530-5

Clinical and Laboratory Standards Institute (CLSI) (2007) Analysis of body fluids in clinical chemistry: approved guideline, CLSI document C49-A. CLSI, Wayne, PA

Clinical and Laboratory Standards Institute (CLSI), formery NCCLS (2001) Urinalysis and collection, transportation of urine specimens; approved guideline GP16-A2, 2nd edn. NCCLS, Wayne, PA. (https://clsi.org)

Clinical Laboratory Improvements of 1988, final rule, Federal Register, Feb. 28, 1992. Clinical Laboratory Improvements of 1988, Final Rule. 42 CFR. Subpart K, 493.1201

Cohen AS, Goldenberg D (1985) Synovial fluid. In: Laboratory diagnostic procedures in the rheumatic diseases, 3rd edn. Grune & Stratton, New York

Cohen EP, Lemann J (1991) The role of the laboratory in evaluation of kidney function. Clin Chem 37:785–796

Colborn T, Dumanoski D, Myers JP (1996) Our stolen future: are we threatening our fertility, intelligence, and survival?: a scientific detective story. Dutton, New York. 306 p. isbn:0-452-27414-1

Department of Health and Human Services (2003) Medicare, Medicaid, and CLIA programs; laboratory requirements relating to quality systems and certain personnel qualifications. Final rule. Fed Regist 68:3639–3714

Graff L (1983) A handbook of routine urinalysis. Lippincott, Williams & Wilkins, Philadelphia, pp 2–65

Harmening DM (1997) Clinical hematology and fundamentals of hemostasis, 3rd edn. F.A. Davis, Philadelphia

Hughes C, Roebuck MJ (2003) Evaluation of the IRIS 939 UDx flow microscope as a screening system for urinary tract infection. J Clin Pathol 56(11):844–849

Kjeldsberg CR, Knight JA (1986) Body fluids, 2nd edn. American Society of Clinical Pathologists Press, Chicago

© Springer International Publishing AG, part of Springer Nature 2018
J. W. Ridley, *Fundamentals of the Study of Urine and Body Fluids*,
https://doi.org/10.1007/978-3-319-78417-5

Kjeldsberg CR, Knight JA (1993) Synovial fluid. In: Body fluids, 3rd edn. American Society of Clinical Pathologists Press, Chicago

Krieg AF, Kjeldsberg CR (1991) Cerebrospinal fluid and other body fluids. In: Henry JB (ed) Clinical diagnosis and management of laboratory methods. WB Saunders, Philadelphia

Lu J, Chen F, Xu H, Huang Y, Lu N (2007) Comparison of three sperm-counting methods for the determination of sperm concentration in human semen and sperm suspensions. Lab Med 38(4):232

McBride LJ (1998) Textbook of urinalysis and body fluids. Lippincott, Williams & Wilkins, Hagerstown, MD

Murray PR, Hampton CM (1980) Recovery of pathogenic bacteria from cerebrospinal fluid. J Clin Microbiol 12:554–557

Mynahan C (1984) Evaluation of macroscopic urinalysis as a screening procedure. Lab Med 15(3):176

National Committee for Clinical Laboratory Standards (2001) Proposed guidelines for evaluation of linearity of quantitative analytic methods document no. EP6-P2. NCCLS, Villanova, PA

National Institutes of Health Clinical Center, Bethesda, MD 20892. Questions about the NIH Clinical Center? http://www.cc.nih.gov/comments.shtml. 02/2016 PVCS (Nursing)

Novak RW (1984) Lack of validity of standard corrections for white cell counts of blood contaminated cerebrospinal fluid in infants. Am J Clin Pathol 82:95–97

Occupational Safety and Health Administration. Healthcare Wide hazards: (Lack of) Universal Precautions. http://www.osha.gov/SLTC/etools/hospital/hazards/univprec/univ.html. Accessed 27 Sept 2016

Occupational Safety and Health Administration. Laboratory Safety Guidance. OSHA; 3904-11R 2011. http://www.osha.gov/Publications/laboratory/OSHA3404laboratory-safety-guidance. pdf. Accessed 27 Sept 2016

Package inserts—Multistix, Clinitest, Acetest, and Ictotest, Bayer/Ames Company

Pels RJ, Bor DH, Woolhandler S et al (1989) Dipstick urinalysis screening of asymptomatic adults for urinary tract disorders. II. Bacteriuria. JAMA 262:1221–1224

Phipps W, Long B, Woods N, Cassmeyer V (1991) Tests of gastric function; gastric analysis; tube and tubeless gastric analysis. In: Medical-surgical nursing concepts, 4th edn. Mosby, St. Louis, MO

Physician office laboratory policy and procedure manual, Northfield, IL, 1993, College of American Pathologists, Section 4, p. 1

iQ200 Operators Manual, 300-4400 Rev A/2005. IRIS Diagnostics Division, IRIS International Inc

Ridley J (2011) Essentials of clinical laboratory science, 1st edn. Delmar Cengage Learning, Clifton Park, NY

Ringsrud KM, Linne JJ (1995) Urinalysis and body fluids: a color text and atlas, 1st edn. Mosby, St. Louis, MO

Rittenouse-Olson K, De Nardin E (2013) Contemporary clinical immunology and serology, 1st edn. Pearson, Upper Saddle River, NJ

Saladin K (2001) Anatomy and physiology: the unity of form and function, 2nd edn. McGraw Hill, New York

Simco V (1981) Fecal fat microscopy. Am J Gastroenterol 75(3):204–208

Simerville JA, Maxted WC, Pahira JJ (2005) Urinalysis: a comprehensive review. Am Fam Physician 71(6):1153–1162

Simmers L, Simmers-Nartker K, Simmers-Kobelak S (2009) Introduction to health science technology, 5th edn. Delmar Cengage Learning, Clifton Park, NY

Sterile pyuria. http://www.gpnotebook.co.uk/cache/1986723880.htm. Accessed 14 Nov 2005

Strasinger SK, DiLorenzo MS (2008a) Urinalysis and body fluids, 5th edn. FA Davis Company, Philadelphia, PA, pp 93–121

Strasinger SK, DiLorenzo MS (2008b) Urinalysis and body fluids, 5th edn. FA Davis Company, Philadelphia, PA, pp 93–121

Thorne D, O'Brien C (2000) Diagnosing chronic pancreatitis. Advance 12(14):8–12

Urinalysis. Available at: http://www-medlib.med.utah.edu/WebPath/TUTORIAL/URINE/URINE. html. Accessed 29 Aug 2005

Wah DT, Wises PK, Butch AW (2005) Analytic performance of the iQ200 automated urine microscopy analyzer and comparison with manual counts using Fuchs-Rosenthal cell chambers. Am J Clin Pathol 123(2):290–296

Westgaard JO (1981) Precision and accuracy: concepts and assessment by method evaluation testing. CRC Crit Rev Clin Lab Sci 13(4):283–330

Index

Printed in the United States
By Bookmasters